Allergic and Non-Allergic Systemic Reactions including Anaphylaxis

Editors

PANIDA SRIAROON
DENNIS K. LEDFORD
RICHARD F. LOCKEY

IMMUNOLOGY AND ALLERGY CLINICS OF NORTH AMERICA

https://www.immunology.theclinics.com/

February 2022 • Volume 42 • Number 1

ELSEVIER

1600 John F. Kennedy Boulevard • Suite 1800 • Philadelphia, Pennsylvania, 19103-2899
http://www.theclinics.com

IMMUNOLOGY AND ALLERGY CLINICS OF NORTH AMERICA Volume 42, Number 1
February 2022 ISSN 0889-8561, ISBN-13: 978-0-323-85015-5

Editor: Katerina Heidhausen
Developmental Editor: Jessica Cañaberal

Immunology and Allergy Clinics of North America (ISSN 0889–8561) is published quarterly by Elsevier Inc., 360 Park Avenue South, New York, NY 10010-1710. Months of issue are February, May, August, and November. Periodicals postage paid at New York, NY and additional mailing offices. Subscription prices are $354.00 per year for US individuals, $844.00 per year for US institutions, $100.00 per year for US students and residents, $432.00 per year for Canadian individuals, $100.00 per year for Canadian students, $861.00 per year for Canadian institutions, $456.00 per year for international individuals, $861.00 per year for international institutions, $220.00 per year for international students. To receive student/resident rate, orders must be accompanied by name of affiliated institution, date of term, and the *signature* of program/residency coordinator on institution letterhead. Orders will be billed at individual rate until proof of status is received. Foreign air speed delivery is included in all *Clinics* subscription prices. All prices are subject to change without notice. **POSTMASTER:** Send address changes to *Immunology and Allergy Clinics of North America,* Elsevier Health Sciences Division, Subscription Customer Service, 3251 Riverport Lane, Maryland Heights, MO 63043. **Customer Service: 1-800-654-2452 (U.S. and Canada); 314-447-8871 (outside U.S. and Canada). Fax: 314-447-8029. E-mail: journalscustomerservice-usa@elsevier.com (for print support); journalsonlinesupport-usa@elsevier.com (for online support).**

Reprints. For copies of 100 or more, of articles in this publication, please contact the Commercial Reprints Department, Elsevier Inc., 360 Park Avenue South, New York, New York 10010-1710. Tel. 212-633-3874, Fax: 212-633-3820, E-mail: reprints@elsevier.com.

Immunology and Allergy Clinics of North America is covered in MEDLINE/PubMed (Index Medicus), Current Contents/Life Sciences, Science Citation Index, ISI/BIOMED, Chemical Abstracts, and EMBASE/Excerpta Medica.

Contributors

EDITORS

PANIDA SRIAROON, MD
Associate Professor of Medicine and Pediatrics, Associate Chief, Division of Allergy and Immunology, Department of Pediatrics, University of South Florida Morsani College of Medicine, Tampa; Director, Food Allergy Clinic, Johns Hopkins All Children's Hospital, St Petersburg, Florida, USA

DENNIS K. LEDFORD, MD
Professor of Medicine and Pediatrics, Division of Allergy and Immunology, Department of Internal Medicine, University of South Florida Morsani College of Medicine; Ellsworth and Mabel Simmons Professor of Allergy and Immunology, James A. Haley Veterans' Hospital, Tampa, Florida, USA

RICHARD F. LOCKEY, MD
Distinguished University Health Professor, Joy McCann Culverhouse Chair of Allergy and Immunology, University of South Florida Morsani College of Medicine; Professor of Medicine, Pediatrics and Public Health, Director, Division of Allergy and Immunology, Department of Internal Medicine, James A. Haley Veterans' Hospital, Tampa, Florida

AUTHORS

KARLA E. ADAMS, MD
Associate Professor of Pediatrics, Allergy & Immunology Division, Department of Medicine, Wilford Hall Ambulatory Surgical Center, San Antonio, Texas, USA

CEM AKIN, MD, PhD
Department of Internal Medicine, Division of Allergy and Clinical Immunology, University of Michigan, Ann Arbor, Michigan, USA

ERNIE AVILLA, MBA
Department of Medicine, Clinical Immunology and Allergy, McMaster University, Hamilton, Ontario, Canada

ADRIANA G. BAGOS-ESTEVEZ, BS
MD Student, University of South Florida, Morsani College of Medicine, Tampa, Florida, USA

DAVID I. BERNSTEIN, MD
Professor Emeritus, Division of Immunology, Allergy and Rheumatology, University of Cincinnati College of Medicine, Cincinnati, Ohio, USA

RONNA L. CAMPBELL, PhD, MD
Professor of Emergency Medicine, Department of Emergency Medicine, Mayo Clinic, Rochester, Minnesota, USA

MARIANA CASTELLS, MD, PhD
Division of Allergy and Clinical Immunology, Department of Medicine, Brigham and Women's Hospital, Harvard Medical School, Boston, Massachusetts, USA

JAMES C. COLLIE, MD
Resident Physician, Department of Internal Medicine, University of South Florida, Tampa, Florida, USA

HEATHER CRUIKSHANK, BA
Department of Medicine, Clinical Immunology and Allergy, McMaster University, Hamilton, Ontario, Canada

YASHU DHAMIJA, MD
Fellow, Division of Immunology, Allergy and Rheumatology, University of Cincinnati College of Medicine, Cincinnati, Ohio, USA

TIMOTHY E. DRIBIN, MD
Division of Emergency Medicine, Cincinnati Children's Hospital Medical Center, Department of Pediatrics, University of Cincinnati College of Medicine, Cincinnati, Ohio, USA

TOLLY E.G. EPSTEIN, MD, MS
Adjunct Associate Professor, Division of Immunology, Allergy and Rheumatology, University of Cincinnati College of Medicine, Cincinnati, Ohio; Allergy Partners of Central Indiana, Indianapolis, Indiana, USA

JOSHUA FOWLER, MD
Resident Physician, Internal Medicine, University of Tennessee College of Medicine, Memphis, Tennessee, USA

THEO GÜLEN, MD, PhD
Department of Respiratory Medicine and Allergy, Karolinska University Hospital, Huddinge; Department of Medicine Solna, Immunology and Allergy Unit, Karolinska Institutet and Karolinska University Hospital; Mastocytosis Centre Karolinska, Karolinska University Hospital and Karolinska Institutet, Stockholm, Sweden

DAVID B.K. GOLDEN, MDCM
Associate Professor of Medicine, Johns Hopkins University, Owings Mills, Maryland, USA

MARGARET M. KUDER, MD, MPH
Department of Allergy and Clinical Immunology, Respiratory Institute, Cleveland Clinic, Cleveland, Ohio, USA

DAVID M. LANG, MD
Department of Allergy and Clinical Immunology, Respiratory Institute, Cleveland Clinic, Cleveland, Ohio, USA

DENNIS K. LEDFORD, MD
Ellsworth and Mabel Simmons Professor of Allergy and Immunology and VA Section Chief of Allergy/Immunology, University of South Florida, Morsani College of Medicine, Tampa, Florida, USA

JAMES T. LI, PhD, MD
Professor of Medicine, Division of Allergic Diseases, Mayo Clinic, Rochester, Minnesota, USA

PHIL LIEBERMAN, MD
Clinical Professor of Medicine and Pediatrics, University of Tennessee College of Medicine, Memphis, Tennessee, USA

RICHARD F. LOCKEY, MD
Distinguished University Health Professor, Joy McCann Culverhouse Chair of Allergy and Immunology, University of South Florida Morsani College of Medicine; Professor of Medicine, Pediatrics and Public Health, Director, Division of Allergy and Immunology, Department of Internal Medicine, James A. Haley Veterans' Hospital, Tampa, Florida

MEGAN S. MOTOSUE, MD
Department of Allergy and Immunology, Kaiser Honolulu Clinic, Honolulu, Hawaii, USA

AISHWARYA NAVALPAKAM, MD
Division of Allergy, Immunology and Rheumatology, Department of Pediatrics, Children's Hospital of Michigan, Central Michigan University College of Medicine, Detroit, Michigan, USA

AMBER N. PEPPER, MD
Division of Allergy and Immunology, Department of Internal Medicine, University of South Florida Morsani College of Medicine, Tampa, Florida, USA

MITCHELL M. PITLICK, MD
Fellow, Division of Allergic Diseases, Mayo Clinic, Rochester, Minnesota, USA

PAVADEE POOWUTTIKUL, MD
Associate Professor of Pediatrics, Division of Allergy, Immunology and Rheumatology, Department of Pediatrics, Children's Hospital of Michigan, Central Michigan University College of Medicine, Detroit, Michigan, USA

NICOLE RAMSEY, MD, PhD
Instructor of Pediatrics, Jaffe Food Allergy Institute, Icahn School of Medicine at Mount Sinai, New York, New York, USA

RUCHI H. SHAH, MD
Department of Allergy and Clinical Immunology, Respiratory Institute, Cleveland Clinic, Cleveland, Ohio, USA

ANITA SHAH, HBSC
Research Assistant, Department of Medicine, Clinical Immunology and Allergy, McMaster University, Hamilton, Ontario, Canada

NARIN THANAPUTKAIPORN, MD
Division of Allergy, Immunology and Rheumatology, Department of Pediatrics, Children's Hospital of Michigan, Central Michigan University College of Medicine, Detroit, Michigan, USA

JAMES M. TRACY, DO
Associate Clinical Professor of Pediatrics, University of Nebraska College of Medicine; Allergy, Asthma and Immunology Associates, Omaha, Nebraska, USA

GERALD W. VOLCHECK, MD
Professor of Medicine, Division of Allergic Diseases, Mayo Clinic, Rochester, Minnesota, USA

JULIE WANG, MD
Professor of Pediatrics, Jaffe Food Allergy Institute, Icahn School of Medicine at Mount Sinai, New York, New York, USA

SUSAN WASERMAN, MSc, MDCM, FRCPC
Professor, Department of Medicine, Clinical Immunology and Allergy, McMaster University, Hamilton, Ontario, Canada

EMMA WESTERMANN-CLARK, MD, MA
Division of Allergy and Immunology, Department of Internal Medicine, University of South Florida Morsani College of Medicine, Tampa, Florida, USA

Contents

There are many definitions of anaphylaxis in the medical literature. The authors propose a modified definition of anaphylaxis to be used for clinical decision making that promotes the early utilization of intramuscular epinephrine. Anaphylaxis can be a result of an allergic or nonallergic mechanism. In general, allergic reactions are more severe; however, any type of anaphylaxis can result in death and improve with IM epinephrine. The World Allergy Organization's Grading Criteria for allergic systemic reactions are adapted as a guide to identify manifestations that may progress to anaphylaxis. The intent is to promote and encourage the use of IM epinephrine in the health care setting before the progression of manifestations and the onset of life-threatening respiratory or cardiovascular dysfunction generally recognized as meeting the definition of anaphylaxis.

Anaphylaxis-related emergency department (ED) visits and hospitalizations are increasing. Triggers for anaphylaxis include food, medications, and stinging insects. Idiopathic anaphylaxis accounts for 30% to 60% of cases of anaphylaxis in adults and up to 10% of cases in children with novel allergens such as galactose-α-1,3 galactose reclassifying these cases. Recent practice guidelines have recommended against the routine use of systemic corticosteroids and antihistamines for the prevention of biphasic reactions and recommend an extended observation, up to 6 hours, for those with risk factors for biphasic anaphylaxis and those with lack of access to epinephrine and to emergency medical services.

There is a myriad of immunologic and nonimmunologic pathways by which the clinical phenotype of anaphylaxis can be produced. An understanding of these pathways is essential for the prevention as well as the treatment of anaphylactic episodes.

There is strong evidence of an association between severe anaphylaxis, especially hymenoptera venom induced, and mast cell (MC) disorders. It has been thought that intrinsic abnormalities in MCs, including the presence of the activating KIT D816V mutation in mastocytosis or of genetic trait, hereditary alpha-tryptasemia, may influence susceptibility to severe anaphylaxis. This article evaluates the potential mechanisms leading to severe MC activation, as well as the differential diagnosis of and range of symptoms attributable to MC mediator release. Also, we offer a global classification for disorders related to MC activation.

The key to managing anaphylaxis is early epinephrine administration. This can improve outcomes and prevent progression to severe and fatal anaphylaxis. Delayed or lack of administration of epinephrine is associated with fatal reactions. Positioning in a recumbent supine position, airway management, and intravenous fluids are essential in its management. Antihistamines and glucocorticosteroids should not be prescribed in place of epinephrine. β-adrenergic agonists by inhalation are indicated for bronchospasm associated with anaphylaxis despite optimal epinephrine treatment. Long-term management of anaphylaxis includes the identification and avoidance of triggers; identification of cofactors, such as mast cell disorders; patient, parent, and caregiver education, and interventions to reduce allergen sensitivity, such as the use of venom immunotherapy for Hymenoptera hypersensitivity. Long-term management is covered in other articles. Consultation with an allergist/immunologist is recommended when necessary.

Anaphylaxis is a systemic allergic reaction that can be caused by food, drugs, insect bites, or unknown triggers in infants and toddlers. Anaphylaxis rates are increasing. Infants and toddlers may have increased exposure to known and unknown allergens, decreased ability to describe their symptoms, and an expanded differential diagnosis for consideration on presentation. The most common symptoms in these age groups are cutaneous and gastrointestinal. Age-specific language may be helpful for caregivers to identify and describe the symptoms of anaphylaxis in infants and toddlers. Long-term management of anaphylaxis includes allergy evaluation to guide avoidance and assess prognosis and education on allergic reaction management; this incorporates the prescription of epinephrine autoinjector and provision of an allergy emergency plan.

Given the increasing prevalence of food allergy, schools and food service establishments must have procedures in place to accommodate those with the condition. Training staff on allergy management has been shown to improve knowledge and skills, although more research is needed to better understand its benefits. Furthermore, although there are challenges involved in maintaining unassigned stock epinephrine programs, they have the potential to reduce morbidity and mortality associated with anaphylaxis by improving access to potentially life-saving medication. Finally, food bans in schools may not be an effective part of food allergy management, and other measures should be considered instead.

Subcutaneous allergen immunotherapy (SCIT) is a proven treatment of allergic rhinitis, asthma, atopic dermatitis, and prevention of Hymenoptera venom anaphylaxis. The known benefit of SCIT, however, must be considered in each patient relative to the potential risks of systemic allergic reactions (SRs). A mean of 1 SR per 1000 injection visits (0.1%) was estimated to occur between 2008 and 2018. Life-threatening anaphylactic events are estimated to occur in 1/160,000 injection visits. The factors that contribute to SRs and fatal reactions (FRs) are reviewed. Risk management strategies are proposed to prevent and decrease future SCIT associated with SRs, anaphylaxis, and FR.

Anaphylaxis is a multi-system syndrome resulting from the release of mediators from mast cells and basophils. Drugs are common causes. Anaphylaxis to certain drugs, vaccines, and biological agents present clinical challenges, and merit referral to a board-certified allergist/immunologist for further evaluation and management.

Perioperative anaphylaxis is a potentially life-threatening and under-recognized event most commonly caused by antibiotics, neuromuscular blocking agents, dyes, latex, and disinfectants. This review provides updates in the epidemiology and pathogenesis of perioperative anaphylaxis, discusses culprit agents, and highlights the tenets of management including a comprehensive allergy evaluation.

Hymenoptera stinging insects are common culprits for allergic reactions. Anaphylaxis to insect stings can be life threatening and is associated with a significant risk of recurrence. Insect allergy requires referral to an allergist/immunologist for education and for diagnostic evaluation that will direct further management and treatment. Venom immunotherapy is safe and effective; it prevents sting anaphylaxis in up to 98% of patients. Potential risk factors for side effects during testing and treatment should be assessed for every patient to mitigate risk and to guide treatment recommendations and the duration of immunotherapy.

IMMUNOLOGY AND ALLERGY CLINICS OF NORTH AMERICA

FORTHCOMING ISSUES

May 2022
Drug Hypersensitivity
Elizabeth J. Phillips, *Editor*

RECENT ISSUES

November 2021
Pediatric Immunology and Allergy
Elizabeth Secord, *Editor*

SERIES OF RELATED INTEREST

Medical Clinics
https://www.medical.theclinics.com/

Preface

Anaphylaxis Is a Continuum and Should Be Treated with Epinephrine Early

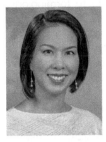
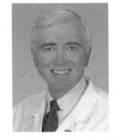
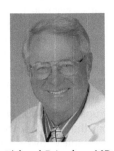

Panida Sriaroon, MD   Dennis K. Ledford, MD   Richard F. Lockey, MD

Editors

Anaphylaxis is an acute, systemic syndrome, usually affecting multiple organs, with clinical features consistent with those that follow allergen exposure, typically by ingestion or injection, of an allergic individual. The absence of a gold standard for diagnosis or a universally accepted definition of this syndrome complicates real-time clinical management. Anaphylaxis is relevant to all clinicians.

Severity of anaphylaxis, for example, evidence of cardiovascular collapse or respiratory distress, is utilized by some to distinguish acute systemic reactions from anaphylaxis. A definition based on severity is useful for research and epidemiologic studies but is less useful for treatment decisions, since epinephrine treatment is more effective when administered prior to the onset of severe manifestations (ie, cardiovascular collapse and/or respiratory distress). The unpredictable potential and pace of progression from mild anaphylaxis, or systemic reactions, to life-threatening anaphylaxis further complicate decision making.

There is debate as to the clinical value of dividing systemic reactions from anaphylaxis due to the following:

1. Efficacy of intramuscular (IM) epinephrine in both systemic reactions and anaphylaxis
2. Greater efficacy of IM epinephrine administered in the early phase of anaphylaxis, when it is more difficult to distinguish from a systemic reaction, compared with administration in the more severe stage of anaphylaxis
3. Variability in the rate of progression from mild anaphylaxis, or a systemic reaction, to life-threatening manifestations
4. Negligible toxicity of IM epinephrine therapy at a dose of 0.01 mg/kg

The editors of this issue prefer the concept of anaphylaxis as a continuum, extending from a grade 1 systemic reaction (cutaneous or upper respiratory without cutaneous) to

Immunol Allergy Clin N Am 42 (2022) xiii–xv
https://doi.org/10.1016/j.iac.2021.10.003
0889-8561/22/© 2021 Published by Elsevier Inc.

immunology.theclinics.com

grade 4/5 (cardiovascular collapse and/or respiratory distress).[1] The intent is that all grades should be assessed and judged by circumstance as to advisability of the early intervention with IM epinephrine rather than withholding epinephrine treatment until severe manifestations occur. All grade 1 reactions do not progress, and all anaphylaxis episodes do not start with grade 1 and progress in a stepwise fashion. This unpredictable variability challenges even the most experienced clinician to assess the potential for severe anaphylaxis. Uncertainty of outcome coupled with an unjustified safety concern of IM epinephrine, utilized in recommended doses, may result in unnecessary treatment delay. The editors acknowledge that there is a debate with respect to terminology, but we advocate for a clinical definition of anaphylaxis as a *continuum* rather than a binary, yes/no definition. Epinephrine should be used at the onset of the reaction and not delayed until the patient has hypotension and/or respiratory difficulty.

This issue begins with articles devoted to *Definition*, *Epidemiology*, and *Pathophysiology*. This introduction is followed by articles devoted to causes of systemic reactions or anaphylaxis, such as *Mast Cell Disorders*, *Food Allergy*, *Allergen Immunotherapy*, *Drugs*, including *Biologics* and *Perioperative Agents*, and *Stinging Insect Venom*. Next, the *Management of Anaphylaxis* is discussed with a separate article for the unique challenges of recognizing and treating *Anaphylaxis in Infants and Toddlers*. The final articles include *Data Gaps and Research Needs*, as well as *Patient Communications*. The intent is to provide the reader summaries of high-yield topics relevant to clinical practice. The authors utilized the most up-to-date literature in their reviews. The editors thank the authors for their contributions and the support of the publisher, Elsevier, for making this issue possible.

Panida Sriaroon, MD
Division of Allergy and Immunology
Department of Pediatrics
University of South Florida
Morsani College of Medicine
140 7th Avenue South, CRI 4008
St. Petersburg, FL 33701, USA

Dennis K. Ledford, MD
Division of Allergy and Immunology
Department of Internal Medicine
University of South Florida
Morsani College of Medicine
13000 Bruce B. Downs Boulevard, 111D
c/o VA Medical Center
Tampa, FL 33612, USA

Richard F. Lockey, MD
Division of Allergy and Immunology
Department of Internal Medicine
University of South Florida
Morsani College of Medicine
13000 Bruce B. Downs Boulevard, 111D
c/o VA Medical Center
Tampa, FL 33612, USA

E-mail addresses:
psriaroo@usf.edu (P. Sriaroon)

dledford@usf.edu (D.K. Ledford)
rlockey@usf.edu (R.F. Lockey)

REFERENCE

1. Cox LS, Sanchez-Borges M, Lockey RF. World Allergy Organization systemic allergic reaction grading system: is a modification needed? J Allergy Clin Immunol Pract 2017;5:58–62.

Anaphylaxis
Definition, Epidemiology, Diagnostic Challenges, Grading System

Adriana G. Bagos-Estevez, BS[a], Dennis K. Ledford, MD[a,b],*

KEYWORDS

- Anaphylaxis • Epinephrine • Allergic reactions • Systemic reactions

KEY POINTS

- Anaphylaxis is a syndrome without a universally accepted definition.
- A more sensitive definition of anaphylaxis is offered to promote the early administration of epinephrine.
- The incidence and prevalence of anaphylaxis have increased in the last 2 decades.
- IM epinephrine is the only effective therapy for anaphylaxis and is more effective with use at the earliest point in the development of anaphylaxis.
- Most anaphylaxis events resolve spontaneously but progression to a serious reaction is not consistently predictable supporting the use of IM epinephrine before the development of life-threatening signs.

INTRODUCTION

Medical definitions serve 2 purposes: to improve communication and facilitate clinical decision making. Anaphylaxis is a syndrome lacking a universally accepted definition. Most anaphylaxis definitions focus on specificity, to avoid mislabeling nonlife threatening, systemic reactions as anaphylaxis. For real-time, clinical decision making, the authors of this article prefer a more sensitive definition to encourage early treatment and monitoring of reactions that *may* become life-threatening. This approach uses the World Allergy Organization Grading Criteria for Systemic Allergic Reactions, shown in **Table 1**, to identify manifestations that may progress to more serious reactions.[1] The acute allergic reaction grading system proposed by Dribin and colleagues also uses a similar scoring system and provides caveats that the grade may change rapidly and the grading system does not dictate or direct management decisions.[2]

[a] University of South Florida, Morsani College of Medicine, 13000 Bruce B Downs Boulevard, VAR 111D, Tampa, FL 33612, USA; [b] Division of Allergy and Immunology, Department of Internal Medicine, James A. Haley VA Hospital, Tampa, FL, USA
* Corresponding author. 13000 Bruce B Downs Boulevard, VAR 111D, Tampa, FL 33612.
E-mail address: dledford@usf.edu

Immunol Allergy Clin N Am 42 (2022) 1–11
https://doi.org/10.1016/j.iac.2021.09.001
0889-8561/22/© 2021 Elsevier Inc. All rights reserved.

Table 1
Modified WAO grading for systemic allergic reactions

	Grades				
				Confirmed Anaphylaxis	
Grade 1	Grade 2	Grade 3	Grade 4	Grade 5	
Symptom(s)/sign(s) from one organ system	Symptom(s)/sign(s) From ≥ 2 organ symptoms listed in grade 1	Lower airway • Mild bronchospasm (cough, wheezing, shortness of breath) which responds to treatment And/or Gastrointestinal • Abdominal cramps and/or vomiting/diarrhea Other • Uterine cramps • Any symptom(s)/sign(s) from grade 1 would be included	Lower airway • Severe bronchospasm not responding or worsening in spite of treatment And/or Upper airway • Laryngeal edema with stridor • Any symptom(s)/sign(s) from grades 1 or 3 would be included	Lower or upper airway • Respiratory failure And/or Cardiovascular • Collapse/hypotension And/or • Loss of consciousness (vasovagal excluded) • Any symptom(s)/sign(s) from grades 1,3, or 4 would be included	
Cutaneous • Urticaria and/or erythema-warmth and/or pruritus other than localized at the injection site And/or • Lip tingling or itching or • Angioedema (not laryngeal) Or Upper respiratory • Nasal Symptoms: sneezing, rhinorrhea, pruritus, and/or nasal congestion And/or • Throat clearing (itchy throat) And/or • Cough not related to bronchospasm Or Conjunctival • Erythema, pruritus, tearing Or Other • Nausea • Metallic taste					

The final grade of the reaction is not determined until the event is over, regardless of the medication administered to treat the reaction. The final report should include the first symptom(s)/sign(s) and the time of onset after the causative agent exposure and a suffix reflecting if and when epinephrine was or was not administered: a, ≤5 min; b, greater than 5 min to≤10 min; c, greater than 10 to≤20 min; d, greater than 20 min; z, epinephrine not administered. Final report: Grade 1 to 5; a-d, or z; First symptom(s)/sign(s); Time of onset of first symptom(s)/signs(s).

Modified from Cox LS, Sanchez-Borges M, Lockey RF. World Allergy Organization Systemic Allergic Reaction Grading System: Is a Modification Needed? J Allergy Clin Immunol Pract. 2017 Jan-Feb;5(1):58-62 e5

Our intent is to inform health care management decisions and to advocate for the utilization of intramuscular (IM) epinephrine, a therapy with very little risk, before serious physiologic dysfunction; dysfunction that fulfills criteria for most definitions of anaphylaxis. There are limited data to prove epinephrine treatment before serious manifestations are always beneficial, and all clinicians do not agree that systemic hypersensitivity reactions progress to anaphylaxis with sufficient frequency to justify the anticipatory use of epinephrine. Early epinephrine administration does not imply treatment before symptoms or signs but rather with manifestation onset, in the anticipation of potential progression. Concerns about early or premature epinephrine use in an unsupervised setting do not necessarily apply to treatment in a health care environment.[3] Epinephrine is the most effective treatment of anaphylaxis; however, it is underutilized.[4] Delayed epinephrine administration is cited as a contributor to anaphylaxis fatality.[5] Therefore, the authors of this article prefer to encourage epinephrine use before severe respiratory or cardiovascular dysfunction. Whether milder reactions are labeled as "mild anaphylaxis" or lower grades of systemic hypersensitivity or allergic reactions is only of semantic concern if epinephrine is used before life-threatening signs.

DEFINITION

Anaphylaxis is a syndrome with potentially multiple features. Validating specific findings, severity, or system involvement required for the diagnosis is problematic, as double-blind studies without epinephrine therapy are not ethical and there is overlap between systemic hypersensitivity reactions and anaphylaxis.[2] Thus, most definitions are evaluated in retrospective cohorts or registries and not prospectively.[1] The absence of prospective data adds to the controversy concerning the optimal definition.

The editors of this book prefer an inclusive anaphylaxis definition and an expansion of the grading system for systemic allergic reactions developed by the World Allergy Organization.[1] A broader, clinical anaphylaxis definition for clinical decision making encourages epinephrine for all grades of systemic reactions. Grade 5 is life-threatening and would be accepted as anaphylaxis by all definitions. Anaphylaxis is a potentially life-threatening syndrome; however, life-threatening manifestations are *not necessary* to justify IM epinephrine.[3,6] The treatment of choice for lower grades of systemic hypersensitivity reactions is IM epinephrine, before life-threatening features, unless the clinical situation clearly provides reassurance that progression is extremely unlikely. Features that predict more severe systemic reactions help in the assessment as to the need for epinephrine during milder signs and symptoms.[6] Factors that predict more severe anaphylaxis include onset in close proximity to the time of allergen exposure, injected culprit antigen (eg, medications, insect allergens) as opposed to ingested, a history of mast cell disorders, advanced age, beta-blockers, and angiotensin pathway inhibitor therapy, and asthma.[6] The authors indicate that IM epinephrine 0.01 mg/kg is sufficiently safe to administer in almost all systemic hypersensitivity reactions, whether milder manifestations are defined as mild anaphylaxis or systemic reactions.

Variability in Current Definitions

Definitions of anaphylaxis currently in the medical literature are listed in **Table 2**.[7] The words serious or severe, life-threatening, rapid, and systemic are common terms to all definitions. Hypersensitivity is preferred to allergy in 5 of the 6, most likely because anaphylaxis is not dependent on a specific immune response. The National Institute

Table 2
Definitions of anaphylaxis currently in the medical literature

WAO 2011	EAACI 2013	AAAAI/ACAAI 2010	ASCIA 2016	NIAID 2006	WHO ICD-11 2019
A serious life-threatening generalized or systemic hypersensitivity reaction. A serious allergic reaction that is, rapid in onset and might cause death	A severe life-threatening generalized or systemic hypersensitivity reaction. An acute, potentially fatal, multi-organ system, allergic reaction	An acute life-threatening systemic reaction with varied mechanisms, clinical presentations, and severity that results from the sudden release of mediators from mast cells and basophils	Any acute onset illness with typical skin features (urticarial rash or erythema/flushing, and/or angioedema), PLUS involvement of respiratory and/or cardiovascular and/or persistent severe gastrointestinal symptoms; or Any acute onset of hypotension or bronchospasm or upper airway obstruction whereby anaphylaxis is considered possible, even if typical skin features are not present.	Anaphylaxis is a serious allergic reaction that involves more than one organ system (for example skin, respiratory tract, and/or gastrointestinal tract). It can begin very rapidly, and symptoms may be severe or life-threatening	Anaphylaxis is a severe, life-threatening systemic hypersensitivity reaction characterized by being rapid in onset with potentially life-threatening airway, breathing, or circulatory problems and is usually, although not always associated with skin and mucosal changes.

Abbreviations: AAAAI/ACAAI, American Academy of Allergy; Asthma and Immunology/American College of Allergy, Asthma; and Immunology; ASCIA, Australasian Society of Clinical Immunology and Allergy; EAACI, European Academy of Allergy and Clinical Immunology; NIAID, National Institute Of Health And Infectious Diseases; WAO, World Allergy Organization; WHO ICD-11, World Health Organization International Classification of Diseaes 11th edition.

From Cardona V, Ansotegui IJ, Ebisawa M, El-Gamal Y, Fernandez Rivas M, Fineman S, Geller M, Gonzalez-Estrada A, Greenberger PA, Sanchez Borges M, Senna G, Sheikh A, Tanno LK, Thong BY, Turner PJ, Worm M. World allergy organization anaphylaxis guidance 2020. World Allergy Organ J. 2020 Oct 30;13(10):100472.

of Allergy and Infectious Disease (NIAID) definition does specify allergy. Skin manifestations are mentioned in 3 of the 6, and the other 3 state that multiple systems are involved. Five of the 6 state that anaphylaxis is life-threatening although the World Health Organization definition, 1 of the 5, subsequently states it is "potentially life-threatening." Two of the 6 state that mediators of basophils and mast cells are involved, and the NIAID definition implies this as allergic or immunologic anaphylaxis depends on mast cells and/or basophils. A definition that classifies anaphylaxis as presenting in more than one system would not include cases of severe anaphylaxis that present with the involvement of only 1 system, for example, cardiovascular collapse in perianesthetic anaphylaxis without evident cutaneous, respiratory, or gastrointestinal manifestations.[8] To define anaphylaxis as a serious life-threatening event is too limited. Fatal and near-fatal anaphylaxis events are extremely rare.[7,9] More than 90% to 99% of anaphylactic reactions or suspected reactions resolve without treatment.[10] However, it is nearly impossible to accurately predict the likelihood of the clinical progression of hypersensitivity reactions or mild anaphylaxis.

The World Allergy Organization (WAO) classifies anaphylaxis as a serious life-threatening generalized or systemic hypersensitivity reaction. WAO grades systemic hypersensitivity reactions on a scale of 1 to 5, whereby 4/5 on the scale is classified as anaphylaxis (see **Table 1**). A Delphi process has been used for acute allergic reactions across a spectrum between mild and life-threatening allergic reactions that can be anaphylactic or nonanaphylactic.[11,12] Thus, anaphylaxis is either a continuum, with milder forms, or is the end result of a systemic hypersensitivity reaction. Both approaches are acceptable if epinephrine is used as the preferred therapy in all but the very mildest systemic hypersensitivity reactions.

Proposed Definition

The anaphylaxis definition the editors propose for this book is the following:

Anaphylaxis is a potentially serious, systemic reaction, either immunologic or non-immunologic, that is usually rapid in onset, is of variable severity, is responsive to the timely administration of epinephrine, and rarely causes death. Severe anaphylaxis is characterized by the compromise of breathing and/or circulation and most often, but not always, progresses from and is preceded by milder signs/symptoms. Cutaneous manifestations, including generalized pruritus, flushing, and urticaria, are the most common initial features of anaphylaxis

The authors support epinephrine 0.01 mg/kg IM as the primary treatment of systemic hypersensitivity reactions Grades 1 to 3, alternatively termed mild anaphylaxis, before the development of life-threatening manifestations of Grade 4/5. Antihistamine therapy or observation may be considered for Grade I or 2 hypersensitivity reactions, although grades can change rapidly, and antihistamine therapy is of little or no use other than to eventually eliminate the symptoms of itching. An antihistamine is not a substitute for epinephrine. Epinephrine should be administered when such symptoms and signs appear rapidly following a known allergen injection or if there is any doubt as to the potential risk of the reaction becoming more severe.

ALLERGIC VERSUS NONALLERGIC

The term anaphylaxis was first used in 1902 by Paul Portier and Charles Richet based on the specific, aberrant allergic reaction of dogs to Portuguese man-of-war toxin injections (*Portier P, Richet C. De l'action anaphylactique de certains venins. C R Séances Soc Biol 1902;54:170*). Prior investigators in the mid to late nineteenth century had described similar adverse immune effects in different animals using egg albumin, diphtheria toxin, heterologous animal sera, and eel extracts, but they did not recognize the specific immune characteristics. Observations from these early studies revealed variability in the physiologic presentation, or shock organ, in various animals experiencing anaphylaxis. This historical connection with allergy has resulted in a frequent, erroneous assumption that all anaphylaxis is an allergic event due to specific IgE triggering mast cell or basophil granule mediator release. Retrospective cohorts do show that most of the anaphylaxis in children and adults is allergic.[13,14]

Nonallergic anaphylaxis is attributed to the degranulation of mast cells or basophils via mechanisms not dependent on a specific immune response. These nonallergic forms of anaphylaxis include idiopathic, exercise-dependent, radiocontrast reactions, and some drug reactions, including most forms of nonsteroidal anti-inflammatory drug (NSAID) anaphylaxis.[15,16] Because both allergic and nonallergic anaphylaxis are related to mast cell/basophil degranulation, albeit by differing mechanisms, supports the same treatment of both allergic and nonallergic anaphylaxis. The prior term for nonallergic anaphylaxis is *anaphylactoid*; however, as the treatments for the 2 mechanisms are the same, the current preference is to use the term "nonallergic anaphylaxis" rather than "anaphylactoid."

There is a limited value of pretreatment with antihistamine and/or corticosteroid in reducing the occurrence or severity of anaphylaxis despite the importance of mast cell and basophil mediators, including histamine. The use of ineffective therapy, such as antihistamines, following the onset of anaphylaxis or systemic hypersensitivity reactions, may delay the use of more effective IM epinephrine.[7] Antihistamine pretreatment is more likely beneficial in nonallergic anaphylaxis.[17] Antihistamines, both H1 and H2, and corticosteroid therapy do not sufficiently block the number of mediators from mast cells/basophils to prevent anaphylaxis in IgE-mediated reactions.

Allergic anaphylaxis is more likely to be life-threatening than nonallergic, but both may cause death and are treated with IM epinephrine.[8] The major advantage in a thorough assessment of prior anaphylaxis by an allergist/immunologist is to identify culprits that may be avoided or to determine if allergen immunotherapy or desensitization could reduce future risk.

BIPHASIC, PERSISTENT, AND REFRACTORY ANAPHYLAXIS

Definitions of anaphylaxis focus on the rapid onset, within minutes and rarely up to hours, after exposure to the culprit allergen or circumstances responsible for anaphylaxis. Biphasic anaphylaxis is defined as a reoccurrence of anaphylaxis signs and symptoms without additional exposure to the provocateur.[18] The time between initial symptom/sign resolution and the reoccurrence of signs/symptoms is variable for biphasic anaphylaxis, but the range of 1 to 48 hours was accepted by Dribin and colleagues.[2] The variability in biphasic anaphylaxis occurrence, 1% to 19%, probably reflects the lack of consistently applied diagnostic criteria. Accurately predicting biphasic anaphylaxis is not generally possible. However, delay in the first dose of epinephrine shows an odds ratio of 2.29 (confidence interval (CI): 1.09–4.79) in predicting the occurrence of biphasic anaphylaxis.[19]

Persistent anaphylaxis is a term used to describe anaphylaxis that persists for more than 4 hours after onset, independent of management of the initial reaction; whereas, refractory anaphylaxis is persistent anaphylaxis despite treatment with IM epinephrine 0.01 mg/kg or a maximum single dose of 0.5 mg.[2] The number of doses or total dose of epinephrine sufficient to categorize anaphylaxis as persistent again is variable, with a Delphi process concluding that 3 or more "doses" or the use of intravenous (IV) epinephrine without resolution is sufficient to identify refractory anaphylaxis. Additional medical management, such as inhaled beta-agonists, oxygen, and high volume IV colloid should be used as indicated, in addition to the epinephrine, to qualify as refractory anaphylaxis. In contrast to biphasic anaphylaxis, there is no evidence that the early utilization of epinephrine is beneficial in preventing persistent or refractory anaphylaxis, but common sense would dictate it is likely to be beneficial.

EPIDEMIOLOGY

The incidence and prevalence of anaphylaxis have increased during the past 10 to 20 years. Whether the higher incidences of anaphylaxis are due to an actual increase in anaphylaxis or due to improvement in the identification of the syndrome by clinicians remains debatable.[20] The variability in anaphylactic definitions limits consistency among epidemiologic studies. Both under-recognition and over-diagnosis will obfuscate studies of a syndrome without a defining characteristic[9] Publications document the latest incidence of anaphylaxis between 50 and 112 episodes per 100,000 persons in 1 year. Prevalence is documented between 0.3% and 5.1%.[10]

Childhood Anaphylaxis

Anaphylaxis in childhood is more common in younger children between the ages of 0 and 4 years. Pediatric anaphylaxis more commonly occurs after the ingestion of foods by an allergic individual, with cow's milk, peanut, and hen egg being the most common allergens.[10] Insect allergy follows food allergy as the next common cause in childhood, when the geographic location is taken into account.[21]

Adult Anaphylaxis

Anaphylaxis in adults is most commonly attributed to drug allergy and insect sting allergy. Notably, reactions differ between young adults and older adults.[22] Administration of drugs by parenteral routes increases the risk of fatality. Some retrospective studies suggest that idiopathic anaphylaxis is the most common cause of adult cases[23]. The recognition of delayed anaphylaxis from the ingestion of alpha-

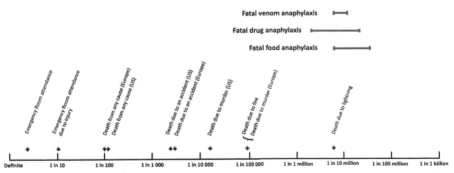

Fig. 1. Estimated rates of fatal drug, food, and venom anaphylaxis compared with other risks for the general population. Reference risks are for the US population unless otherwise stated. Colored bars represent the range of estimates from recent population-based studies of fatal anaphylaxis. (*From* Turner PJ, Jerschow E, Umasunthar T, Lin R, Campbell DE, Boyle RJ. Fatal Anaphylaxis: Mortality Rate and Risk Factors. J Allergy Clin Immunol Pract. 2017 Sep-Oct;5(5):1169-1178.)

Annual incidence of fatal anaphylaxis in food or venom allergic individuals

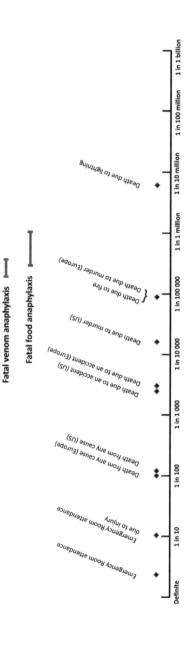

Fig. 2. Estimated rates of fatal food and venom anaphylaxis for people with known food allergy or insect venom allergy. Reference risks are for the US population unless otherwise stated. Data shown for individuals with food allergy are the 95% confidence interval of fatal food anaphylaxis risk, derived from the systematic review of.[27] Data shown for individuals with insect venom anaphylaxis were calculated using the range of estimates from recent population-based studies of fatal venom anaphylaxis, and an estimated 3% population prevalence of insect venom allergy.[26] (*From* Turner PJ, Jerschow E, Umasunthar T, Lin R, Campbell DE, Boyle RJ. Fatal Anaphylaxis: Mortality Rate and Risk Factors. J Allergy Clin Immunol Pract. 2017 Sep-Oct;5(5):1169-1178.)

galactose-D-galactose, a carbohydrate found in most mammalian meat (pork, beef, mutton) but not present in catarrhine mammals (humans and old world primates), fish, or fowl. The anaphylaxis from this carbohydrate occurs 4 to 6 hours after ingestion in allergic subjects and is an IgE-mediated allergic reaction.[24] The delay in the anaphylaxis originally limited the recognition of this allergen as a cause. Following the characterization of this syndrome, many of the idiopathic cases in adult anaphylaxis surveys are now attributed to alpha-galactose-D-galactose allergy.[13] Evidence demonstrates that tick bites in the United States are responsible for the exposure to alpha-galactose-D-galactose resulting in specific IgE responsible for the allergic reaction to red meat.[25] The rationale for the delay in symptoms is not clear.

Fatal Anaphylaxis

The incidence of anaphylaxis death in the general population is rare, and the mortality incidence among subjects with known allergy or prior anaphylaxis is uncommon.[5] Estimates of mortality from anaphylaxis in the general population approximate the risk of death from lightning strikes, about 1:9,000,000, **Fig. 1**.[5] Mortality in the population with documented allergy to insect venom or food approximates the death rate from fire or murder in Europe, about 1:500 to 900,000, **Fig. 2**.[5] Fatal anaphylaxis from insect stings is more common in subjects over 60 years, whereas fatal anaphylaxis from food allergens is more common in the second and third decades of life.[22] Older adults with comorbidities, particularly cardiovascular disease, are at increased risk of death in general, particularly to medications and insect stings.[5] Also, the mortality of anaphylaxis in the perioperative setting is greater than other scenarios, likely due to physiologic dysfunction associated with anesthesia and surgery.[8] Many, but not all, deaths from anaphylaxis were preceded by nonfatal episodes.[10] The correct diagnosis, counseling of affected subjects, and provision of epinephrine auto-injectors are important to limit fatalities.[3]

SUMMARY

Definitions of syndromes are problematic as there are no definitive tests or findings to prove or exclude the diagnosis. Anaphylaxis is usually sudden in onset, not expected, and not amenable to blinded, evidentiary human studies. The definition of anaphylaxis should be clinically useful and understandable for all or most stakeholders, including health professionals, the public, and policy makers. Regardless of the strategy to define the condition, the prompt use of safe and effective IM epinephrine is essential. Early recognition of potential anaphylaxis, monitoring of vital signs and symptoms, and prompt use of epinephrine optimize acute outcomes. Identification of the culprit is important to avoid or limit subsequent occurrences of this potentially life-threatening condition.

CLINICS CARE POINTS

- When monitoring patients for manifestations that indicate possible anaphylaxis be vigilant for generalized urticaria, pruritus, nasal congestion and rhinorrhea, nausea, abdominal cramps, chest tightness, throat clearing, and cough. A vague sensation of an impending problem is not unusual at the onset. Children may demonstrate vomiting as a primary manifestation.

- Hypotension without skin symptoms is suggestive of a mast cell disorder predisposing to anaphylaxis.

- Risk factors for a greater likelihood of progression to severe anaphylaxis include allergen exposure by injection, symptom onset in close proximity to causal exposure, preexisting asthma, mast cell disorder, and delay in the administration of IM epinephrine following the onset of symptoms.
- Anaphylaxis mortality is associated with older age, cardiovascular disease, treatment with beta-blockers or angiotensin inhibiting drugs and mast cell disorders.

DISCLOSURE

The authors have nothing to disclose that has a direct financial interest in the subject matter or materials discussed.

REFERENCES

1. Barg W, Medrala W, Wolanczyk-Medrala A. Exercise-induced anaphylaxis: an update on diagnosis and treatment. Curr Allergy Asthma Rep 2011;11(1):45–51.
2. Cardona V, Ansotegui IJ, Ebisawa M, et al. World allergy organization anaphylaxis guidance 2020. World Allergy Organ J 2020;13(10):100472.
3. Commins SP, James HR, Kelly LA, et al. The relevance of tick bites to the production of IgE antibodies to the mammalian oligosaccharide galactose-α-1,3-galactose. J Allergy Clin Immunol 2011;127(5):1286–93.e6.
4. Commins SP, Satinover SM, Hosen J, et al. Delayed anaphylaxis, angioedema, or urticaria after consumption of red meat in patients with IgE antibodies specific for galactose-alpha-1,3-galactose. J Allergy Clin Immunol 2009;123(2):426–33.
5. Cox LS, Sanchez-Borges M, Lockey RF. World allergy organization systemic allergic reaction grading system: is a modification needed? J Allergy Clin Immunol Pract 2017;5(1):58–62.e5.
6. Dribin TE, Schnadower D, Spergel JM, et al. Severity grading system for acute allergic reactions: a multidisciplinary Delphi study. J Allergy Clin Immunol 2021; 148(1):173–81.
7. Farnam K, Chang C, Teuber S, et al. Nonallergic drug hypersensitivity reactions. Int Arch Allergy Immunol 2012;159(4):327–45.
8. Hogan SP. Severity grading system for acute allergic reactions-time for validation and assessment of best practices. J Allergy Clin Immunol 2021;148(1):86–8.
9. Mali S. Anaphylaxis during the perioperative period. Anesth Essays Res 2012; 6(2):124–33.
10. Pattanaik D, Lieberman P, Lieberman J, et al. The changing face of anaphylaxis in adults and adolescents. Ann Allergy Asthma Immunol 2018;121(5):594–7.
11. Prince BT, Mikhail I, Stukus DR. Underuse of epinephrine for the treatment of anaphylaxis: missed opportunities. J Asthma Allergy 2018;11:143–51.
12. Tanno LK, Bierrenbach AL, Simons FER, et al. Critical view of anaphylaxis epidemiology: open questions and new perspectives. Allergy Asthma Clin Immunol 2018;14:12.
13. Tejedor Alonso MA, Moro Moro M, Múgica García MV. Epidemiology of anaphylaxis. Clin Exp Allergy 2015a;45(6):1027–39.
14. Tejedor-Alonso MA, Moro-Moro M, Múgica-García MV. Epidemiology of anaphylaxis: contributions from the last 10 years. J Investig Allergol Clin Immunol 2015b;25(3):163–75 [quiz follow 174–165].
15. Trcka J, Schmidt C, Seitz CS, et al. Anaphylaxis to iodinated contrast material: nonallergic hypersensitivity or IgE-mediated allergy? AJR Am J Roentgenol 2008;190(3):666–70.

16. Turner PJ, Baumert JL, Beyer K, et al. Can we identify patients at risk of life-threatening allergic reactions to food? Allergy 2016;71(9):1241–55.
17. Turner PJ, DunnGalvin A, Hourihane JO. The emperor has no symptoms: the risks of a blanket approach to using epinephrine autoinjectors for all allergic reactions. J Allergy Clin Immunol Pract 2016;4(6):1143–6.
18. Turner PJ, Gowland MH, Sharma V, et al. Increase in anaphylaxis-related hospitalizations but no increase in fatalities: an analysis of United Kingdom national anaphylaxis data, 1992-2012. J Allergy Clin Immunol 2015;135(4):956–63.e1.
19. Turner PJ, Jerschow E, Umasunthar T, et al. Fatal anaphylaxis: mortality rate and risk factors. J Allergy Clin Immunol 2017;5(5):1169–78.
20. Webb LM, Lieberman P. Anaphylaxis: a review of 601 cases. Ann Allergy Asthma Immunol 2006;97(1):39–43.
21. Worm M, Moneret-Vautrin A, Scherer K, et al. First European data from the network of severe allergic reactions (NORA). Allergy 2014;69(10):1397–404.
22. Wright CD, Longjohn M, Lieberman PL, et al. An analysis of anaphylaxis cases at a single pediatric emergency department during a 1-year period. Ann Allergy Asthma Immunol 2017;118(4):461–4.
23. Alqurashi W, Stiell I, Chan K, et al. Epidemiology and clinical predictors of biphasic reactions in children with anaphylaxis. Ann Allergy Asthma Immunol 2015;115(3):217–23.e2.
24. Dribin TE, Sampson HA, Camargo CA Jr, et al. Persistent, refractory, and biphasic anaphylaxis: a multidisciplinary Delphi study. J Allergy Clin Immunol 2020;146(5):1089–96.
25. Lee S, Peterson A, Lohse CM, et al. Further evaluation of factors that may predict biphasic reactions in emergency department anaphylaxis patients. J Allergy Clin Immunol Pract 2017;5(5):1295–301.
26. Golden DBK. Anaphylaxis to insect stings. Immunol Allergy Clin North Am 2015; 35(2):287–302.
27. Umasunthar T, Leonardi-Bee J, Hodes M, et al. Incidence of fatal food anaphylaxis in people with food allergy: a systematic review and meta-analysis. Clin Exp Allergy 2013;43(12):1333–41.

Anaphylaxis
Epidemiology and Differential Diagnosis

Megan S. Motosue, MD[a],*, James T. Li, PhD, MD[b],
Ronna L. Campbell, PhD, MD[c]

KEYWORDS

- Anaphylaxis • Epidemiology • Differential Diagnosis

KEY POINTS

- Allergic reactions and anaphylaxis occur on a severity continuum from mild and self-limited to potentially life-threatening or fatal reactions.
- The most common causes of anaphylaxis are food, medications, and stinging insects.
- Rates of anaphylaxis-related emergency department visits and hospitalizations are increasing though fatal anaphylaxis is rare.

INTRODUCTION

Anaphylaxis is a potentially life-threatening allergic reaction. Since its initial description by Charles Richet and Paul Portier in 1902,[1] our understanding of anaphylaxis has grown in terms of its epidemiology and underlying causes.

ANAPHYLAXIS EPIDEMIOLOGY

The overall global incidence of anaphylaxis is reported to be between 50 and 112 episodes per 100,000 person-years[2] and the global incidence among children has been estimated to range from 1 to 761 per 100,000 person-years.[3] The lifetime prevalence of anaphylaxis ranges from 0.3% to 5.1%.[2,4] Data from Europe reported that more than a quarter of anaphylaxis cases occurred in those younger than 18 years of age.[5]

Time Trends

In the United States (US), a retrospective study[6] based on administrative claims data found that emergency department (ED) visits for anaphylaxis increased by 101% between 2005 and 2014. During that same time frame, hospitalizations for anaphylaxis in

[a] Department of Allergy and Immunology, Kaiser Honolulu Clinic, 1010 Pensacola Street, Honolulu, HI, USA; [b] Division of Allergic Diseases, Mayo Clinic, 200 First Street Southwest Mayo Clinic, Rochester, MN, USA; [c] Department of Emergency Medicine, Mayo Clinic, 200 First Street Southwest Generose Building G-410, Rochester, MN, USA
* Corresponding author.
E-mail address: Megan.S.Motosue@kp.org

Immunol Allergy Clin N Am 42 (2022) 13–25
https://doi.org/10.1016/j.iac.2021.09.010
0889-8561/22/© 2021 Elsevier Inc. All rights reserved.

immunology.theclinics.com

the US increased by 37.6%.[7] This mirrors global trends whereby increasing anaphylaxis-related hospitalizations have been reported in Europe,[8,9] the United Kingdom (UK),[10] and Australia.[11] Hospital admission rates differ by country with the highest rates in Australia and lowest rates in the US and Spain. In the US, less than 20% of anaphylaxis-related ED visits are admitted (observation or hospital ward).[7] This is likely due to differences in admission thresholds between countries and the emergence of observation units, particularly in the US, which may not be coded as an admission.[12]

Despite increases in anaphylaxis hospitalizations, anaphylaxis fatalities in the US have been low and stable at about 0.63 to 0.75 per million adults per year. Overall, anaphylaxis-related fatalities account for an estimated 1% of hospitalizations and 0.1% of ED visits for anaphylaxis.[13] The top 3 causes of fatal anaphylaxis in adults are medications (38%–58.8%),[11,14] insect venom (15.2%-18%),[11,14] and foods (6.7%).[11,14] African American ethnicity and older age have been associated with fatal anaphylaxis, with fatal venom-related anaphylaxis more common in males and Caucasians.[13]

Common Triggers

Food is the most common trigger for anaphylaxis-related hospitalizations and highest in the pediatric population (age <18 years). The most common specific food trigger varies by age group with cow's milk more common in infants, peanuts in children, and shellfish and tree nuts in young adults and adults.[15] In the US, ED visits for food-induced anaphylaxis increased by 214% ($P < .001$) from 2005 to 2014 with the highest rates reported in infants and toddlers (age 0–2 years).[6] This supports other studies published in Spain[9] and Canada[16] whereby rates of anaphylaxis in children ages 0 to 4 years were 3 times greater than those among older age groups. Pediatric patients represent a vulnerable patient population as the diagnosis of food induced anaphylaxis in infants and children can be very challenging. Younger patients also may not have a prior diagnosis of food allergy and may present either with a subtle or delayed clinical presentation. Consequently, caregivers and health care providers must maintain a high level of suspicion when evaluating pediatric patients for reactions in the context of a food exposure.[17]

Mediations are another common trigger for anaphylaxis. Adverse drug reactions occur in up to 10% of the general population and of those 10% are drug hypersensitivity reactions.[18] The most common drug triggers in the US are antibiotics (penicillin, cephalosporins, and sulfonamides), nonsteroidal anti-inflammatory drugs (NSAIDs), biologics, and immunomodulators.[19–21] Medications are the most common cause of fatal anaphylaxis in the US[14] and elsewhere including Brazil, New Zealand, Australia, and the UK. In contrast to other allergic triggers, rates of fatal medication-induced anaphylaxis are increasing.[14] Data from the UK fatal anaphylaxis registry reported that many of those with fatal drug anaphylaxis had no prior indication of drug allergy suggesting that the first reaction can be fatal.[22,23]

Stinging insects are a common trigger in both pediatric and adult patient populations. Systemic reactions to insect stings may affect up to 0.8% of children and 3% of adults with at least 40 fatal stings per year nationally.[24] The most common insect triggers include hymenopterans (yellow jacket, hornet, wasp, honeybee and imported fire ant). Venom specific triggers differ by region with wasp more common in Austria, Germany, and central Europe[5] whereas honeybee is more common in South Korea.[25] The incidence of insect allergy has increased in some areas and decreased in others, which experts have attributed to multiple factors including insect migration, climate change, and the encroachment of humans into new habitats.[26] Although insect allergy is more common in young adults, fatal anaphylaxis due to insect stings is more likely to occur in adults older than 45 years of age, likely related to comorbidities and impaired compensatory mechanisms.[27] Similar to drug induced reactions, published data from the UK fatal anaphylaxis registry[22,23] suggest that the initial venom-induced anaphylactic reaction can be fatal.

Differential Diagnosis

Anaphylaxis phenotypes

Castells[28] published a new classification scheme for anaphylaxis based on phenotypic presentations and on underlying endotypes. The phenotypes are defined by clinical presentation into 4 types: (1) type I-like reactions, (2) cytokine storm-like reactions, (3) mixed reactions, and (4) complement reactions (**Fig. 1**). Type I-like reactions present with a spectrum of signs and symptoms including pruritus, hives, flushing, shortness of breath, vomiting, and cardiovascular collapse and may be due to both immunoglobulin E (IgE)- and non–IgE-mediated mechanisms. Typical IgE-mediated triggers include foods, medications, and Hymenoptera venoms. Non–IgE-mediated reactions may occur through mast cell mediator release via the Mas-related G protein-coupled receptor X2 (MRGPRX2), a newly described G-coupled receptor

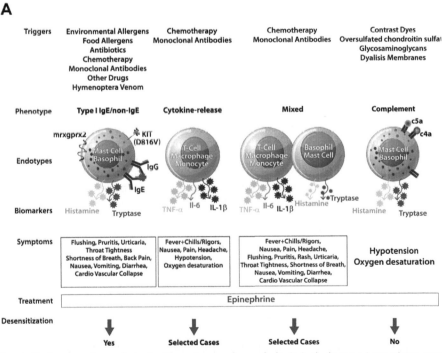

Fig. 1. Pathways of anaphylaxis. Phenotypes of anaphylaxis include type I reactions, cytokine storm-like reactions, and mixed reactions. Endotypes of anaphylaxis include IgE- and non–IgE-mediated reactions, direct mast cell and basophil activation, cytokine release, and mixed reactions. Biomarkers include tryptase, histamine, and other mast cell/basophil mediators, as well as cytokines, such as TNF-α, IL-1β, and IL-6. Desensitization is indicated in type I reactions and selected cases of cytokine storm and mixed reactions but not in direct mast cell/basophil release. (*From* Castells M. Diagnosis and management of anaphylaxis in precision medicine. J Allergy Clin Immunol. 2017 Aug;140(2):321 to 333.)

expressed on mast cells. Drugs with tetrahydroisoquinoline (THIQ) motifs, which include quinolone antibiotics (eg, levofloxacin and ciprofloxacin) along with neuromuscular-blocking agents (eg, atracurium and rocuronium) have been shown to directly activate mast cells via the MRGPRX2 receptor. IgG-dependent pathways is another mechanism of non–IgE-mediated reactions as animal models and human observational studies have shown that IgG alone and in immune complexes can activate mast cells and contribute to anaphylactic reactions.[29] Rituximab and other chimeric IgG monoclonal antibodies can trigger histamine and tryptase release potentially supporting the role of IgG in anaphylactic reactions.[28]

In contrast, cytokine storm-like reactions, the second type of anaphylaxis in the aforementioned scheme, present with fever, chills, headache, malaise and may be followed by hypotension, oxygen desaturation, and myocardial dysfunction. Severe cases may lead to disseminated intravascular coagulation and multi-organ failure. Such reactions are due to the release of proinflammatory mediators IL-1β, IL-6, and TNF-α. Monoclonal antibodies and chemotherapy agents such as oxaliplatin are triggers for these types of reactions. Corticosteroid and COX-1 inhibitor pretreatment do not prevent severe reactions but have been used to decrease intensity. When reactions present with a combination of type 1 and cytokine storm like reactions (eg, hives, swelling, fever, chills, hypotension, and desaturations), they are labeled as mixed reactions (type 3). Monoclonal antibodies and chemotherapy agents are causes of mixed reactions.

The fourth anaphylaxis phenotype is due to direct mast cell activation as can occur with vancomycin or through complement activation by contrast dyes, oversulfated chondroitin sulfate, and glycosaminoglycans. Patients with this phenotype may present with hives, oxygen desaturation, and hypotension.

Exercise-induced anaphylaxis
In addition to foods, drugs, and Hymenoptera venom, exercise is another important trigger for anaphylaxis. Exercise-induced anaphylaxis (EIA) reportedly occurs in up to 3% of all anaphylaxis cases.[30] EIA is subcategorized into (1) drug-dependent exercise-induced anaphylaxis (DDEIA), (2) food-independent exercise-induced anaphylaxis (FIEIA), and (3) food-dependent exercise-induced anaphylaxis (FDEIA) with and without IgE sensitivity. In terms of its natural history, for most patients with EIA the frequency of attacks tends to stabilize (46%) or decrease (47%).[31]

In cases of FIEIA, exercise is the only trigger with the most common reported exercise activities being running, brisk walking, biking, racquet sports, intense gardening, and vigorous dancing.[30] In DDEIA, the combination of drug intake with exercise triggers anaphylaxis. The most common drug triggers are NSAIDs with cases of cephalosporins reported.[30]

FDEIA is a disorder in which anaphylaxis develops when exercise takes place within a few hours of ingesting a specific food. Frequently cited food triggers in Western populations include wheat with the major protein epitope omega-5-gliadin, other grains, and nuts. In Asian populations, wheat and shellfish are most common though other foods including seeds, vegetables, fruits, meats, cow's milk, and egg have been reported.[32] Whether exercise increases the absorption of the allergen[33] or lowers the activation threshold of mast cells and basophils[34] remains unclear, as the specific mechanism of FDEIA has not been elucidated. FDEIA is considered a postprandial event and patients are recommended to avoid exercise for to 4 to 6 hours after eating a known food trigger, to lower exercise intensity after eating, to avoid exercising in extreme temperatures, and to carry an epinephrine autoinjector when exercising.[32]

Recently, the induction of anaphylaxis has been described with the combination of food ingestion and nonexercise augmenting factors. These observations have given rise to the concept of "augmentation factor-triggered food allergy,[35]" and highlight the importance of cofactors in facilitating anaphylaxis.[32,36] Augmenting factors include alcohol, menstruation, acute infections, and medications specifically NSAIDs and antacids. As these factors may lower the reaction threshold and increase reaction severity, cases of anaphylaxis should be evaluated for augmenting factors as they play an important role in the development of allergic reactions.[36]

Idiopathic anaphylaxis
When no trigger is identified, anaphylaxis is classified as idiopathic. Idiopathic anaphylaxis (IA) accounts for up to 30% to 60% of cases of anaphylaxis in adults and up to 10% of cases in children.[37–39] IA occurs more commonly in women than in men.[37] Those with IA have a high frequency of atopy as 48% of IA patients have food allergy, allergic rhinitis, or other atopic condition.[40] It is a diagnosis of exclusion as systemic mastocytosis and other mast cell disorders need to be ruled out. In addition, over the last decade, sensitivity to novel allergens such as the oligosaccharide galactose-alpha-(1,3)-galactose (α-gal) have reclassified previous cases of IA.[41]

α-Gal anaphylaxis
Sensitization to α-gal has been classically associated with 2 distinct presentations: (1) immediate hypersensitivity reaction to cetuximab and (2) delayed anaphylaxis to red meat (noncatarrhine mammalian meat). The unique delayed reaction is thought to be due to the digestive processes required to expose the carbohydrate moiety.[42] Cases of α-gal have been reported in the US and worldwide including Australia, Japan, Africa, and Europe.[43] Sensitization to α-gal occurs via tick bites with the lone star tick (*Amblyomma americanum*) being the relevant tick species in the US (**Fig. 2**).[43] In a single center retrospective study, α-gal was the most common cause of anaphylaxis. On a follow-up report from the same center, the percentage of IA cases decreased from 59% in their previous report to 35%, which the authors attributed to the recognition of α-gal cases.[39,41] Additional research is needed to identify additional novel allergens to further clarify cases of IA.

Non-allergic mimics of anaphylaxis
The differential diagnosis of anaphylaxis is broad and includes flushing syndromes (pheochromocytoma, carcinoid tumor, medullary carcinoma of the thyroid, and vasovagal reactions), restaurant syndromes (scombroidosis and monosodium glutamate ingestion reactions), and nonorganic disease (Munchausen stridor, vocal cord dysfunction, and panic attack).[15] A more comprehensive list of nonallergic differential diagnoses is listed in **Box 1**.

Diagnostic Challenges

Anaphylaxis is underrecognized and underdiagnosed.[44,45] Anaphylaxis is frequently missed in patients seen in the ED, undergoing anesthesia and surgery, and those treated with biologic agents such as monoclonal antibodies and chemotherapy.[28] This is likely due to the myriad of associated diagnostic challenges and the spontaneous recovery of the majority of affected individuals. Anaphylaxis lacks a clinically useful definition and a reliable, diagnostic biomarker. There exists a disconnect in how anaphylaxis has been defined traditionally based on IgE, mast cells, and basophils and how the diagnosis of anaphylaxis is applied clinically. In fact, a round table meeting[46] of ED providers concluded, "the traditional mechanistic definition of anaphylaxis is not useful."

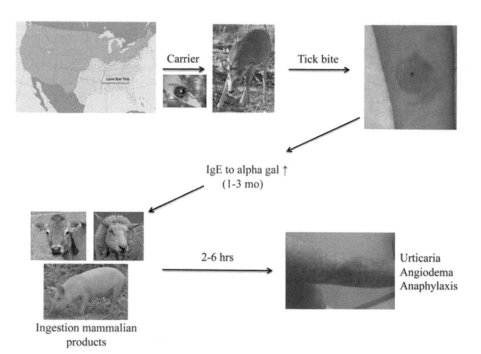

Carrier

Tick bite

IgE to alpha gal ↑
(1-3 mo)

2-6 hrs

Urticaria
Angiodema
Anaphylaxis

Ingestion mammalian
products

Fig. 2. Summary of α-Gal sensitization leading to clinical symptoms of red meat allergy. The southeastern section of the US is where most of the reactions to meat derived from non-primate mammals (eg, beef, lamb, or pork) have been reported. This region overlaps with the distribution of the Lone Star tick, **Amblyomma americanum**. The current hypothesis is that people are bitten by Lone Star ticks carried by deer into rural and urban areas. Following a period of time, IgE to α-Gal develops. Once specific-IgE to α-Gal reaches sufficient levels, ingestion of red meat can trigger reactions. (*Adapted from* Steinke JW, Platts-Mills TA, Commins SP. The alpha-gal story: lessons learned from connecting the dots. J Allergy Clin Immunol. 2015 Mar;135(3):589-96; quiz 597.)

In addition, although there have been numerous national and international guidelines published, the lack of consensus between these guidelines compounds current challenges. For example, a food-induced reaction that results in persistent vomiting and dyspnea (without bronchospasm) would constitute anaphylaxis under NIAID/FAAN criteria.[47] However, under guidelines published in the UK[48] and Australia,[49] these presenting symptoms would not meet anaphylaxis criteria given the absence of mucocutaneous manifestations.[50] Refinements to the NIAID/FAAN clinical criteria were recently proposed by the WAO Anaphylaxis Committee[51] but the impact on clinical management is unknown.

In addition, beyond establishing consensus guidelines, efforts to disseminate these recommendations to address knowledge, and practice gaps are needed. In a cross-sectional survey of over 3000 paramedics in the US, 98% correctly identified a "classic case" in which a patient presented with urticaria, itching, and angioedema after exposure to penicillin. However, only 2.9% were able to identify an atypical case without the usual skin findings or a known allergen exposure.

A lack of available point of care testing represents another diagnostic challenge. Although anaphylaxis is a clinical diagnosis, the use of biomarkers may support the diagnosis and assist clinicians in differentiating anaphylaxis from potential mimics.

Box 1
Differential diagnosis of anaphylaxis

Neurologic/autonomic dysregulation
1. Vasovagal and vasodepressor reactions
2. Postural orthostatic tachycardia syndrome
3. Seizure
4. CVA

Cardiovascular
1. Cardiogenic shock
2. Hemorrhagic shock
3. Vasodilatory/distributive/endotoxic shock
4. Capillary leak syndrome (hypovolemic shock)
5. Pulmonary embolus

Endocrine/flushing
1. Carcinoid
2. Pheochromocytoma
3. VIP-secreting tumors
4. Thyroid medullary carcinoma
5. Menopause (flushing, hot flashes)
6. Hypoglycemia

Iatrogenic/drugs
1. Vancomycin (Red Man syndrome)
2. Niacin (flushing)
3. General and spinal anesthetics (hypotension)

Toxic
1. "Restaurant syndromes"
   a. Scombroidosis
   b. MSG
2. Alcohol
3. Sulfites

Hematologic/malignant
1. Systemic mastocytosis
2. Urticaria pigmentosa
3. Basophil leukemia
4. Acute promyelocytic leukemia with tretinoin treatment

Immunologic
1. Bradykinin-mediated angioedema

Infection
1. Hydatid cyst (*Echinococcus granulosus*)
2. Sepsis/septic shock

Psychosomatic/functional disorders
1. Panic attack
2. Factitious anaphylaxis
   a. Munchausen stridor
3. Undifferentiated somatoform anaphylaxis
4. Vocal cord dysfunction

Abbeeviations: C1, complement 1; C4, complement 4; CBC, complete blood count; CVA, cerebrovascular accident; EtOH, ethanol; FSH, follicle-stimulating hormone; 5-HIAA, urine 5-hydroxy indole acetic acid; LH, luteinizing hormone; MSG, monosodium glutamate; RHC, right heart catheterization; TTE, transthoracic echocardiogram; VIP, vasoactive intestinal peptide.

Adapted from LoVerde D, Iweala OI, Eginli A, Krishnaswamy G. Anaphylaxis. Chest. 2018 Feb;153(2):528-543.

The main biomarker currently available is serum tryptase.[20] Serum tryptase is increased 30 minutes following the onset of a reaction, peaks 1 to 2 hours after reaction onset, and remains elevated up to 6 to 8 hours.[28] However, although tryptase is recommended by current guidelines, it is not useful for ED providers as results are typically not available in time to guide clinical decision-making. In addition, although its positive predictive value is high (93%), total serum tryptase has a low negative predictive value.[52] Moreover, tryptase is often not elevated in cases of food-induced anaphylaxis. Additional biomarkers, such as platelet activating factor, chymase, chemokine ligand-2, and carboxypeptidase A3, are being studied but are difficult to measure.[53] Future studies are needed to identify additional candidate biomarkers along with examining the sensitivity and specificity of using combinations of biomarkers. In addition, the barrier of obtaining timely biomarker results to facilitate clinical decision making needs to be addressed.

New Advances in Anaphylaxis

Updated anaphylaxis treatment recommendations were published in 2020. Based on a recently updated Joint Task Force on Practice Parameters (JTFPP),[19] routine use of postevent glucocorticoids and antihistamines is no longer recommended as an intervention to prevent biphasic anaphylaxis. The benefit of glucocorticoids and antihistamines in the acute management of anaphylaxis and in the prevention of biphasic anaphylaxis has not been established.[54,55] In addition, studies have raised concerns

---

Box 2
Clinical criteria for diagnosing persistent, refractory, and biphasic anaphylaxis

Persistent anaphylaxis is highly likely when the following criterion is fulfilled: [a]
1. Presence of symptoms/examination findings that fulfil the 2006 NIAID/FAAN anaphylaxis criteria that persist for at least 4 h[1]

Refractory anaphylaxis is highly likely when both of the following 2 criteria are fulfilled: [b]
1. Presence of anaphylaxis following appropriate epinephrine dosing and symptom-directed medical management (eg, IV fluid bolus for hypotension).
2. The initial reaction must be treated with 3 or more appropriate doses of epinephrine (or initiation of an IV epinephrine infusion). [c]

Biphasic anaphylaxis is highly likely when all of the following 4 criteria are fulfilled: [d]
1 New/recurrent symptoms/examination findings must fulfil the 2006 NIAID/FAAN anaphylaxis criteria.[1]
2. Initial symptoms/examination findings must completely resolve before the onset of new/recurrent symptoms/examination findings.
3. There cannot be allergen reexposure before the onset of new/recurrent symptoms/examination findings.
4. New/recurrent symptoms/examination findings must occur within 1–48 h from complete resolution of initial symptoms/examination findings.

[a] The diagnosis of persistent anaphylaxis is independent of the management of the initial reaction.

[b] Refractory anaphylaxis is not dependent on the duration of symptoms/examination findings.

[c] Appropriate epinephrine dosing: 0.01 mg/kg IM epinephrine, maximum single dose 0.5 mg. Also includes manufacturer recommended dosing for epinephrine auto-injectors.

[d] The diagnosis of biphasic anaphylaxis is independent of the management of the initial reaction.

From Dribin TE, Sampson HA, Camargo CA, Jr., et al. Persistent, refractory, and biphasic anaphylaxis: A multidisciplinary Delphi study. J Allergy Clin Immunol 2020;146(5):1089-96.

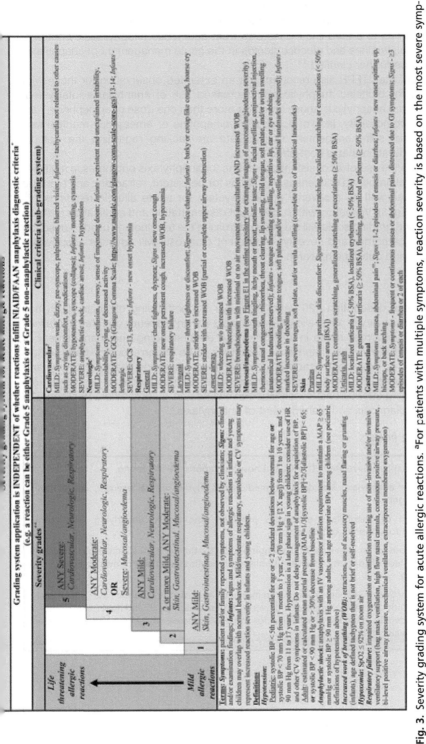

Fig. 3. Severity grading system for acute allergic reactions. [a]For patients with multiple symptoms, reaction severity is based on the most severe symptom; symptoms that constitute more severe grades always supersede symptoms from less severe grades. The grading system can be used to assign reaction severity at any time during the course of reactions; reactions may progress rapidly (within minutes) from one severity grade to another. The grading system does not dictate management decisions; reactions of any severity grade may require treatment with epinephrine. [b]Patients with severe cardiovascular and/or neurologic involvement may have urinary or stool incontinence. However, the significance of incontinence as an isolated symptom is unclear, and it is therefore not included as a symptom in the subgrading system. [c]Abdominal pain may also result from uterine cramping. (*From* Dribin TE, Schnadower D, Spergel JM, et al. Severity grading system for acute allergic reactions: A multidisciplinary Delphi study [published online ahead of print, 2021 Jan 19]. J Allergy Clin Immunol. 2021;S0091-6749(21)00047-6.)

regarding the harmful effects of glucocorticoids.[56] The most recent European Academy of Allergy and Clinical Immunology guidelines[57] have moved antihistamines from second line to a third line measure to treat cutaneous anaphylaxis symptoms. The role antihistamines and glucocorticoids in the acute management of anaphylaxis will need to be further clarified.[12]

In addition, the JTFPP also recommends an extended observation for those with risk factors for biphasic anaphylaxis or increased risk of anaphylaxis fatality (eg, resolved severe anaphylaxis, those requiring more than one dose of epinephrine, cardiovascular comorbidity, lack of access to epinephrine or emergency medical services, or poor self-management skills). Data are lacking regarding the optimal observation duration that is cost-effective.

To address the use of inconsistent definitions for anaphylaxis outcomes, a multidisciplinary panel proposed consensus definitions for persistent, refractory, and biphasic anaphylaxis as well as a severity grading system for acute allergic reactions[58,59] (**Box 2** and **Fig. 3**). Validation with subsequent dissemination and application of these definitions and grading scale will aid in standardizing the terminology used to describe anaphylaxis outcomes and severity. Consistent diagnosis will advance anaphylaxis clinical care and outcome research.

SUMMARY

Since its initial description 120 years ago, our understanding of anaphylaxis has grown. The discovery of novel allergens such as α-gal and recently updated guidelines exemplify the progress made in improving our understanding and management of anaphylaxis. However, as anaphylaxis continues to be underrecognized and underdiagnosed, it is likely that anaphylaxis is far more common than previously and currently reported. Efforts to address deficiencies such as the need for biomarkers and establishing international consensus definitions and guidelines are necessary to improve the diagnosis and management of anaphylaxis.

CLINICS CARE POINTS

- Rates of anaphylaxis-related ED visits and hospitalizations are increasing.
- Triggers for anaphylaxis include food, medications, Hymenoptera, exercise, and a novel allergen α-gal.
- Recognition of anaphylaxis endotypes provides insight into underlying mechanisms responsible for anaphylaxis phenotypes.
- The diagnosis of anaphylaxis is challenging due to the lack of a universally accepted definition, lack of consensus between published guidelines, and lack of available point of care testing.
- Recent practice guidelines have recommended against the routine use of systemic corticosteroids and antihistamines to prevent biphasic anaphylaxis and have recommended an extended observation for those with increased risk of a biphasic reaction or anaphylaxis fatality.

DISCLOSURE

R.L. Campbell is an author for UpToDate and a consultant for Bryn Pharma. All other authors declare no conflicts of interest.

REFERENCES

1. Cohen SG, Zelaya-Quesada M. Portier, Richet, and the discovery of anaphylaxis: a centennial. J Allergy Clin Immunol 2002;110(2):331–6.
2. Tejedor Alonso MA, Moro Moro M, Mugica Garcia MV. Epidemiology of anaphylaxis. Clin Exp Allergy 2015;45(6):1027–39.
3. Wang Y, Allen KJ, Suaini NHA, et al. The global incidence and prevalence of anaphylaxis in children in the general population: A systematic review. Allergy 2019;74(6):1063–80.
4. Wood RA, Camargo CA Jr, Lieberman P, et al. Anaphylaxis in America: the prevalence and characteristics of anaphylaxis in the United States. J Allergy Clin Immunol 2014;133(2):461–7.
5. Worm M, Moneret-Vautrin A, Scherer K, et al. First European data from the network of severe allergic reactions (NORA). Allergy 2014;69(10):1397–404.
6. Motosue MS, Bellolio MF, Van Houten HK, et al. Increasing Emergency Department Visits for Anaphylaxis, 2005-2014. J Allergy Clin Immunol Pract 2017;5(1): 171–175 e3.
7. Motosue MS, Bellolio MF, Van Houten HK, et al. Outcomes of Emergency Department Anaphylaxis Visits from 2005 to 2014. J Allergy Clin Immunol Pract 2018; 6(3):1002–1009 e2.
8. Jeppesen AN, Christiansen CF, Froslev T, et al. Hospitalization rates and prognosis of patients with anaphylactic shock in Denmark from 1995 through 2012. J Allergy Clin Immunol 2016;137(4):1143–7.
9. Tejedor-Alonso MA, Moro-Moro M, Mosquera Gonzalez M, et al. Increased incidence of admissions for anaphylaxis in Spain 1998-2011. Allergy 2015;70(7): 880–3.
10. Turner PJ, Gowland MH, Sharma V, et al. Increase in anaphylaxis-related hospitalizations but no increase in fatalities: an analysis of United Kingdom national anaphylaxis data, 1992-2012. J Allergy Clin Immunol 2015;135(4):956–963 e1.
11. Liew WK, Williamson E, Tang ML. Anaphylaxis fatalities and admissions in Australia. J Allergy Clin Immunol 2009;123(2):434 42.
12. Turner PJ, Campbell DE, Motosue MS, et al. Global Trends in Anaphylaxis Epidemiology and Clinical Implications. J Allergy Clin Immunol Pract 2020;8(4): 1169–76.
13. Turner PJ, Jerschow E, Umasunthar T, et al. Fatal Anaphylaxis: Mortality Rate and Risk Factors. J Allergy Clin Immunol Pract 2017;5(5):1169–78.
14. Jerschow E, Lin RY, Scaperotti MM, et al. Fatal anaphylaxis in the United States, 1999-2010: temporal patterns and demographic associations. J Allergy Clin Immunol 2014;134(6):1318–1328 e7.
15. Poowuttikul P, Seth D. Anaphylaxis in children and adolescents. Pediatr Clin North Am 2019;66(5):995–1005.
16. Simons FE, Peterson S, Black CD. Epinephrine dispensing patterns for an out-of-hospital population: a novel approach to studying the epidemiology of anaphylaxis. J Allergy Clin Immunol 2002;110(4):647–51.
17. Samady W, Trainor J, Smith B, et al. Food-induced anaphylaxis in infants and children. Ann Allergy Asthma Immunol 2018;121(3):360–5.
18. Lazarou J, Pomeranz BH, Corey PN. Incidence of adverse drug reactions in hospitalized patients: a meta-analysis of prospective studies. JAMA 1998;279(15): 1200–5.
19. Shaker MS, Wallace DV, Golden DBK, et al. Anaphylaxis-a 2020 practice parameter update, systematic review, and Grading of Recommendations, Assessment,

Development and Evaluation (GRADE) analysis. J Allergy Clin Immunol 2020; 145(4):1082–123.

20. Cardona V, Ansotegui IJ, Ebisawa M, et al. World allergy organization anaphylaxis guidance 2020. World Allergy Organ J 2020;13(10):100472.

21. Simons FE, Ardusso LR, Dimov V, et al. World Allergy Organization Anaphylaxis Guidelines: 2013 update of the evidence base. Int Arch Allergy Immunol 2013; 162(3):193–204.

22. Pumphrey R. Anaphylaxis: can we tell who is at risk of a fatal reaction? Curr Opin Allergy Clin Immunol 2004;4(4):285–90.

23. Pumphrey RS. Lessons for management of anaphylaxis from a study of fatal reactions. Clin Exp Allergy 2000;30(8):1144–50.

24. Graft DF. Insect sting allergy. Med Clin North Am 2006;90(1):211–32.

25. Cho H, Kwon JW. Prevalence of anaphylaxis and prescription rates of epinephrine auto-injectors in urban and rural areas of Korea. Korean J Intern Med 2019;34(3):643–50.

26. Barne C, Alexis NE, Bernstein JA, et al. Climate change and our environment: the effect on respiratory and allergic disease. J Allergy Clin Immunol Pract 2013;1(2): 137–41.

27. Tankersley MS, Ledford DK. Stinging insect allergy: state of the art 2015. J Allergy Clin Immunol Pract 2015;3(3):315–22, quiz 323.

28. Castells M. Diagnosis and management of anaphylaxis in precision medicine. J Allergy Clin Immunol 2017;140(2):321–33.

29. Cianferoni A. Non-IgE-mediated anaphylaxis. J Allergy Clin Immunol 2021; 147(4):1123–31.

30. Geller M. Clinical Management of Exercise-Induced Anaphylaxis and Cholinergic Urticaria. J Allergy Clin Immunol Pract 2020;8(7):2209–14.

31. Shadick NA, Liang MH, Partridge AJ, et al. The natural history of exercise-induced anaphylaxis: survey results from a 10-year follow-up study. J Allergy Clin Immunol 1999;104(1):123–7.

32. Feldweg AM. Food-Dependent, Exercise-Induced Anaphylaxis: Diagnosis and Management in the Outpatient Setting. J Allergy Clin Immunol Pract 2017;5(2): 283–8.

33. Matsuo H, Morimoto K, Akaki T, et al. Exercise and aspirin increase levels of circulating gliadin peptides in patients with wheat-dependent exercise-induced anaphylaxis. Clin Exp Allergy 2005;35(4):461–6.

34. Kivity S, Sneh E, Greif J, et al. The effect of food and exercise on the skin response to compound 48/80 in patients with food-associated exercise-induced urticaria-angioedema. J Allergy Clin Immunol 1988;81(6):1155–8.

35. Brockow K, Kneissl D, Valentini L, et al. Using a gluten oral food challenge protocol to improve diagnosis of wheat-dependent exercise-induced anaphylaxis. J Allergy Clin Immunol 2015;135(4):977–984 e4.

36. Niggemann B, Beyer K. Factors augmenting allergic reactions. Allergy 2014; 69(12):1582–7.

37. Ditto AM, Harris KE, Krasnick J, et al. Idiopathic anaphylaxis: a series of 335 cases. Ann Allergy Asthma Immunol 1996;77(4):285–91.

38. Kemp SF, Lockey RF, Wolf BL, et al. Anaphylaxis. A review of 266 cases. Arch Intern Med 1995;155(16):1749–54.

39. Webb LM, Lieberman P. Anaphylaxis: a review of 601 cases. Ann Allergy Asthma Immunol 2006;97(1):39–43.

40. Tejedor Alonso MA, Sastre DJ, Sanchez-Hernandez JJ, et al. Idiopathic anaphylaxis: a descriptive study of 81 patients in Spain. Ann Allergy Asthma Immunol 2002;88(3):313–8.
41. Pattanaik D, Lieberman P, Lieberman J, et al. The changing face of anaphylaxis in adults and adolescents. Ann Allergy Asthma Immunol 2018;121(5):594–7.
42. Steinke JW, Platts-Mills TA, Commins SP. The alpha-gal story: lessons learned from connecting the dots. J Allergy Clin Immunol 2015;135(3):589–96, quiz 597.
43. Platts-Mills TAE, Li RC, Keshavarz B, et al. Diagnosis and Management of Patients with the alpha-Gal Syndrome. J Allergy Clin Immunol Pract 2020;8(1): 15–23 e1.
44. Sclar DA, Lieberman PL. Anaphylaxis: underdiagnosed, underreported, and undertreated. Am J Med 2014;127(1 Suppl):S1–5.
45. Tuttle KL, Wickner P. Capturing anaphylaxis through medical records: Are ICD and CPT codes sufficient? Ann Allergy Asthma Immunol 2020;124(2):150–5.
46. Nowak R, Farrar JR, Brenner BE, et al. Customizing anaphylaxis guidelines for emergency medicine. J Emerg Med 2013;45(2):299–306.
47. Sampson HA, Munoz-Furlong A, Campbell RL, et al. Second symposium on the definition and management of anaphylaxis: summary report–second National Institute of Allergy and Infectious Disease/Food Allergy and Anaphylaxis Network symposium. Ann Emerg Med 2006;47(4):373–80.
48. Panesar SS, Javad S, de Silva D, et al. The epidemiology of anaphylaxis in Europe: a systematic review. Allergy 2013;68(11):1353–61.
49. Brown SG, Mullins RJ, Gold MS. Anaphylaxis: diagnosis and management. Med J Aust 2006;185(5):283–9.
50. Anagnostou K, Turner PJ. Myths, facts and controversies in the diagnosis and management of anaphylaxis. Arch Dis Child Jan 2019;104(1):83–90.
51. Turner PJ, Worm M, Ansotegui IJ, et al. Time to revisit the definition and clinical criteria for anaphylaxis? World Allergy Organ J 2019;12(10):100066.
52. Buka RJ, Knibb RC, Crossman RJ, et al. Anaphylaxis and Clinical Utility of Real-World Measurement of Acute Serum Tryptase in UK Emergency Departments. J Allergy Clin Immunol Pract 2017;5(5):1280–1287 e2.
53. Beck SC, Wilding T, Buka RJ, et al. Biomarkers in Human Anaphylaxis: A Critical Appraisal of Current Evidence and Perspectives. Front Immunol 2019;10:494.
54. Choo KJ, Simons FE, Sheikh A. Glucocorticoids for the treatment of anaphylaxis. Evid Based Child Health 2013;8(4):1276–94.
55. Gabrielli S, Clarke A, Morris J, et al. Evaluation of Prehospital Management in a Canadian Emergency Department Anaphylaxis Cohort. J Allergy Clin Immunol Pract 2019;7(7):2232–8, e3.
56. Campbell DE. Anaphylaxis Management: Time to Re-Evaluate the Role of Corticosteroids. J Allergy Clin Immunol Pract 2019;7(7):2239–40.
57. Muraro A, Halken S, Arshad SH, et al. EAACI food allergy and anaphylaxis guidelines. Primary prevention of food allergy. Allergy 2014;69(5):590–601.
58. Dribin TE, Sampson HA, Camargo CA Jr, et al. Persistent, refractory, and biphasic anaphylaxis: A multidisciplinary Delphi study. J Allergy Clin Immunol 2020;146(5):1089–96.
59. Dribin TE, Schnadower D, Spergel JM, et al. Severity grading system for acute allergic reactions: A multidisciplinary Delphi study. J Allergy Clin Immunol 2021. https://doi.org/10.1016/j.jaci.2021.01.003.

Pathophysiology of Immunologic and Nonimmunologic Systemic Reactions Including Anaphylaxis

Joshua Fowler, MD*, Phil Lieberman, MD[1]

KEYWORDS

- Anaphylaxis • Anaphylactic reaction • Anaphylaxis mechanism of production
- Anaphylaxis mediators

KEY POINTS

- Anaphylaxis is more a syndrome than a specific condition.
- Episodes may be immunologically or nonimmunologically induced.
- There are numerous pathophysiologic pathways that can participate in the production of anaphylactic episodes.

INTRODUCTION

Anaphylaxis is an acute and potentially life-threatening systemic reaction that occurs rapidly on the introduction of a given trigger. But what causes anaphylaxis? Classically, the term anaphylaxis was used to describe an allergen-driven process in which particular IgE antibodies were induced on exposure to an antigen, causing mast cell (MC) activation via cross-linking of IgE receptors. The centralized role of the MC in anaphylactic events has been well known for decades. And it is the activation of the MC that leads to the degranulation of its many diverse mediators including histamine, PAF-1, prostaglandins, leukotrienes, and tryptase, to name a few. These mediators induce the typical clinical signs associated with anaphylaxis including bronchoconstriction, vasodilation, and hypovolemia. The potential result of this constellation of systemic manifestations could be fatal by cardiac failure and/or asphyxiation.[1,2]

Over time, however, it has become clear that non–IgE-mediated pathways exist in relation to MC activation and that these pathways can lead to the same clinical symptoms defined by classic anaphylaxis. To offer a clear view into the many pathways and

University of Tennessee College of Medicine, Memphis, TN, USA
[1] Present address: 6139 Chapelle Circle West, Memphis, TN 38120.
* Coresponding author. 1270 Isle Bay Drive, Memphis, TN 38103.
E-mail address: jfowle40@uthsc.edu

Immunol Allergy Clin N Am 42 (2022) 27–43
https://doi.org/10.1016/j.iac.2021.09.011
0889-8561/22/© 2021 Elsevier Inc. All rights reserved.

interwoven mechanisms involved in anaphylactic events, it will be helpful to distinguish the MC as the chief effector cell. The mechanisms involved in MC activation can then be divided into immunologic and nonimmunologic mechanisms, as seen in **Fig. 1**. The immunologic mechanisms include the classic IgE-mediated pathway as well as an IgG-mediated pathway. The nonimmunologic mechanisms include direct MC activation via a multitude of receptors including PAF and opioid receptors.[3] Also of note is the human G-protein-coupled receptor, MRGPRX2, found on MC that has been found to be a receptor for certain drugs and cationic proteins that can cause direct MC degranulation and subsequent anaphylactic events.[1]

Finally, there is the non–MCcell-mediated mechanism causing anaphylactic episodes. An example being over sulfate chondroitin sulfate contamination of heparin which results in identical clinical symptoms associated with anaphylaxis by direct activation of the contact system and/or complement with likely no involvement of MCs.[1] It is these varying pathways and mechanisms that we will further explore in the discussion later in discussion.

HISTORY/BACKGROUND

Anaphylaxis is an intriguing phenomenon in that many could recognize its presentation, especially when its occurrence is rapid and dramatic, whereas also being difficult to clearly define when pressed. Therefore, we feel it important to trace the term anaphylaxis back to its origins and follow the ever-evolving criteria needed to establish its diagnosis today. The term "anaphylaxis" was first established by Charles Richet and Paul Portier in 1901 when attempts were made to induce prophylaxis to the venom of a sea anemone but inadvertently invoked the opposite reaction. There initial goal was to inoculate or immunize certain animals to the venom of the sea anemone species but in fact the animals were acquiring an increased sensitivity to the venom.

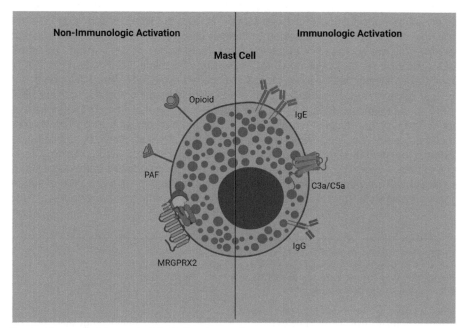

Fig. 1. Mast cell. (*Created with* BioRender.com).

They noted that on the readministration of the venom the animal subjects would often experience fatal reactions, reactions that appeared systematically different from the venom administered at lethal doses. And from this realization came the term "anaphylaxis" ("ana" being Greek for "opposite," "phylaxis" being Greek for "protection").[1,4,5]

By 1925, the term anaphylaxis was becoming more widespread in the clinical setting though it was still unclear whether humans could be grouped with the animal models whereby anaphylactic sensitization had been seen. Within the next 20 years, the use of medications was becoming more common and with that, it had become apparent that humans were indeed subject to experiencing anaphylactic reactions. And in 1945, anaphylaxis was formally defined for the first time by Robert Cooke in his classic text "Allergy in Theory and Practice" as "a special or particular immunologic type of induced protein (or hapten) sensitivity and may in for experimental animals and may properly be considered as a subdivision of allergy."[4,6,7] It is also interesting to highlight that during this time the relationship of anaphylaxis with the MC was not yet known.

The MC was first discovered by Paul Ehrlich in 1877. However, the MC's function remained a mystery for the better part of a century until 1952 when J. F. Riley and G. B. West uncovered the fact that a significant source of histamine came from the MC. And thus, the connection was established between the MC and anaphylaxis.

As time passed, we saw the advent of polypharmacy and with it an increased prevalence in anaphylactic events. It was not long after the discovery of immunoglobulin E (IgE) that a clear mechanism of anaphylaxis came into view and that was by the way of IgE activation of MCs via cross-linking of IgE receptors residing on MCs and basophils. But in keeping with the evolution of anaphylaxis as a term, more and more endotypes surfaced which only deepened the complexity involved with distinguishing a set criterion for anaphylaxis. By the 1970s, the updated definition of anaphylaxis was "a systemic, immediate hypersensitivity reaction caused by IgE-mediated immunologic release of mediators from MCs and basophils." But the recognition that different endotypes exist beyond the IgE-mediated mechanism borne a new term, anaphylactoid reaction. "The term 'anaphylactoid reaction' refers to a clinically similar event not mediated by IgE."[8-11]

Objections arose to this distinction in 2003 when the World Allergy Organization suggested that all events, whether IgE-mediated or not, should be labeled as "anaphylactic episodes." It was also proposed to further classify the mechanism of production of these episodes into immunologic and nonimmunologic. The nonimmunologic events would be synonymous with the term "anaphylactoid" and the immunologic events were further categorized into IgE-mediated and non-IgE mediated.[9]

This now leads us to the most current definition of anaphylaxis which is a modification of the WAO definition: "Anaphylaxis is a potentially serious, systemic reaction, either immunologic or nonimmunologic, that is usually rapid in onset, of variable severity, and may cause death. Severe anaphylaxis is characterized by either compromise of breathing and/or circulation and most often is preceded by milder signs/symptoms and occasionally occurs without such symptoms."[12]

DISCUSSION

To fully understand the intricacies and interwoven mechanisms that propagate an anaphylactic event let us first begin with the principal effector cell, the MC. It is important to point out that there has been multiple effector cells identified in relation to the different mechanisms of anaphylaxis though the MC has been studied the most extensively and is intimately related to the IgE-mediated mechanism. MCs are now considered to be highly versatile immune cells involved with many physiologic and pathologic states. MCs function as immunomodulators and in homeostatic processes in the epithelium, endothelium, and nervous system. Over time it has also become more apparent that the way in which MCs mature and function has a direct correlation with the microenvironment they inhabit. These local microenvironments impact the way MCs react to various stimuli through the release of a range of biologically active mediators. Their dispersal into a vast array of different tissues allows MCs to participate in many biological processes such as angiogenesis and tissue repair as well as involvement in innate and adaptive immunity.[4] But whereby do MCs originate? And how do they arrive at their varied destinations?

There has been much debate on the origin of the MC with some earlier studies pointing to the liver and yolk sac as sites of embryonic MC origin, but there was simply no way to distinguish between MC precursors and pluripotent stem cells. We now know, due to the work of Kitamura and colleagues, that human MCs are derived from a common pluripotent hematopoietic progenitor originating in the bone marrow. But unlike other cells of hematopoietic origin, which mature in the bone marrow before being released into circulation, MCs travel as immature progenitor cells through the circulation to designated tissues whereby they complete their maturation process.[1,4]

The mechanisms involved in the recruitment of progenitor MCs to peripheral tissues during physiologic and inflammatory states have not been completely revealed. Several studies from the past decade highlight the importance of some integrins, adhesion molecules, chemokines, and their receptors, as well as cytokines and growth factors as important players in the directed migration of MCs to specific locations under normal and pathologic circumstances. They tend to settle in areas found at the border between the host and the external environment. These sites have the highest entry potential of pathogens or contact with harmful substances and include the skin, respiratory mucosa, and gastrointestinal tract. These microenvirons foster phenotypic changes which effect function, contents, structure, and the response to endogenous stimuli and drugs.[4]

The capacity of MCs to promptly interact with the microenvironment and respond through the release of an array of biologically active mediators is in a delicate balance, whereby the insufficient regulation of MC functions can lead to distressing effects. Because of this, MCs have been implicated in the pathogenesis of several chronic allergic/inflammatory disorders, as well as acute events such as anaphylaxis. The mechanisms by which MCs, as well as the other effector cells that will be addressed, mediate an anaphylactic event can be further categorized into immunologic and nonimmunologic.[1,4]

Immunologic Mechanisms

IgE-mediated pathway

The first immunologic pathway that we will discuss is the classic IgE-mediated pathway. As previously stated, the chief effector cell in this pathway is the MC. And to a lesser extent the basophil can participate. This pathway is characterized by the formation of allergen-specific IgE and subsequent binding of this IgE to the FcεRI receptor primarily on MCs. After re-exposure to the allergen, there is a cross-linking of IgE/FcεRI complexes, as seen in **Fig. 2**.[13] The formation of these complexes leads to a dimerization of the receptor. Downstream signaling activates a series of tyrosine kinases which then phosphorylase tyrosine residues in the intracellular portion of the IgE receptor. After this, a second protein kinase comes to further phosphorylate the chain. This action triggers a sequence leading to the activation of Inositol triphosphate (IP3) which results in an influx of extracellular calcium

IgE Cross-linking Induces Mast Cell Activation and Degranulation

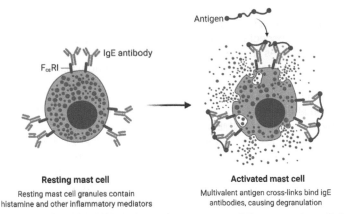

Resting mast cell
Resting mast cell granules contain histamine and other inflammatory mediators

Activated mast cell
Multivalent antigen cross-links bind igE antibodies, causing degranulation

Fig. 2. Mast cell activation and degranulation. (*Reprinted from* "IgE Cross-linking Induces Mast Cell Activation and Degranulation" by BioRender.com (2021)).

into the cell.[1] Granules containing preformed mediators such as histamine, tryptase, and PAF are then released from the cells, whereas the de novo synthesis of other inflammatory mediators such as leukotrienes, prostaglandins, and cytokines occurs as well. The result is the smooth muscle contraction and increased vascular permeability associated with anaphylaxis.[13]

The importance of this process was illustrated decades ago, when it was determined that purified IgE was capable of transferring skin reactivity from sensitized human subjects to naive hosts.[14-17] Similarly, transfer of antigen-specific IgE into naive mice sensitizes the animals to have anaphylaxis on subsequent exposure to that allergen.[18,19] Such IgE-mediated anaphylaxis is absent in mice that lack the high-affinity IgE receptor FcεRI, as well as in MC-deficient mice, further signifying the importance of IgE-mediated MC activation in such models of anaphylaxis.[20-23]

IgG-mediated pathway

Until recently, only the IgE-mediated pathway had been universally accepted as the mechanistic explanation of anaphylaxis induction. But there is now more and more evidence emerging in line with the possibility that human MC activation via FcgRI-IgG can produce anaphylactic events. Both animal models and human observational studies point to the fact that IgG alone or in immune complexes (ICs) can activate MCs and either initiate or contribute to the severity of anaphylactic reactions.[2] IgG antibodies recognize and bind to Fc gamma receptors (FcgRs), which have different affinities and are expressed on multiple cell types.[2,24,25] Among the many receptor types involved with activation signaling, FcgRI is the only one that binds with high affinity to monomeric IgG, primarily IgG1 and IgG3. It is expressed on both MCs and neutrophils. FcgRI binding to specific IgG1 can lead to activation of MCs.[2,24-30] Both IgG1 and IgG3 can instead activate FcgRI expressed on monocytes and macrophages. Although FcgRI receptors are normally occupied by monomeric IgG, this does not prevent their activation by IgG ICs. The latter has higher binding affinity and can therefore displace monomeric IgG and trigger hypersensitivity responses. In mouse models, it has been shown that antigens can induce macrophages, basophils, and neutrophils to release PAF by activating FcgRIII or FcgRIV.[31,32] With these models, IgG seemed to require higher levels of specific IgG antibodies and antigens, in contrast to IgE-mediated anaphylaxis, which can be seen in **Fig. 3**. This is likely due to the lower affinity of FcgRs compared with FcεRI.

Another good example of the IgG–neutrophil/macrophage-mediated pathway comes from a multicenter prospective study conducted on 86 patients who experienced anaphylaxis to an NBMAs received during anesthesia. There were 86 matched controls.[33] NMBA is a low-molecular-weight antigen that is administered via IV in rather large quantities which favors IC formation and circulation. In this study, 31% of patients with anaphylaxis had no biomarkers of IgE–dependent anaphylaxis. These data validate the notion that an alternative pathway independent of IgE exists in patients who experienced anaphylactic events to NMBA. The research also showed that the more severe the reaction, the higher the concentration of anti-NMBA IgG, aPAF, neutrophil activation markers, as well as markers for FCγR activation. It was also revealed that neutrophils became increasingly more activated and underwent the release of neutrophil elastase and developed elevated neutrophil extracellular traps. This occurred soon after anaphylaxis onset, particularly in patients without any evidence of IgE-dependent anaphylaxis. This demonstrates the importance of this pathway separate from the classic IgE mediated pathway. Ultimately this study shows it is possible that an IgG-mediated pathway could compound the severity of an anaphylactic event coupled with the activation of the IgE pathway and induce anaphylaxis in the absence of IgE.[2,33]

Complement activation

The final pathway belonging to the immunologic mechanism of anaphylaxis is complement activation. The initiation of the complement cascade occurs via a multitude of stimuli and results in the formation of C3a, C4a, C5a. These mediators are referred to as anaphylatoxins.[1,34] Several sources of evidence have highlighted the production of C3a, C5a as well the depletion of complement levels in human anaphylaxis. This suggests that these anaphylatoxins can be involved in anaphylaxis.[1,35–37]

On complement activation, C3a, C5a are released which subsequently triggers the activation of MCs, basophils, endothelial cells, and smooth muscles via their particular

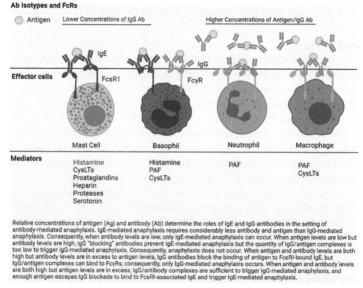

Relative concentrations of antigen (Ag) and antibody (Ab) determine the roles of IgE and IgG antibodies in the setting of antibody-mediated anaphylaxis. IgE-mediated anaphylaxis requires considerably less antibody and antigen than IgG-mediated anaphylaxis. Consequently, when antibody levels are low, only IgE-mediated anaphylaxis can occur. When antigen levels are low but antibody levels are high, IgG "blocking" antibodies prevent IgE-mediated anaphylaxis but the quantity of IgG/antigen complexes is too low to trigger IgG-mediated anaphylaxis. Consequently, anaphylaxis does not occur. When antigen and antibody levels are both high but antibody levels are in excess to antigen levels, IgG antibodies block the binding of antigen to FcεRI-bound IgE, but IgG/antigen complexes can bind to FcγRs; consequently, only IgG-mediated anaphylaxis occurs. When antigen and antibody levels are both high but antigen levels are in excess, IgG/antibody complexes are sufficient to trigger IgG-mediated anaphylaxis, and enough antigen escapes IgG blockade to bind to FcεRI-associated IgE and trigger IgE-mediated anaphylaxis.

Fig. 3. IgE versus IgG mediated activation. (*Created with* BioRender.com).

receptors. It has been shown that C3a has a direct effect on MC activation in rat, human MC line HMC-1, and in CD34-derived human MCs.[38,39] These potent inflammatory mediators have also been shown to directly induce vascular permeability and smooth muscle contraction. The phenotypic response elicited from an IgE-mediated reaction can be indistinguishable from that produced by complement activation. But complement induced events may differ from IgE reactions in that they can present on the initial exposure.[2]

ICs have been shown to activate the complement system, generating anaphylatoxins such as C3a that can then further activate MCs and basophils.[40] There are also instances whereby complement activation occurs independently from IC formation. An example of this has occurred in reactions to drugs solubilized in therapeutic liposomes and lipid-based excipients like the diluents used for preparations of propofol and paclitaxel. Cremophor EL, the diluent previously used, was able to activate complement under physiologic conditions, forming large micelles with serum lipids and cholesterol.[41–43]

Another example of complement activation producing anaphylactic reactions has been seen in events to dextran and von Willebrand factor (vWF).[44,45] Keeping in line with some of the hallmark features of complement reactions, they can occur on the first infusion and can be prevented by pretreatment with antihistamines, steroids, and NSAIDs.

Dextran is a polysaccharide with a repetitive structure that can be immunogenic. In a small subpopulation of individuals with high titers of preformed dextran-reactive antibodies (DRAs) of IgG class, the infusion of dextran generates harmful ICs. They activate complement and cause the aggregation of leukocytes and platelets. The aggregated material is sequestered in the lung, and the release of vasoactive mediators leads to signs and symptoms associated with anaphylaxis.[44]

In a clinical prospective study, a patient with severe von Willebrand disease was found to have IgG alloantibodies against vWF along with a history of posttransfusion anaphylaxis. During an 18-day period, the patient was treated with factor VIII-vWF concentrate and with recombinant factor VIII. Complement system activation and plasma levels of antibodies to vWF and complement-fixing IgG–vWF complexes were evaluated. IgE, IgA, and IgM antibodies to vWF were not found.[45] During this study the patient experienced symptoms of anaphylaxis when IgG antibodies to vWF were measured at days 1 and 6 after replacement with factor VIII-vWF concentrate. This observation suggested a cause-effect relationship between the formation of IgG–vWF complexes and massive complement activation in posttransfusion non–IgE-mediated anaphylactic reactions to vWF.[45] In this patient, there was no indication of MC activation or the contact phase of the coagulation cascade. Therefore, it was concluded that the clinical syndrome was a direct effect of complement anaphylatoxins on vascular permeability and smooth muscle contraction.[2,46]

Nonimmunologic Mechanisms

There are several agents capable of inciting MC degranulation by directly binding to cell surface receptors[1,13] Such agents include neuropeptides such as substance P (SP), certain polycationic molecules, stem cell factor, cytokines, opioids, and several different drugs. It has also been found that physical factors such as heat, cold, or exercise can incite MC degranulation though the mechanisms underlying these events are less clear.[1,13,47]

It is, however, the more recent discovery of the MRGPRB2 receptor found on mice MCs that has garnered much attention.[1,13] This mouse MC receptor was determined to be the ortholog of human MRGPRX2 via reverse-transcriptase in mouse peritoneal

MCs. Both MRGPRB2 and MRGPRX2 share similar characteristics. They reside on, MCtc, and respond to similar ligands. Analyses conducted by McNeil et al. revealed that certain drugs containing structural patterns called tetrahydroisoquinoline (THIQ) were capable of activating MRGPRB2. These structural patterns are present on certain drugs such as icatibant, several fluoroquinolones, and neuromuscular blocking drugs (NMBDs). Drugs within these classes can promote Ca2+ mobilization in HEK293 cells that express the MRGPRX2 receptor thereby stimulating MC degranulation and inducing the release of histamine, TNF, and PD2, which is illustrated in **Fig. 4.**[48] It is interesting to note that whereby these ortholog receptors differ is in the concentration of agonist required for activation. Studies have suggested that the differences in the amino acid sequences of MRGPRX2 and MrgprB2 influence the ability of peptide ligands to activate these receptors.[49,50]

The range of drugs known to induce MRGPRX2-dependent MC pathway is continuing to expand. For instance, in mouse models, passive cutaneous anaphylaxis was induced with iodinated contrast, and a clear association with MCs and MRGPRB2 was found. However, capacity for receptor-induced activation by these peptidergic drugs does not fully account for the unpredictable severity of reactions. It is becoming clearer that distinct receptor levels, as well as the overall functionality of the receptor may be the key to gaining further insight into the different reactions of certain individuals than others.[51] Evidence is accumulating to support the notion that genetic alterations to the MRGPRX2 protein do influence the response of the receptor to identifiable triggers. A specific example includes the results of Reddy and colleagues in which a single amino-acid changed the induction of pruritis through its receptor.[52] Other studies have been investigating the role of MRGPRX2 variants in relation to patients with drug reactions, specifically in regards to the activity of the receptor. Though some of these studies are still ongoing, the specific role of different mutations in regards to clinical epidemiology is yet to be fully understood.[53]

Non–mast Cell-mediated Mechanisms

In addition to these mast-cell-derived mediators of anaphylaxis, there exist other systems of inflammation that can be activated to produce mediators that cause the same signs and symptoms associated with classic anaphylaxis. These systems include coagulation, complement, kallikrein, and platelet-related pathways. It is also important to realize that though these pathways can lead to an anaphylactic event in the absence of MC involvement, MC activation can also recruit and activate these same pathways leading to a synergistic escalation in the clinical features associated with anaphylaxis.[1,13]

The hallmark example of a non–MC cell-mediated mechanism is the over-sulfated chondroitin sulfate (OSCS) contaminated unfractionated heparin. A brief background will be offered to help explain how these mechanisms were discovered. In January 2008, health authorities in the United States began receiving reports of groups of acute hypersensitivity reactions in patients undergoing dialysis that had been occurring since November 2007. The symptoms associated with these reactions included hypotension, facial swelling, tachycardia, urticaria, and nausea. Though initial investigations yielded no obvious answer, an investigation conducted by the CDC revealed a common thread to these reactions; heparin sodium used for injection. Once this link was established the contaminant was then identified to be OSCS. Though the culprit was made known, a biological link between OCSC and adverse clinical events remained elusive.[54]

But then a study was conducted by Kishimoto and colleagues to attempt to determine this missing biological connection. And their results revealed that OSCS found in

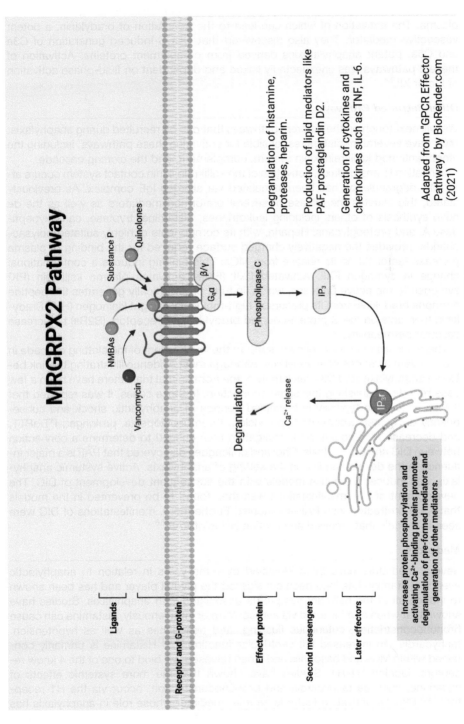

Fig. 4. MGRPX2 pathway. (*Adapted from "GPCR Effector Pathway", by BioRender.com (2021)).*

contaminated lots of unfractionated heparin, as well as a synthetically generated OSCS reference standard, directly activated the kinin–kallikrein pathway in human plasma. The activation of which can lead to the generation of bradykinin, a potent vasoactive mediator. They also discovered that OSCS induced generation of C3a and C5a, potent anaphylatoxins derived from complement proteins. Activation of these 2 pathways was unexpectedly linked and dependent on fluid-phase activation of factor XII.[54]

Other Recruited Pathways

We will next touch on the different pathways that can be recruited during anaphylaxis. MCs have several mediators responsible for activating these pathways, including the aforementioned kallikrein–kinin system, complement, and the clotting cascade.

In relation to anaphylaxis, activation of the kallikrein–kinin contact system occurs after MC degranulation has been stimulated via allergen/IgE complex. As previously stated, this initiates the release of several preformed mediators as well as the de novo synthesis of others including leukotrienes, histamine, tryptase, carboxypeptidase A, and proteoglycans. Heparin, with its components of highly sulfated polysaccharide, provides the negatively charged surface required for the binding of plasma protease factor XII on its release from MCs. This binding induces a conformational change in zymogen FXII. Activated FXII (FXIIa) activates plasma kallikrein (PK) zymogen to the active protease, which, in turn, proteolytically generates the peptide hormone bradykinin from its precursor, high-molecular-weight kininogen (HK). Bradykinin then acts on the G protein-coupled bradykinin B2 receptors (B2Rs) to increase vascular permeability.[55]

There has also been evidence to support the involvement of the clotting cascade in more severe episodes of anaphylaxis. Although most evidence illustrating the link between anaphylaxis and DIC has largely come from animal trials there have been a few case reports establishing this same connection. In these cases, it was reported that the patients were typically in sustained periods of anaphylactic shock and subsequently developed worsening hypotension, thrombocytopenia, prolonged PT/aPTT, and decreased fibrinogen. An investigation then ensued to determine a connection between DIC and anaphylaxis. Choi and colleagues discovered that PAF is a major influence in the developing DIC in the setting of anaphylaxis. Active systemic anaphylaxis was induced in mouse models with the subsequent development of DIC. The development of DIC manifestations was then found to be prevented in the models that were pretreated with PAF-antagonist. Furthermore, manifestations of DIC were seen in models that received an injection bolus of PAF.[56]

Mediators

Several mediators have been identified over the years in relation to anaphylactic events. Histamine has long been considered the pivotal player and has been shown to induce all of the hallmark symptoms associated with anaphylaxis. Studies have shown that when administered via aerosol form or intravenously, histamine can cause bronchoconstriction, cutaneous flushing, and headaches as well as hypotension, tachycardia, an increased left ventricular function.[57,58] Histamine is primarily contained within MCs and basophils and when released will bind to one of the 4 know receptors, labeled H1-H4. Studies have shown that the more systemic effects of histamine, such as tachycardia and bronchoconstriction, occur via the H1 receptor.[57,58] Platelet-activating factor is another mediator whose role in anaphylaxis has been under more recent review. PAF is a very potent phospholipid-derived mediator that can activate a variety of cells expressing the PAF-receptor (PAF-R).[59,60] These

Table 1
Mast cell mediators and their pathophysiologic activities

Mediators	Pathophysiologic Activities	Clinical Manifestations	Comments
Histamine	Contraction of smooth muscle, vasodilatation, increased vascular permeability, mucus secretion, and activation of nociceptive neuronal receptors	Wheezing, flushing, urticaria, pruritus, rhinorrhea, abdominal pain, diarrhea, and angioedema	Works through both H1 and H2 receptors. Although accounting for a large portion of the clinical manifestations, blockade of its activity does not control all manifestations completely
Prostaglandin	Smooth muscle spasm, affects platelet adherence, and vasodilatation	Wheezing, diarrhea, cramping abdominal pain, and hypotension	
Leukotriene	Smooth muscle contraction, increased vasopermeability	Probable main effect is wheezing with bronchoconstriction, possible hypotension	
Platelet Activating Factor	Activation of platelets, vasodilatation	May contribute to intravascular coagulation with platelet activation, probable hypotension, and shock	Levels have been directly correlated with the severity of events and fatalities, also levels of platelet-activating hydrolase, the enzyme responsible for its degradation, have been inversely correlated with severity and fatalities as well
Interleukins	Not well defined	Not well defined	In spite of lack of knowledge of exact effects, levels of some interleukins have been associated with the severity of episodes
Chymase	Possibly recruits complement by cleaving C3, may have a beneficial effect by inactivation of neuropeptides, can recruit contact system	Not well defined	Levels have been associated with direct activation of the contact system and thus indirectly associated with the severity of events

(continued on next page)

Table 1
(continued)

Mediators	Pathophysiologic Activities	Clinical Manifestations	Comments
Tryptase	Not well defined	Not well defined	Used as a biomarker to diagnose events
Tumor Necrosis Factor	Not well defined	Not well defined	Levels have been associated with severity of events
Neuropeptides	Not well defined	Not well defined	Can magnify events by further degranulating mast cells
Recruited Pathways	Activation of the coagulation pathway has been associated with decreased Factor V, decreased Factor VIII, and decreased fibrinogen. Activation of complement cascade has been demonstrated by decreased levels of complement components 3 and 4 as well as the formation of C3a. Activation of the contact system has been demonstrated by the formation of kallikrein C1 inhibitor complexes as well as elevated levels of kinins.	Disseminated intravascular coagulation and hypotension	Levels of activation have been shown to correlate with the severity of episodes

From Lieberman P, Garvey LH. Mast Cells and Anaphylaxis. Curr Allergy Asthma Rep. 2016 Mar;16(3):20; with permission.

include endothelium, smooth muscle, and MCs.[61,62] PAF is very similar to histamine in their physiologic effects. It can induce vascular permeability, decrease cardiac output, induce smooth muscle contraction of the central airways and gastrointestinal tract, and lead to vasodilation with consequent circulatory collapse.[2,63,64] PAF is inactivated by PAF acetylhydrolase (PAF-AH) and has a half-life of 3 to 13 minutes. In relation to anaphylaxis, PAF induces a potent mediator in anaphylaxis pathogenesis such as PGE2, as well as nitric oxide.[64,65] MC-derived PAFs appear to be important in IgE-mediated reactions in humans as demonstrated by the severe anaphylaxis in patients with high levels of PAF and decreased PAF-AH activity, with the lowest levels of PAF-AH activity being associated with a 27-fold higher risk of severe or fatal anaphylaxis compared with the risk in patients with normal levels of PAF-AH activity.[66,67]

Other important mediators include CysLTs, tryptase, prostaglandins, and various cytokines/chemokines (IL-2,IL-6,IL-10, TNF) whose pathophysiologic activity and clinical manifestations can be found detailed in **Table 1**. Of note, it has been described by Brown and colleagues that these cytokines mentioned have been associated with severe anaphylactic reactions.[68]

SUMMARY

Anaphylaxis remains one of the most urgent medical emergencies, in which immediate recognition and prompt intervention can be the difference between life and death. Our understanding of the antibodies, effector cells, and mediators that contribute to the manifestations seen in anaphylaxis has continued to evolve and progress. Despite the knowledge gained in these mechanisms, the clinical management of anaphylaxis has remained the same for years. As we've discussed, most of the anaphylactic events are due to systemic MC degranulation. This degranulation process was initially thought to be primarily IgE-mediated. But over time it has become more apparent that a significant number of anaphylactic events occur by multiple different mechanisms either synergistically or independently. An example includes the discovery of the IgG-mediated pathway in inducing MC degranulation. There is also direct MC degranulation independent of IgE via PAF and opioid receptors as well as the human G-protein-coupled receptor, MRGPRX2, that has been found to be the receptor for many drugs and cationic proteins capable of producing direct MC degranulation and anaphylactic events. Our hope is that as we continue to advance in our understanding of the pathophysiology of anaphylaxis in all of its interconnected mechanisms, greater efforts to develop more effective approaches for preventing anaphylactic events as well as provide more effective options for prompt diagnosing and effective treatment will become more available.

CLINICS CARE POINTS

- Understanding of the complexities of anaphylaxis will result in better diagnosis with biomarkers, improved avoidance or pretreatment strategies, and more effective, individualized therapies.
- The remarkable efficacy of IM epinephrine enables effective therapy of anaphylaxis, regardless of pathways responsible.

DISCLOSURE

Sanofi (Consultant).

REFERENCES

1. Lieberman P, Garvey LH. Mast cells and anaphylaxis. Curr Allergy Asthma Rep 2016;16:20.
2. Cianferoni A. Non-IgE mediated anaphylaxis. J Allergy Clin Immunol 2021;147: 1123–31.
3. Bruhns P, Chollet-Martin S. Mechanisms of human drug-induced anaphylaxis. J Allergy Clin Immunol 2021;147:1133–42.
4. Zayas E, da Silva M, Jamur MC, et al. Mast cell function: a new vision of an old cell. J Histochem Cytochem 2014;62(10):698–738.
5. Samter M. Excerpts from classics in allergy. Columbus (OH): Ross Laboratories; 1969:32–33. Library of Congress Catalog Number 70-77908. Published for the 25th Anniversary of the American Academy of Allergy.
6. Simons FER. Anaphylaxis, killer allergy: long-term management in the community. J Allergy Clin Immunol 2006;117:367–77.
7. Cooke RA. Allergy in theory and practice, 5. Philadelphia (PA): W. B. Saunders Company; 1945.
8. Lieberman P. Anaphylaxis and anaphylactoid reactions. In: Middleton E, Ellis EF, Yunginger JW, et al, editors. Allergy: principles and practice, II, 5th edition. St. Louis (MO): Mosby-Year Book, Inc.; 1998. p. 1079–92.
9. Johansson SJO, Bieber T, Dahl R, et al. Revised nomenclature for allergy for global use: report of the nomenclature review committee of the World Allergy Organization. J Allergy Clin Immunol 2004;113:832–6.
10. Lieberman P. Anaphylaxis. In: Atkinson F, Bochner B, Busse W, et al, editors. Allergy: principles and practice. 7th edition. Philadelphia (PA): Mosby; 2009. p. 1027–51.
11. Webb L, Lieberman P. Anaphylaxis: a review of 601 cases. Ann Allergy Asthma Immunol 2006;97(1):39–43.
12. Cox LS, Sanchez-Borges M, Lockey RF. World Allergy Organization systemic allergic reaction grading system Is a modification needed? J Allergy Clin Immunol Pract 2017;5:58–62.
13. Reber LL, Hernandez JD, Galli SJ. The pathophysiology of anaphylaxis. J Allergy Clin Immunol 2017;140:335–48.
14. Stanworth DR, Humphrey JH, Bennich H, et al. Specific inhibition of the Prausnitz-Kustner reaction by an atypical human myeloma protein. Lancet 1967;2:330–2.
15. Ishizaka K, Ishizaka T, Richter M. Effect of reduction and alkylation on allergen-combining properties of reaginic antibody. J Allergy 1966;37:135–44.
16. Ribatti D. The discovery of immunoglobulin E. Immunol Lett 2016;171:14.
17. Oettgen HC. Fifty years later: emerging functions of IgE antibodies in host defense, immune regulation, and allergic diseases. J Allergy Clin Immunol 2016; 137:1631–45.
18. Wershil BK, Mekori YA, Murakami T, et al. ^{125}I-fibrin deposition in IgE-dependent immediate hypersensitivity reactions in mouse skin. Demonstration role mast cells using genetically mast cell-deficient mice locally reconstituted cultured mast cells. J Immunol 1987;139:2605–14.
19. Dombrowicz D, Flamand V, Brigman KK, et al. Abolition of anaphylaxis by targeted disruption of the high affinity immunoglobulin E receptor alpha chain gene. Cell 1993;75:969–76.
20. Feyerabend TB, Weiser A, Tietz A, et al. Cre-mediated cell ablation contests mast cell contribution in models of antibody- and T cell-mediated autoimmunity. Immunity 2011;35:832–44.

21. Oka T, Kalesnikoff J, Starkl P, et al. Evidence questioning cromolyn's effectiveness and selectivity as a 'mast cell stabilizer' in mice. Lab Invest 2012;92:1472–82.

22. Lilla JN, Chen CC, Mukai K, et al. Reduced mast cell and basophil numbers and function in Cpa3-Cre; Mcl-1fl/fl mice. Blood 2011;118:6930–8.

23. Dombrowicz D, Flamand V, Brigman KK, et al. of anaphylaxis by targeted disruption of the high affinity immunoglobulin E receptor alpha chain gene. Cell 1993; 75:969–76.

24. Bruhns P. Properties of mouse and human IgG receptors and their contribution to disease models. Blood 2012;119:5640–9.

25. Bruhns P, Iannascoli B, England P, et al. Specificity and affinity of human Fcgamma receptors and their polymorphic variants for human IgG subclasses. Blood 2009;113:3716–25.

26. Woolhiser MR, Okayama Y, Gilfillan AM, et al. IgG-dependent activation of human mast cells following up-regulation of FcgammaRI by IFN-gamma. Eur J Immunol 2001;31:3298–307.

27. Okayama Y, Kirshenbaum AS, Metcalfe DD. Expression of a functional highaffinity IgG receptor, Fc gamma RI, on human mast cells: up-regulation by IFNgamma. J Immunol 2000;164:4332.

28. Mancardi DA, Albanesi M, Jonsson F, et al. The high-affinity human IgG receptor FcgammaRI (CD64) promotes IgG-mediated inflammation, anaphylaxis, and anti-tumor immunotherapy. Blood 2013;121:1563–73.

29. Woolhiser MR, Brockow K, Metcalfe DD. Activation of human mast cells by aggregated IgG through FcgammaRI: additive effects of C3a. Clin Immunol 2004;110: 172–80.

30. Tkaczyk C, Okayama Y, Woolhiser MR, et al. Activation of human mast cells through the high affinity IgG receptor. Mol Immunol 2002;38:1289–93.

31. Jonsson F, Mancardi DA, Kita Y, et al. Mouse and human neutrophils induce anaphylaxis. J Clin Invest 2011;121:1484–96.

32. Finkelman FD, Khodoun MV, Strait R. Human IgE-independent systemic anaphylaxis. J Allergy Clin Immunol 2016;137:1674–16780, 1.

33. Jonsson F, de Chaisemartin L, Granger V, et al. An IgG-induced neutrophil activation pathway contributes to human drug induced anaphylaxis. Sci Transl Med 2003;40:643–72.

34. Klos A, Tenner AJ, Johswich KO, et al. The role of the anaphylatoxins in health and disease. Mol Immunol 2009;46:2753–66.

35. Brown SG, Stone SF, Fatovich DM, et al. Anaphylaxis: clinical patterns, mediator release, and severity. J Allergy Clin Immunol 2013;132:1141–9, e5.

36. Gorski JP, Hugli TE, Muller-Eberhard HJ. C4a: the third anaphylatoxin of the human complement system. Proc Natl Acad Sci USA 1979;76:5299–302.

37. Smith PL, Kagey Sobotka A, Bleecker ER, et al. Physiologic manifestations of human anaphylaxis. J Clin Invest 1980;66:1072–80.

38. Yancey KB, Hammer CH, Harvath L, et al. Studies of human C5a as a mediator of inflammation in normal human skin. J Clin Invest 1985;75:486–95.

39. Zwirner J, Gotze O, Sieber A, et al. The human mast cell line HMC-1 binds and responds to C3a but not C3a(desArg). Scand J Immunol 1998;47:19–24.

40. Wolbing F, Fischer J, Koberle M, et al. About the role and underlying mechanisms of cofactors in anaphylaxis. Allergy 2013;68:1085–92.

41. Weiszhar Z, Czucz J, Revesz C, et al. Complement activation by polyethoxylated pharmaceutical surfactants: Cremophor-EL, Tween80 and Tween-20. Eur J Pharm Sci 2012;45:492–8.

42. Szebeni J, Muggia FM, Alving CR. Complement activation by Cremophor EL as a possible contributor to hypersensitivity to paclitaxel: an in vitro study. J Natl Cancer Inst 1998;90:300–6.

43. Khodoun M, Strait R, Orekov T, et al. Peanuts can contribute to anaphylactic shock by activating complement. J Allergy Clin Immunol 2009;123:342–51.

44. Hedin H, Richter W, Messmer K, et al. Incidence, pathomechanism and prevention of dextran-induced anaphylactoid/anaphylactic reactions in man. Dev Biol Stand 1980;48:179–89.

45. Bergamaschini L, Mannucci PM, Federici AB, et al. Posttransfusion anaphylactic reactions in a patient with severe von Willebrand disease: role of complement and alloantibodies to von Willebrand factor. J Lab Clin Med 1995;125:348–55.

46. Bergamaschini L, Santangelo T, Fariicciotti A, et al. Study of complement-mediated anaphylaxis in humans. The role of IgG subclasses (IgG1 and/or IgG4) in the complement-activating capacity of immune complexes. J Immunol 1996;156:1256–61.

47. Asero R, Piantanida M, Pravettoni V. Allergy to LTP: to eat or not to eat sensitizing foods? A follow-up study. Eur Ann Allergy Clin Immunol 2018;50:156–62.

48. McNeil BD, Pundir P, Meeker S, et al. Identification of a mast-cell-specific receptor crucial for pseudo-allergic drug reactions. Nature 2015;519:237–41.

49. Katritch V, Cherezov V, Stevens RC. Diversity and modularity of G protein-coupled receptor structures. Trends Pharmacol Sci 2012;33:17–27.

50. Reddy VB, Graham TA, Azimi E. A single amino acid in MRGPRX2 necessary for binding and activation by pruritogens. J Allergy Clin Immunol 2017;140:1726–8.

51. Babina M, Guhl S, Artuc M, et al. Allergic FcεRI- and pseudo-allergic MRGPRX2-triggered mast cell activation routes are independent and inversely regulated by SCF. Allergy Eur J Allergy Clin Immunol 2018;73:256–60.

52. Porebski G, Kwiecien K, Pawica M, et al. Mas-related G protein-coupled Receptor-X2 (MRGPRX2) in drug hypersensitivity reactions. Front Immunol 2018;9:3027.

53. Ayudhya CC, Roy S, Alkanfari I, et al. Identification of gain and loss of function missense variants in MRGPRX2's transmembrane and intracellular domains for mast cell activation by substance p. Int J Mol Sci 2019;20:5247.

54. Kishimoto TK, Viswanathan K, Ganguly T, et al. Contaminated heparin associated with adverse clinical events and activation of the contact system. N Engl J Med 2008;358:2457–67.

55. Sala-Cunill A, Bjorkqvist J, Senter R, et al. Plasma contact system activation drives anaphylaxis in severe mast cell-mediated allergic reactions. J Allergy Clin Immunol 2015;135:1031–43, e6.

56. Borahay MA, Harirah HM, Olson G, et al. Disseminated intravascular coagulation, hemoperitoneum, and reversible ischemic neurological deficit complicating anaphylaxis to prophylactic antibiotics during cesarean delivery: a case report and review of literature. AJP Rep 2011;1:15–20.

57. Kaliner M, Sigler R, Summers R, et al. Effects of infused histamine: analysis of the effects of H-1 and H-2 histamine receptor antagonists on cardiovascular and pulmonary responses. J Allergy Clin Immunol 1981;68:365–71.

58. Vigorito C, Russo P, Picotti GB, et al. Cardiovascular effects of histamine infusion in man. J Cardiovasc Pharmacol 1983;5:531–7.

59. Cao C, Tan Q, Xu C, et al. Structural basis for signal recognition and transduction by platelet-activating-factor receptor. Nat Struct Mol Biol 2018;25:488–95.

60. Triggiani M, Schleimer RP, Warner JA, et al. Differential synthesis of 1-acyl-2-acetyl-sn-glycero-3-phosphocholine and platelet-activating factor by human inflammatory cells. J Immunol 1991;147:660–6.

61. Basran GS, Page CP, Paul W, et al. Platelet-activating factor: a possible mediator of the dual response to allergen? Clin Allergy 1984;14:75–9.
62. Cuss FM, Dixon CM, Barnes PJ. Effects of inhaled platelet activating factor on pulmonary function and bronchial responsiveness in man. Lancet 1986;2:189–92.
63. Stafforini DM, McIntyre TM, Zimmerman GA, et al. Platelet-activating factor, a pleiotrophic mediator of physiological and pathological processes. Crit Rev Clin Lab Sci 2003;40:643–72.
64. Gill P, Jindal NL, Jagdis A, et al. Platelets in the immune response: revisiting platelet-activating factor in anaphylaxis. J Allergy Clin Immunol 2015;135: 1424–32.
65. Vadas P. The platelet-activating factor pathway in food allergy and anaphylaxis. Ann Allergy Asthma Immunol 2016;117:455–7.
66. Vadas P, Perelman B. Effect of epinephrine on platelet-activating factor-stimulated human vascular smooth muscle cells. J Allergy Clin Immunol 2012;129: 1329–33.
67. Vadas P, Gold M, Perelman B, et al. Platelet-activating factor, PAF acetylhydrolase, and severe anaphylaxis. N Engl J Med 2008;358:28–35.
68. Brown, et al. J Allergy Clin Immunol 2009;1244(4):786–92, e4.

Anaphylaxis and Mast Cell Disorders

Theo Gülen, MD, PhD[a,b,c],*, Cem Akin, MD, PhD[d]

KEYWORDS

- Anaphylaxis • Mastocytosis • Mast cell hyperreactivity • D816 V mutation
- Tryptase • Mast cell activation syndromes • Hereditary alpha-tryptasemia

KEY POINTS

- Patients with mastocytosis have a high risk of developing severe anaphylaxis, not only when suffering from venom allergy but also in the absence of a clear trigger/allergy.
- The severity and frequency of anaphylactic reactions in patients with mastocytosis may depend on hyperreleasability of mast cells due to their inherent state of hyperreactivity, and due to the potential influence of occult or overt IgE-dependent allergies.
- Comprehensive management of patients with mastocytosis with anaphylaxis can be complex and requires special knowledge about disease pathogenesis and special considerations in prophylactic measures; patient care should therefore be implemented in specialized centers or in close collaboration with experts.

INTRODUCTION

Mast cells (MCs) are granulated, tissue-fixed effector cells that reside in almost all vascularized tissues.[1,2] The multifunctional capacity of MCs originates from their ability to detect triggers of internal or external stress or danger, which leads to the release of a spectrum of mediators.[3,4] Both the number of MCs and their activation in the tissue increase with inflammation, but it remains elusive how the MC reactivity is regulated.

MCs are well known for their role as the effector cells of immediate-type hypersensitivity reactions; however, they also play a crucial role in the pathogenesis of MC disorders, such as mastocytosis. MC activation may occur at the local level, such as in urticaria, or systemically with clinical signs and symptoms of anaphylaxis.[3,5,6] Although IgE-mediated reaction, through the cross-linking of IgE molecules bound to the MC surface by FcεRI receptors, is thought to be the most common pathway, non-IgE-mediated mechanisms involving activation of complement C3a/C5a

[a] Department of Respiratory Medicine and Allergy, Karolinska University Hospital, Huddinge; [b] Department of Medicine Solna, Immunology and Allergy Unit, Karolinska Institutet and Karolinska University Hospital; [c] Mastocytosis Centre Karolinska, Karolinska University Hospital and Karolinska Institutet, Stockholm, Sweden; [d] Department of Internal Medicine, Division of Allergy and Clinical Immunology, University of Michigan, Ann Arbor, MI, USA
* Correspondence author. Department of Respiratory Medicine and Allergy, K85, Karolinska University Hospital Huddinge, Stockholm SE-141 86, Sweden.
E-mail addresses: theo.gulen@ki.se; tgulen@gmail.com

Immunol Allergy Clin N Am 42 (2022) 45–63
https://doi.org/10.1016/j.iac.2021.09.007
immunology.theclinics.com
0889-8561/22/© 2021 The Authors. Published by Elsevier Inc.

receptors[6,7] or the Mas-related G protein receptor-X2 (MRGPRX2) have also been proposed.[8] Upon activation, MCs release granule-stored and newly formed cell membrane-derived lipid mediators and cytokines into the extracellular space. These mediators include histamine, proteases, proteoglycans, eicosanoids, and cytokines such as tumor necrosis factor-α.[9,10] Blood basophils may also participate in allergic and other inflammatory reactions in the same way as MCs[11,12]; nevertheless, not all hypersensitivity reactions involve both cell types, even if the reaction is systemic. Notably, some of the mediators involved in anaphylactic reactions are produced and released primarily by MCs, but not by basophils. Inappropriate release of MC mediators causes the so-called mast cell mediator-related symptoms.

ANAPHYLAXIS

Anaphylaxis can be defined as an acute, severe, systemic hypersensitivity reaction and represents an example of excessive MC activation resulting in an abundant release of various mediators (see definition of anaphylaxis in Adriana G. Bagos-Estevez and Dennis K. Ledford's article, "Anaphylaxis: Definition, Epidemiology, Diagnostic Challenges, Grading System," in this issue). Anaphylaxis concurrently affects multiple organ systems and presents with a broad array of symptoms and signs. Data about the prevalence and incidence of anaphylaxis are limited and often inconsistent.[13–17] It is, however, widely accepted that anaphylaxis is a relatively rare condition. Studies from the United Kingdom indicate an increase in hospital admissions due to anaphylaxis over the last 2 decades.[18] The diagnosis of anaphylaxis is based on a constellation of different signs and symptoms, and the current diagnostic criteria require concurrent occurrence of a minimum of 2 organ systems that generally include the cutaneous, gastrointestinal (GI), respiratory, and cardiovascular systems[19,20] (**Table 1**). For information regarding the grading system, epidemiology, and differential diagnosis of anaphylaxis, see Adriana G. Bagos-Estevez and Dennis K. Ledford's article, "Anaphylaxis: Definition, Epidemiology, Diagnostic Challenges, Grading System," in this issue and Motosue and colleagues' article, "Anaphylaxis: Epidemiology and Differential Diagnosis," in this issue.

Thus, anaphylaxis presently remains a clinical entity and its understanding for an allergist remains limited with respect to factors determining severity and underlying intracellular effector mechanisms. Anaphylaxis comprises a heterogeneous group of conditions regarding the nature and route of exposure to triggers, organ involvement, severity, and time course. Hence, it would be reasonable to consider anaphylaxis as a syndrome, in which different phenotypes and endotypes may be described instead of defining the condition as a "single clinical entity." For instance, food-induced systemic reaction is a leading cause of anaphylaxis in children, whereas venom- or drug-induced reactions account for most adult cases.[16,21–23] The distinctions not only are limited to triggers but also are applicable to the clinical manifestations. In addition, mortality occurs mostly in adult patients due to cardiovascular failure, whereas this manifestation is rare in children.[24,25]

From this perspective, severe anaphylaxis (SA) seems to be a distinct anaphylaxis phenotype, because all these observations cannot be merely explained by a random phenomenon. At present, the clinical and biological features of SA are not yet well characterized, although these patients usually present with hypotension and/or loss of consciousness. It is therefore crucial to gain deep insight into the underlying mechanisms. In this regard, subjects with MC activation disorders (MCAD), including mastocytosis, provide a unique disease model to investigate specific features of SA, because the existing evidence indicates a strong association between these 2 conditions.[26–28]

Table 1
Criteria for the diagnosis of anaphylaxis and related disorders of severe mast cell activation

Disorder	Diagnostic Criteria
Anaphylaxis	Anaphylaxis is highly likely when any one of the following 3 criteria is fulfilled:
1	Acute onset of an illness (minutes to several hours) with involvement of the skin, mucosal tissue, or both (eg, generalized hives, itching or flushing, swollen lips-tongue-uvula) AND at least one of the following:
A	Respiratory compromise (eg, dyspnea, wheeze-bronchospasm, stridor, reduced peak flow, hypoxia)
B	Cardiovascular compromise (eg, hypotension, syncope, collapse, incontinence)
2	Two or more of the following that occur rapidly after exposure to a *likely allergen* for that patient (minutes to several hours):
A	Involvement of the skin or mucosal tissue
B	Respiratory compromise
C	Cardiovascular compromise
D	Persistent gastrointestinal symptoms (eg, crampy abdominal pain, vomiting)
3	Hypotension after exposure to a *known allergen* for that patient (minutes to several hours)
SM	Diagnosis requires presence of major and 1 minor criterion or presence of 3 minor criteria in extracutaneous organ biopsy specimens, preferably bone marrow:
Major criterion	Multifocal aggregates of MCs ($\geq$15 MCs per cluster) in biopsy sections
Minor criteria	
1	In MC infiltrates in extracutaneous biopsy sections, >25% of the MCs (CD117+) are spindle shaped or have atypical morphology
2	Presence of an activating *KIT* mutation at codon 816, generally D816V, in bone marrow, blood, or other extracutaneous organ(s)
3	Detection of aberrant MC clones expressing CD117 with CD25 and/or CD2 in bone marrow or blood or another extracutaneous organs
4	Baseline serum tryptase persistently exceeds $\geq$20 ng/mL
MMAS	Diagnosis requires presence of one or 2 minor criteria of SM:
1	Presence of an activating *KIT* mutation D816V, in bone marrow, blood, or other extracutaneous organ(s) AND/OR
2	Detection of aberrant MC clones expressing CD117 with CD25 in bone marrow or blood or another extracutaneous organ(s)
MCAS	Three criteria are required to fulfill MCAS diagnosis:
1	Severe, episodic symptoms that are attributable to MC activation with concurrent involvement of at least 2 organs including skin, cardiovascular, gastrointestinal, and upper/lower respiratory systems
2	An event-related increase in serum tryptase above the individual's sBT according to formula ($\geq$sBT + 20% of sBT + 2 ng/mL)
3	Appropriate response to drugs directed against MC activation or effects of MC mediators to reduce/suppress symptoms

Abbreviations: MCAS, mast cell activation syndromes; MMAS, monoclonal mast cell activation syndrome; sBT, serum baseline tryptase; SM, systemic mastocytosis.
Data from Refs.[19,20,30,31,37,38]

MAST CELL ACTIVATION DISORDERS

MCAD refer to a heterogeneous group of conditions that may be caused by an increased number of MCs and/or hyperactive MCs.[29] These disorders can vary in severity, but common symptoms include often severe reactions to insect stings, and in rare cases to foods or drugs. MCAD comprise clonal (eg, mastocytosis) and nonclonal (idiopathic) variants.[29] Clonal MC disorders (CMD) are well-characterized by intrinsic MC defects, including *KIT* mutation D816V, and/or expression of aberrant MC receptors, which may cause a "hyperactive" state of MCs leading to excessive release of mediators. **Fig. 1**, schematically illustrates the wide spectrum of disorders related to MC activation.

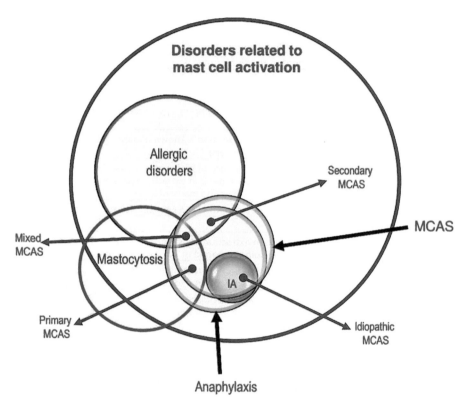

Fig. 1. Spectrum of disorders manifested by mast cell activation. These disorders encompass a broad and heterogeneous group of conditions that can range from very rare (eg, MCAS) to very common (eg, allergic disorders), some of which have an increased number of MCs and/or hyperactive MCs in various organs. It is essential to obtain accurate diagnosis due to the substantial overlapping in clinical presentation of these conditions. Please see the text for further discussion. MCAS, mast cell activation syndromes; IA, idiopathic anaphylaxis.

Mastocytosis

Mastocytosis is characterized by excessive accumulation, proliferation, and activation of abnormal MCs in several organs, including the skin, bone marrow, and GI tract.[30,31] The World Health Organization (WHO) introduced a classification of mastocytosis into 2 main groups: cutaneous mastocytosis (CM) and systemic mastocytosis (SM) involving at least 1 extracutaneous organ.[30] SM has been classified into several subgroups, with more than 85% of affected subjects having indolent SM (ISM) with a good prognosis (**Box 1**). The remaining 15% of affected subjects have more aggressive variants of the disease with a poor prognosis. According to the WHO diagnostic criteria, the diagnosis of SM requires the existence of a major and a minor criterion or 3 minor criteria on extracutaneous biopsy materials, most commonly from the bone marrow[30,31] (see **Table 1**). The incidence and prevalence of mastocytosis are unknown, but evidence suggests that it is a rare condition. In recent studies, the prevalence of ISM is estimated to be 9.6 to 13 in 100,000 and the incidence for all subtypes of SM is predicted to be 0.89 per 100,000 per year.[32,33]

The clinical picture of SM is protean, ranging from asymptomatic disease to a highly aggressive course with multisystem involvement. In patients with ISM, symptoms may be acute or chronic and result from the local or remote effects of excess mediator release from MCs, such as histamine, proteases, leukotrienes, and prostaglandins. Exogenous and endogenous triggers include physical exertion, cold, heat, insect venoms, consumption of alcohol, infections, nonsteroidal anti-inflammatory drugs (NSAIDs), and emotional stress. Specific triggers vary greatly among patients. Individual patients often present a variable and changing pattern of symptoms. These so-called MC mediator-release symptoms and signs include flushing, pruritus, palpitations, dizziness, hypotension, syncope, breathing difficulties, abdominal pain, nausea, vomiting, diarrhea, headache, sweating, lethargy, fatigue, impaired concentration, irritability, anxiety, depression, arthralgia, myalgia, and osteoporosis.[30] Not all patients experience all these manifestations; however, a history of flushing is a cardinal symptom. In addition, some subjects may experience isolated symptoms, whereas others develop a constellation of signs and symptoms resembling an anaphylaxis, which can be life threatening (ie, anaphylactic shock).[26,28] Typically, patients suddenly feel very warm and then experience palpitations, dizziness, and a decrease in blood pressure due to systemic vasodilatation that often leads to syncope.[34] Acute attacks may be brief or prolonged, but duration is usually 15 to 30 minutes.[34] Patients often experience severe fatigue lasting around 24 hours following the spells.[34]

There are also subjects with advanced SM, including aggressive SM, SM with associated hematologic neoplasm, and MC leukemia. Interestingly, the occurrence of anaphylaxis due to the excessive release of MC mediators in these patients is less common compared with that in patients with ISM.

Box 1
WHO classification of mastocytosis 2016[a]

- Cutaneous mastocytosis (CM)
  - Maculopapular CM (MPCM) = Urticaria pigmentosa (UP)
  - Diffuse CM
  - Mastocytoma of skin

- Systemic mastocytosis (SM)
  - Indolent SM
  - Smouldering SM
  - SM with associated hematological neoplasm (AHN)[b]
  - Aggressive SM
  - Mast-cell leukemia

[a]Adapted from[30,31].

[b]The previous term *SM with clonal hematologic non–mast cell-lineage disease.*

Monoclonal Mast Cell Activation Syndrome

Recently, a novel variant of clonal MCAD has been introduced, the so-called monoclonal mast cell activation syndrome (MMAS).[35,36] These patients are also mainly characterized by recurring episodes of anaphylaxis with hypotension and syncope and have clonal MCs expressing the D816V *KIT* mutation and/or CD25+ aberrant surface markers. However, they do not fulfill the WHO criteria for SM diagnosis and lack typical skin changes of mastocytosis (**Table 1**).[35,36]

WHY IS THE RISK OF SEVERE ANAPHYLAXIS INCREASED IN MAST CELL DISORDERS?

The likelihood of MCs to secrete mediators, also known as "releasability" in the context of systemic MC activation and anaphylaxis, depends on several factors including the underlying primary disease.[37,38] Greater severity correlates with the higher burden or number of involved MCs, and the cellular activation level, for example, "hyperactivated" state.[37,38] These factors together result in an increased releasability of MC mediators. There are some additional factors, including level of expression of activated receptors and/or signaling molecules on MCs, genetic predisposition (eg, genetic polymorphisms in IL-10 or IL-13), copy number of the tryptase gene, route of allergen exposure (eg, parenteral route) and type of triggering allergen (eg, insect venom), level of allergen-specific IgE, triggering cofactors, hormonal influences, and the presence of comorbid conditions[38–40] (**Box 2**). Such activation processes culminate in degranulation and release of preformed and newly synthesized membrane lipid mediators, such as histamine, tryptase, prostaglandins, and proinflammatory cytokines. Measurement of acute serum total tryptase is the current gold standard laboratory test to confirm systemic MC activation.

Subjects with mastocytosis, for instance, have a high risk of developing severe, life-threatening anaphylaxis; this may depend on hyperreleasability of MCs in these subjects due to their inherent state of hyperreactivity, often associated with occult or overt IgE-dependent allergies.[37,38] Chronically activated KIT receptor in mastocytosis may be responsible for the hyperreactivity in MCs. Indeed, in almost all subjects with SM, MCs exhibit the *KIT* D816V mutation, and the KIT ligand stem cell factor augments IgE-dependent mediator release in normal MCs.[34] However, not all patients with SM bearing the *KIT* D816V mutation develop anaphylaxis. Therefore, additional

---

Box 2
Potential factors associated to severe mast cell activation

- Increased number of mast cells involved in the reaction
- Increased *releasability* of mast cells
- *Hyperreactive* state of mast cells
- Increased copy number of tryptase gene (ie, hereditary alpha-tryptasemia)
- Presence of cofactors
- Type of allergen
- Route of allergen
- Presence of comorbidities (eg, cardiovascular)
- Gender (male)
- Increased age

genetic polymorphisms or mutations in MC signaling components, other than the activating *KIT* D816V mutation, may contribute to MC dysregulation and the predisposition for anaphylaxis.[41]

Hereditary Alpha-Tryptasemia

Hereditary alpha-tryptasemia (HαT) is another modifying factor that may influence the prevalence and severity of anaphylaxis. HαT is a recently identified autosomal dominant genetic trait that is characterized by excess copies of alpha-tryptase gene, *TPSAB1*.[42,43] Individuals with HαT may have slightly increased numbers of MCs in bone marrow and GI biopsies, and serum baseline tryptase (sBT) levels are typically greater than 8 ng/mL (often $\geq$10 ng/mL).[43] However, they generally do not have increased urinary secretion of other MC mediators, such as prostaglandins and histamine metabolites. HαT is found in approximately 6% of the general population, and there is no consistent clinical phenotype associated with HαT.[44,45] The risk for severe spontaneous and/or insect venom-triggered anaphylaxis in HαT subjects was reported to be increased.[46–48] It is also reported that increased germline copies of α-tryptase are associated with increased severity of venom anaphylaxis and idiopathic anaphylaxis (IA) in SM.[48] Thus, HαT may confer an increased risk for SA, which is independent of the presence of concomitant CMD. However, to date, no studies have shown that MCs in patients with HαT are hyperreactive. In addition, the prevalence of HαT among patients with allergies is the same as that among unselected controls.[44] Therefore, these findings related to HαT need to be confirmed in larger cohorts.

CHARACTERISTIC OF ANAPHYLAXIS IN PATIENTS WITH CLONAL MAST CELL DISORDERS

Distinct features of SA in subjects with SM are the profile of eliciting triggers as well as the clinical course of reactions.

The cause of anaphylaxis in SM may vary; however, Hymenoptera venom is the most common elicitor.[26,27,49] There is a correlation between elevated sBT levels and the severity of systemic reactions to Hymenoptera stings.[50] In a study analyzing 226 patients presenting with anaphylaxis to an emergency care setting, SM was diagnosed in 7.7% of adults and stings from flying insects were the triggers in half of these subjects.[51] Another study reported a 28% overall prevalence of venom-induced anaphylaxis (VIA) among 122 patients with SM, which is clearly higher than in the general population.[27] Interestingly, VIA may be the presenting symptom that may lead to the diagnosis of SM. In this regard, one large study reported that approximately 10% of 379 subjects with systemic reactions to Hymenoptera sting had elevated sBT levels ($\geq$11.4 ng/mL), and most of these subjects had SM or MMAS diagnosed by bone marrow biopsies.[52] Many such patients have evidence of venom-specific IgE in blood, although specific IgE levels may be lower compared with the nonmastocytosis venom-allergic population[53]; this could possibly be due to the binding of IgE onto the increased numbers of MCs, making it less available to be detected in the serum. Notably also, skin prick test reactions to venom extract in SA may be diminished in size or even absent.[54]

Drug- or food-induced reactions were also reported as an elicitor of anaphylaxis in SM[28,55]; however, most of those reactions remain patient reported and unconfirmed. Therefore, interpretations of these data should be made with caution due to the lack of reliable confirmatory in vitro tests and the absence of provocation tests. There are occasional case reports of patients with allergy to foods or preservatives.[56] Another case report presented a patient with more than 10 SA episodes after eating meat, where a provocation test with pork resulted in delayed SA with only low levels of specific IgE to meats and galactose-alpha-1,3-galactose.[57] Further diagnostic workup confirmed an underlying ISM.[57] Most recently, a large, systematic study investigating food hypersensitivity and food-induced anaphylaxis (FIA) in SM subjects found that the prevalence of FIA in SM was at least 10-fold less compared with the prevalence of VIA in SM.[58] Thus cumulative clinical experience suggests that the incidence of IgE-mediated food allergy is not, or not fundamentally, increased in subjects with SM compared with that in the general population.[58] Some patients with SM complain about flushing and GI symptoms triggered by histamine-rich diets, spicy foods, and alcohol; however, these symptoms rarely progress to anaphylaxis.[58]

Likewise, data on patients with drug hypersensitivity and MC disorders are scarce and literature is largely limited to case reports.[59] Remarkably, most of these cases are related to general anesthesia and radiocontrast media exposure.[60,61] Experience suggests that some patients with SM may be at risk for severe non-IgE-mediated reactions, such as those experienced with perioperative muscle relaxants. Such risk is probably lower in patients who have tolerated previous general anesthesia and/or who have no history of anaphylaxis during anesthesia. At present, available data in the literature are scant on this topic, and it is not possible to provide clear recommendations. Some experts suggest premedicating with antihistamines and corticosteroids before anesthesia and recommend perioperative drugs with lower intrinsic MC activation properties. Furthermore, unlike VIA, drug-induced anaphylaxis (DIA) is rarely associated with undetected MC disorder in the literature. In this regard, a study investigating patients with NSAID hypersensitivity and its correlation to occult SM failed to show elevated sBT levels.[62] Thus, it is not known whether the incidence of DIA is increased in SM because there are currently no systematic studies.

By contrast, patients with IA, that is, unexplained anaphylaxis, are more likely to have SM.[26,55] Indeed, there is an intriguing relationship between IA and MCAD. Because CMD can be potentially misdiagnosed as IA, it is, therefore, essential to distinguish it from true IA.[35,63] Akin and colleagues[35] reported the presence of a clonal MC population in 5 of 12 patients with IA in whom there were no features of urticaria pigmentosa or histologic evidence for SM on bone marrow biopsies.[35] Similarly, Gulen and colleagues[63] performed bone marrow examinations in 30 cases of unexplained SA without signs of CM and reported that 47% of these patients were subsequently diagnosed with CMD, both clonal and/or aberrant MC populations. Finally, a recent study investigated 56 subjects with more than 3 episodes/y of unexplained SA. Bone marrow (BM) examination found evidence of MC clonal disease in 14% (8 of 56).[64] The reasons for the discrepancies among these studies may be the differences in diagnostic criteria for IA and referral patterns.

Another suggestive feature of SA in patients with SM is the distinct clinical pattern and course of episodes. Patients with SM with SA frequently present with severe cardiovascular signs and symptoms including hypotensive syncope,[26,28,49] whereas respiratory symptoms, urticaria, and angioedema are rare.[49] For instance, the occurrence of syncope/loss of conciseness has been reported to be 72% during SA among patients with SM regardless of triggers[26]; this is also confirmed in SM with VIA.[53] These observations led to the development of predictive models to distinguish patients presenting with SA and underlying CMD, specifically SM and MMAS. Because the diagnosis of SM requires an extracutaneous biopsy, it may be challenging for clinicians to decide whether to pursue further evaluation in subjects presenting with SA but no other features of SM. In this regard, the Spanish

Network on Mastocytosis (REMA) proposed a scoring tool to predict high-risk patients, which is based on a combined clinical (ie, male gender and clinical symptoms of syncopal episodes in the absence of urticaria/angioedema during SA) and laboratory (elevated sBT levels of $\geq$25 ng/mL) criteria.[49] Thus, the REMA score has been used to screen patients presenting with SA but lack typical signs of CM and showed a sensitivity of 92% and specificity of 81%, regardless of the trigger.[49] A modification of the "REMA score" subsequently has been proposed as the "Karolinska score," using a reduced sBT level of $\geq$20 ng/mL.[63] This modified version resulted in a better sensitivity (93%) and specificity (94%), when retrospectively applied in patients with IA.[63] When available, these tools should be used together with peripheral blood *KIT* D816V mutation analysis, because it is independently a strong indicator of the underlying SM.[65] Finally, further modification of previous tools was proposed—the so-called National Institute of Health Idiopathic Clonal Anaphylaxis Score—by using clinical symptoms, gender, a baseline tryptase cutoff of 11.4 ng/mL, and allele-specific polymerase chain reaction testing to detect the presence or absence of *KIT* D816V mutation in peripheral blood.[64] However, this scoring tool has not been yet validated.

MAST CELL ACTIVATION SYNDROMES

MC activation syndrome (MCAS) may be diagnosed in some patients when the symptoms are systemic and MCAS criteria are fulfilled[37,38,66,67] (see **Table 1**). MCAS can be defined as a disorder of MC activation with various causes all resulting in severe, recurrent, and episodic symptoms due to systemic MC mediator release.[37,38,66,67] Patients with MCAS often present with symptoms of anaphylaxis. However, it is noteworthy that neither all anaphylaxis fulfill diagnostic criteria of MCAS nor do all MCAS episodes reach the severity of anaphylaxis. It is also worth mentioning that MC activation can manifest as a less severe and/or chronic condition, therefore MCAS cannot be diagnosed in these patients. Thus, not all mediator-related and clinically relevant symptoms can be classified as MCAS.[38]

Three sets of criteria are required for an MCAS diagnosis: (1) typical episodic symptoms consistent with MC activation, (2) objective laboratory evidence of MC involvement with a substantial transient increase in validated MC mediators in the serum or in the urine (preferably, an event-related increase in serum tryptase levels according to the formula $\geq 1.2 \times$ sBT + 2 ng/mL within 4 hours of an acute episode), and (3) control of symptoms with MC-directed therapies.[37,38,67] Once a diagnosis of MCAS has been confirmed, further classification is necessary. MCAS has been classified into 3 variants.[37,38] Primary MCAS is defined by the presence of clonal MCs and includes MMAS and mastocytosis (systemic and/or cutaneous) (**Table 2**). Diagnosis of primary (clonal) MCAS can only be made after an extracutaneous biopsy, most often after a bone marrow biopsy.[30,31] Clonal MCAS can present with IA.[35,63,64] Secondary MCAS results in symptoms of MC activation through IgE- and non-IgE-mediated processes, such as food-, drug-, or Hymenoptera venom-induced SA. This variant has no evidence of a clonal MC population. Finally, idiopathic MCAS results in MC activation symptoms without a clear precipitating cause. Patients with IA are the epitome of idiopathic MCAS; therefore, it is essential to evaluate whether the patient meets criteria for IA. However, idiopathic MCAS is a broader entity and may also include patients whose episodes may not fulfill the clinical criteria of IA, such as patients presenting with concomitant skin and GI symptoms causing event-related elevation of serum tryptase.

Table 3 illustrates features of anaphylaxis in various MCADs and HαT.

THERAPEUTIC OPTIONS

Acute episodes of SA in patients with MC disorders should be treated in the same manner as other forms of anaphylaxis.[20,68,69] Roberts and colleagues[70,71] stressed the unique role of epinephrine in the treatment of SA in a patient with SM who was refractory to vasopressor therapy with dopamine, yet quickly improved with epinephrine. Intramuscular (IM) epinephrine is the drug of choice. Evidence suggests that treatment of systemic reactions with epinephrine prevents progression to more severe symptoms.[69] Unfortunately, epinephrine is still underutilized, whereas corticosteroids are widely used as first-line therapy despite the lack of evidence.[72] In refractory cases of severe hypotension not responding to repeated doses of IM epinephrine, or hypotension followed by cardiac arrest, intravenous (IV) epinephrine should be given with continuous monitoring of cardiac response, blood pressure, and oxygen saturation. Supplemental high-flow oxygen and IV fluid (eg, normal saline) replacement should be administered. When cardiovascular status and respiratory function stabilize, second-line medications such as histamine receptor type-1 (HR1) and type-2 (HR2) blockers and corticosteroids are usually recommended.[68] However, the value of corticosteroids in the acute management of anaphylaxis is unclear because there is no substantial evidence to support their proposed effect on the prevention of protracted or biphasic reactions.[73]

With regard to the long-term management and prevention of SA, measures aim to reduce the severity and/or frequency of the acute episodes. Prevention is the most important aspect, therefore all patients with mastocytosis who have a history of anaphylaxis should be prescribed self-injectable epinephrine after receiving adequate information and training on the appropriate use. Information and education should also be extended to the patient's family and caregivers, and an action plan for the management of acute episodes should be implemented.

Although avoidance is the mainstay of the prevention of SA, there is a wide individual variation among patients with mastocytosis. Hence, the general advice to avoid all the literature-reported potential triggers for MC degranulation is not recommended; instead, a tailored management strategy is necessary.[74] When possible, patients should undergo a thorough allergy workup including allergy tests for several known/

Table 2 Classification of mast cell activation syndromes	
Variant of MCAS	**Clinical and Laboratory Findings**

Primary (clonal)	Clonal mast cells found
	a. Established SM: criteria to diagnose SM are fulfilled
	b. Established CM: criteria for CM are fulfilled but the criteria to diagnose SM are not fulfilled
	c. Neither CM nor SM can be diagnosed, but one or both of the following minor SM criteria documenting mast cell clonality found:
	    i. *KIT* D816V or
	    ii. CD25 expression in mast cells

Secondary	An underlying allergic, atopic, inflammatory, or neoplastic disease is found but no monoclonal mast cells are detectable (*KIT* mutation and/or CD25 expression in mast cells not found)
Idiopathic	No underlying allergy or atopy and no monoclonal (*KIT*-mutated and/or CD25+) mast cells are detectable

Data from Refs.[37,38]

Table 3
Features of anaphylaxis in various mast cell activation disorders and hereditary alpha-tryptasemia

	SM	CM	MCAS	HαT
Risk of anaphylaxis increased?	+	+/−	+	+ in a subgroup
Clinical features	Hypotension, flushing, abdominal cramping, less urticarial, and angioedema	Variable	Not all episodes may reach the severity of anaphylaxis. Symptoms may also include urticaria and angioedema; however, it should always involve ≥2 organs	Variable. HαT by itself does not confer a particular clinical phenotype but is thought to amplify symptoms and severity of anaphylaxis
Markers of clonality (KIT D816V, CD25 on MCs)	+	+/−	+ in primary MCAS, whereas − in secondary and idiopathic MCAS	Negative in pure HαT; however, SM is detected more frequently in HαT and patients may have both conditions
Baseline tryptase	>20 ng/mL in most patients	May be normal or elevated	Normal or elevated	>8 ng/mL
Diagnosis	Bone marrow biopsy and checking for WHO criteria	Inspection of skin, Darier sign, skin biopsy	Consensus criteria (see text)	Genetic testing for TPSAB1 copy number

Table 4
Prophylactic therapy in patients with mast cell activation disorders

Drug	Indication	Proposed Mechanism of Action
Histamine receptor type-1 blocker	All patients	Blocks histamine receptor type-1
Histamine receptor type-2 blocker	Patients with gastrointestinal symptoms or those not responding to histamine receptor type-1 blocker	Blocks histamine receptor type-2
Antileukotrienes	Add-on treatment in patients with persistent dermatologic complaints who do not respond adequately to histamine receptor type-1 blocker	Blocks leukotriene receptor
Cromolyn sodium	Patients with persistent gastrointestinal symptoms (eg, crampy abdominal pain, vomiting, diarrhea) and resistance to histamine receptor type-1 and type 2 blockers	Effects on various cell types including MCs; may block IgE-dependent activation of MCs
Ketotifen	In patients with idiopathic anaphylaxis and resistance to histamine receptor-type 1 blockers	Inhibits activation of MCs, inhibits histamine binding to histamine receptor type 1
Aspirin	Patients with severe, recurrent anaphylaxis	Suppresses the generation of prostaglandin D_2 in human MCs
Glucocorticosteroids	Preventive maintenance therapy at low doses for recurrent anaphylaxis not responsive to histamine receptor blockers	Blocks mediator production and cytokine synthesis as well as mediator secretion in MCs
Allergen immunotherapy	In patients with mastocytosis in whom venom allergy is detected, lifelong immune therapy is generally recommended	Effects on various cell types including MCs, and aids development of venom-specific immune tolerance
Omalizumab	Patients with severe, recurrent anaphylaxis	IgE depletion and hyposensitization of MCs through downregulation of nonspecific IgE receptors

(continued on next page)

Table 4 (continued)		
Drug	**Indication**	**Proposed Mechanism of Action**
Interferon-alpha	Generally recommended in patients with aggressive SM but has also been shown to control severe MC activation episodes	Suppresses mast cell function, including histamine release
Cladribine	Patients with aggressive variant of SM and severe, life-threatening anaphylaxis	Causes apoptosis in MCs independent of the presence of the common D816V *KIT* mutation
Midoaustrin	Patients with aggressive variant of SM and in certain cases, indolent SM with severe, life-threatening anaphylaxis	Blocks *KIT* D816V activation and MC proliferation in SM and also inhibits IgE-dependent activation and mediator secretion in MCs
Avapritinib	Patients with aggressive variant of SM and in certain cases, indolent SM with severe, life-threatening anaphylaxis	Selectively inhibits KIT exon 17 mutants, including *KIT* D816V

potential triggers to assess for potential culprit agents. In addition, an allergist evaluation can be used as guidance to map out patients' individual trigger profile to avoid relevant food, medication, and inhalational triggers of MC activation. For instance, eliminations of histamine-rich diets or avoidance of certain drugs including NSAIDs is not routinely recommended. In contrast, Hymenoptera stings seem to be the most frequent cause of anaphylaxis in adult patients with mastocytosis.[26] Thus, those with sting anaphylaxis who are sensitized to Hymenoptera venom should be recommended lifelong venom immunotherapy, which reduces recurrent anaphylaxis risk with stings.[53] At present, there is no consensus among experts whether to prescribe epinephrine to all patients diagnosed with mastocytosis or to prescribe it only to those with a history of anaphylaxis or who are at increased risk for anaphylaxis. This issue has been discussed in a recent study, wherein a risk assessment tool to predict occurrence of anaphylaxis in patients with mastocytosis was developed.[27] This tool may facilitate the determination of "correct" patients with mastocytosis who need epinephrine autoinjectors.

There are currently no randomized studies to show which prophylactic therapy options are superior in mastocytosis. A stepwise approach should therefore be considered in all patients[74] **(Table 4)**. The first step includes HR1 blockers. Doses can be adjusted individually, and doses up to 4 times higher than the recommended doses can be used similar to those in patients with chronic urticaria. In the same manner, HR2 blockers, antileukotrienes, oral cromolyn, and corticosteroids can be additionally given in unresponsive patients. If the combination therapies are ineffective, omalizumab, which is a humanized monoclonal antibody that specifically binds to free IgE, can be used. Omalizumab has been shown to diminish the frequency of anaphylactic episodes in anecdotal reports and case series with varying success.[63,75,76]

Nevertheless, there are presently no randomized, placebo-controlled studies to recommend omalizumab in routine use.

Although it is generally assigned for patients with aggressive SM, in rare, refractory cases, cytoreductive or immunomodulatory therapy including interferon-alpha 2b[77] and cladribine (2-CDA)[78] was historically reported to be beneficial in controlling mediator-related symptoms. Current first-line cytoreductive therapy options include tyrosine kinase inhibitors (TKIs) targeting the MC growth receptor KIT. A recent study provided initial evidence that midostaurin, in addition to reversed organ damage and decreased splenomegaly and bone marrow MC burden in patients with advanced SM,[79] was found to improve mediator-related symptoms and quality of life, suggesting that the drug may also be useful in patients with ISM suffering from severe mediator-related symptoms resistant to conventional therapies.[80,81] Avapritinib is another novel TKI that selectively inhibits *KIT* D816V.[82] Both midostaurin and avapritinib are currently approved for treatment of advanced SM. A recent phase 2 study reported symptom reduction and MC cytoreduction with avapritinib in patients with ISM.[83] Additionally, prompt resolution of recurrent anaphylaxis with the addition of avapritinib was described in a patient with SM-AHN.[84] However, the effects of TKIs on anaphylaxis remain to be explored.

SUMMARY

Anaphylaxis is an important feature of patients with MC disorders. Hence, the presence of underlying CMD should be strongly suspected in patients with VIA as well as patients with recurrent IA; in particular, when these episodes present with severe hypotensive syncope. A bone marrow examination should be considered if the sBT level is elevated ($\geq$11.4 ng/mL) and/or if the peripheral blood *KIT* D816V mutation is present.

Appropriate treatment with IM epinephrine remains underutilized in most cases, despite increased awareness and recognition of anaphylaxis. Expanding knowledge on the presentation and triggers of anaphylaxis among patients with mastocytosis, their relatives, and health care providers will improve its recognition and management and increase patient safety. Moreover, a better understanding of the pathogenesis of SA by exploring the intrinsic changes in MCs of patients will provide important insight into its long-term management. Further research may lead to identification of novel biomarkers[85] to distinguish patients with SA as well as development of new drugs targeting intracellular MC activation mechanisms and mediators.

CLINICS CARE POINTS

- The presence of recurrent hypotensive episodes and/or syncope without urticaria and/or angioedema and/or respiratory symptoms during anaphylaxis increases the odds of underlying CMD.

- Patients with Hymenoptera VIA and elevated baseline serum tryptase level should be investigated for the presence of mastocytosis; particularly if peripheral blood *KIT* D816V mutation is present.

- HαT is a genetic trait and may confer an increased risk for SA, which is independent of the presence of concomitant CMD.

- MCAS may be diagnosed when the symptoms due to MC mediator release are severe, recurrent, and systemic, and MCAS criteria are fulfilled. An event-related increase in sBT is critical to diagnosis.

FUNDING

This study was supported by grants from the Konsul TH C Bergh Foundation, Sweden, and through the regional agreement on medical training and clinical research (ALF) between Stockholm County Council and Karolinska Institutet, Stockholm, Sweden.

DISCLOSURE

T. Gülen has received lecture fees from Thermo Fisher. C. Akin has received consultancy fees from Blueprint Medicines and Novartis and has a patent for LAD2 cells.

REFERENCES

1. Galli SJ, Kalesnikoff J, Grimbaldeston MA, et al. Mast cells as "tunable" effector and immunoregulatory cells: recent advances. Annu Rev Immunol 2005;23:749–86.
2. Galli SJ, Tsai M. Mast cells: versatile regulators of inflammation, tissue remodeling, host defense and homeostasis. J Dermatol Sci 2008;49(1):7–19.
3. Valent P, Akin C, Hartmann K, et al. Mast cells as a unique hematopoietic lineage and cell system: from Paul Ehrlich's visions to precision medicine concepts. Theranostics 2020;10(23):10743–68.
4. Varricchi G, Marone G. Mast cells: fascinating but still elusive after 140 years from their discovery. Int J Mol Sci 2020;21(2):464.
5. Galli SJ, Tsai M. Mast cells in allergy and infection: versatile effector and regulatory cells in innate and adaptive immunity. Eur J Immunol 2010;40(7):1843–51.
6. Kalesnikoff J, Galli SJ. Anaphylaxis: mechanisms of mast cell activation. Chem Immunol Allergy 2010;95:45–66.
7. Iwaki S, Tkaczyk C, Metcalfe DD, et al. Roles of adaptor molecules in mast cell activation. Chem Immunol Allergy 2005;87:43–58.
8. Kelso JM. MRGPRX2 signaling and skin test results. J Allergy Clin Immunol Pract 2020;8(1):426.
9. Gilfillan AM, Beaven MA. Regulation of mast cell responses in health and disease. Crit Rev Immunol 2011;31(6):475–529.
10. Castells M. Mast cell mediators in allergic inflammation and mastocytosis. Immunol Allergy Clin North Am 2006;26(3):465–85.
11. Siracusa MC, Kim BS, Spergel JM, et al. Basophils and allergic inflammation. J Allergy Clin Immunol 2013;132(4):789–801.
12. Korošec P, Gibbs BF, Rijavec M, et al. Important and specific role for basophils in acute allergic reactions. Clin Exp Allergy 2018;48(5):502–12.
13. Lieberman P, Camargo CA Jr, Bohlke K, et al. Epidemiology of anaphylaxis: findings of the American College of Allergy, Asthma and Immunology Epidemiology of Anaphylaxis Working Group. Ann Allergy Asthma Immunol 2006;97(5): 596–602.
14. Worm M. Epidemiology of anaphylaxis. Chem Immunol Allergy 2010;95:12–21.
15. Panesar SS, Javad S, de Silva D, et al. The epidemiology of anaphylaxis in Europe: a systematic review. Allergy 2013;68(11):1353–61.
16. Wood RA, Camargo CA Jr, Lieberman P, et al. Anaphylaxis in America: the prevalence and characteristics of anaphylaxis in the United States. J Allergy Clin Immunol 2014;133(2):461–7.
17. Decker WW, Campbell RL, Manivannan V, et al. The etiology and incidence of anaphylaxis in Rochester, Minnesota: a report from the Rochester Epidemiology Project. J Allergy Clin Immunol 2008;122(6):1161–5.

18. Sheikh A, Hippisley-Cox J, Newton J, et al. Trends in national incidence, lifetime prevalence and adrenaline prescribing for anaphylaxis in England. J R Soc Med 2008;101(3):139–43.
19. Sampson HA, Munoz-Furlong A, Campbell RL, et al. Second symposium on the definition and management of anaphylaxis: summary report–second National Institute of Allergy and Infectious Disease/Food Allergy and Anaphylaxis Network symposium. Ann Emerg Med 2006;47(4):373–80.
20. Simons FE, Ardusso LR, Bilo MB, et al. World allergy organization guidelines for the assessment and management of anaphylaxis. World Allergy Organ J 2011; 4(2):13–37.
21. Braganza SC, Acworth JP, McKinnon DR, et al. Paediatric emergency department anaphylaxis: different patterns from adults. Arch Dis Child 2006;91(2): 159–63.
22. Vetander M, Helander D, Flodstrom C, et al. Anaphylaxis and reactions to foods in children–a population-based case study of emergency department visits. Clin Exp Allergy 2012;42(4):568–77.
23. Worm M, Eckermann O, Dolle S, et al. Triggers and treatment of anaphylaxis: an analysis of 4,000 cases from Germany, Austria and Switzerland. Dtsch Arztebl Int 2014;111(21):367–75.
24. Moneret-Vautrin DA, Morisset M, Flabbee J, et al. Epidemiology of life-threatening and lethal anaphylaxis: a review. Allergy 2005;60(4):443–51.
25. Turner PJ, Jerschow E, Umasunthar T, et al. Fatal anaphylaxis: mortality rate and risk factors. J Allergy Clin Immunol Pract 2017;5(5):1169–78.
26. Gulen T, Hagglund H, Dahlen B, et al. High prevalence of anaphylaxis in patients with systemic mastocytosis - a single-centre experience. Clin Exp Allergy 2014; 44(1):121–9.
27. Gulen T, Ljung C, Nilsson G, et al. Risk factor analysis of anaphylactic reactions in patients with systemic mastocytosis. J Allergy Clin Immunol Pract 2017;5(5): 1248–55.
28. Brockow K, Jofer C, Behrendt H, et al. Anaphylaxis in patients with mastocytosis: a study on history, clinical features and risk factors in 120 patients. Allergy 2008; 63(2):226–32.
29. Akin C. Mast cell activation disorders. J Allergy Clin Immunol Pract 2014;2(3): 252–7.
30. Gulen T, Hagglund H, Dahlen B, et al. Mastocytosis: the puzzling clinical spectrum and challenging diagnostic aspects of an enigmatic disease. J Intern Med 2016;279(3):211–28.
31. Valent P, Akin C, Metcalfe DD. Mastocytosis 2016: updated WHO classification and novel emerging treatment concepts. Blood 2016;129(11):1420–7.
32. van Doormaal JJ, Arends S, Brunekreeft KL, et al. Prevalence of indolent systemic mastocytosis in a Dutch region. J Allergy Clin Immunol 2013;131(5): 1429–31.
33. Cohen SS, Skovbo S, Vestergaard H, et al. Epidemiology of systemic mastocytosis in Denmark. Br J Haematol 2014;166(4):521–8.
34. Gulen T, Hagglund H, Dahlen SE, et al. Flushing, fatigue, and recurrent anaphylaxis: a delayed diagnosis of mastocytosis. Lancet 2014;383(9928):1608.
35. Akin C, Scott LM, Kocabas CN, et al. Demonstration of an aberrant mast-cell population with clonal markers in a subset of patients with "idiopathic" anaphylaxis. Blood 2007;110(7):2331–3.

36. Sonneck K, Florian S, Mullauer L, et al. Diagnostic and subdiagnostic accumulation of mast cells in the bone marrow of patients with anaphylaxis: Monoclonal mast cell activation syndrome. Int Arch Allergy Immunol 2007;142(2):158–64.

37. Valent P, Akin C, Bonadonna P, et al. Proposed diagnostic algorithm for patients with suspected mast cell activation syndrome. J Allergy Clin Immunol Pract 2019; 7(4):1125–33.

38. Gülen T, Akin C, Bonadonna P, et al. Selecting the right criteria and proper classification to diagnose mast cell activation syndromes: a critical review. J Allergy Clin Immunol Pract 2021;22. S2213-2198(21)00676-0.

39. Metcalfe DD, Peavy RD, Gilfillan AM. Mechanisms of mast cell signaling in anaphylaxis. J Allergy Clin Immunol 2009;124(4):639–46.

40. Gilfillan AM, Peavy RD, Metcalfe DD. Amplification mechanisms for the enhancement of antigen-mediated mast cell activation. Immunol Res 2009;43(1–3):15–24.

41. Valent P, Akin C, Arock M. Diagnosis and treatment of anaphylaxis in patients with mastocytosis. Curr Treat Options Allergy 2014;1(3):247–61.

42. Lyons JJ, Sun G, Stone KD, et al. Mendelian inheritance of elevated serum tryptase associated with atopy and connective tissue abnormalities. J Allergy Clin Immunol 2014;133(5):1471–4.

43. Lyons JJ, Yu X, Hughes JD, et al. Elevated basal serum tryptase identifies a multisystem disorder associated with increased TPSAB1 copy number. Nat Genet 2016;48(12):1564–9.

44. Robey RC, Wilcock A, Bonin H, et al. Hereditary alpha-tryptasemia: UK prevalence and variability in disease expression. J Allergy Clin Immunol Pract 2020; 8(10):3549–56.

45. Chollet MB, Akin C. Hereditary alpha tryptasemia is not associated with specific clinical phenotypes. J Allergy Clin Immunol 2021;148(3):889–94.

46. O'Connell MP, Lyons JJ. Hymenoptera venom-induced anaphylaxis and hereditary alpha-tryptasemia. Curr Opin Allergy Clin Immunol 2020;20(5):431–7.

47. Lyons JJ, Chovanec J, O'Connell MP, et al. Heritable risk for severe anaphylaxis associated with increased α-tryptase-encoding germline copy number at TPSAB1. J Allergy Clin Immunol 2021;147(2):622–32.

48. Greiner G, Sprinzl B, Górska A, et al. Hereditary alpha tryptasemia is a valid genetic biomarker for severe mediator-related symptoms in mastocytosis. Blood 2021;137(2):238–47.

49. Alvarez-Twose I, Gonzalez de Olano D, Sanchez-Munoz L, et al. Clinical, biological, and molecular characteristics of clonal mast cell disorders presenting with systemic mast cell activation symptoms. J Allergy Clin Immunol 2010;125(6): 1269–78.

50. Rueff F, Przybilla B, Bilo MB, et al. Predictors of severe systemic anaphylactic reactions in patients with Hymenoptera venom allergy: importance of baseline serum tryptase-a study of the European Academy of Allergology and Clinical Immunology Interest Group on Insect Venom Hypersensitivity. J Allergy Clin Immunol 2009;124(5):1047–54.

51. Oropeza AR, Bindslev-Jensen C, Broesby-Olsen S, et al. Patterns of anaphylaxis after diagnostic workup: a follow-up study of 226 patients with suspected anaphylaxis. Allergy 2017;72(12):1944–52.

52. Bonadonna P, Perbellini O, Passalacqua G, et al. Clonal mast cell disorders in patients with systemic reactions to Hymenoptera stings and increased serum tryptase levels. J Allergy Clin Immunol 2009;123(3):680–6.

53. Jarkvist J, Salehi C, Akin C, et al. Venom immunotherapy in patients with clonal mast cell disorders: IgG4 correlates with protection. Allergy 2020;75(1):169–77.

54. Gulen T, Moller Westerberg C, Lyberg K, et al. Assessment of in vivo mast cell reactivity in patients with systemic mastocytosis. Clin Exp Allergy 2017;47(7): 909–17.

55. Gonzalez de Olano D, de la Hoz Caballer B, Nunez Lopez R, et al. Prevalence of allergy and anaphylactic symptoms in 210 adult and pediatric patients with mastocytosis in Spain: a study of the Spanish network on mastocytosis (REMA). Clin Exp Allergy 2007;37(10):1547–55.

56. Cifuentes L, Ring J, Brockow K. Clonal mast cell activation syndrome with anaphylaxis to sulfites. Int Arch Allergy Immunol 2013;162(1):94–6.

57. Roenneberg S, Bohner A, Brockow K, et al. alpha-Gal-a new clue for anaphylaxis in mastocytosis. J Allergy Clin Immunol Pract 2016;4(3):531–2.

58. Jarkvist J, Brockow K, Gülen T. Low frequency of IgE-mediated food hypersensitivity in mastocytosis. J Allergy Clin Immunol Pract 2020;8(9):3093–101.

59. Bonadonna P, Pagani M, Aberer W, et al. Drug hypersensitivity in clonal mast cell disorders: ENDA/EAACI position paper. Allergy 2015;70(7):755–63.

60. Weingarten TN, Volcheck GW, Sprung J. Anaphylactoid reaction to intravenous contrast in patient with systemic mastocytosis. Anaesth Intensive Care 2009; 37(4):646–9.

61. Renauld V, Goudet V, Mouton-Faivre C, et al. Case report: perioperative immediate hypersensitivity involves not only allergy but also mastocytosis. Can J Anaesth 2011;58(5):456–9.

62. Seitz CS, Brockow K, Hain J, et al. Non-steroidal anti-inflammatory drug hypersensitivity: association with elevated basal serum tryptase? Allergy Asthma Clin Immunol 2014;10(1):19.

63. Gulen T, Hagglund H, Sander B, et al. The presence of mast cell clonality in patients with unexplained anaphylaxis. Clin Exp Allergy 2014;44(9):1179–87.

64. Carter MC, Desai A, Komarow HD, et al. A distinct biomolecular profile identifies monoclonal mast cell disorders in patients with idiopathic anaphylaxis. J Allergy Clin Immunol 2018;141(1):180–8.

65. Kristensen T, Vestergaard H, Bindslev-Jensen C, et al. Sensitive KIT D816V mutation analysis of blood as a diagnostic test in mastocytosis. Am J Hematol 2014; 89(5):493–8.

66. Akin C, Valent P, Metcalfe DD. Mast cell activation syndrome: proposed diagnostic criteria. J Allergy Clin Immunol 2010;126(6):1099–104.

67. Valent P, Akin C, Arock M, et al. Definitions, criteria and global classification of mast cell disorders with special reference to mast cell activation syndromes: a consensus proposal. Int Arch Allergy Immunol 2012;157(3):215–25.

68. Muraro A, Roberts G, Worm M, et al. Anaphylaxis: guidelines from the European Academy of Allergy and Clinical Immunology. Allergy 2014;69(8):1026–45.

69. Lieberman PL. Recognition and first-line treatment of anaphylaxis. Am J Med 2014;127(1 Suppl):S6–11.

70. Roberts LJ 2nd, Turk JW, Oates JA. Shock syndrome associated with mastocytosis: pharmacologic reversal of the acute episode and therapeutic prevention of recurrent attacks. Adv Shock Res 1982;8:145–52.

71. Turk J, Oates JA, Roberts LJ 2nd. Intervention with epinephrine in hypotension associated with mastocytosis. J Allergy Clin Immunol 1983;71(2):189–92.

72. Clark S, Camargo CA Jr. Emergency treatment and prevention of insect-sting anaphylaxis. Curr Opin Allergy Clin Immunol 2006;6(4):279–83.

73. Campbell DE. Anaphylaxis management: time to re-evaluate the role of corticosteroids. J Allergy Clin Immunol Pract 2019;7(7):2239–40.

74. Gulen T, Akin C. Pharmacotherapy of mast cell disorders. Curr Opin Allergy Clin Immunol 2017;17(4):295–303.

75. Carter MC, Robyn JA, Bressler PB, et al. Omalizumab for the treatment of unprovoked anaphylaxis in patients with systemic mastocytosis. J Allergy Clin Immunol 2007;119(6):1550–1.

76. Broesby-Olsen S, Vestergaard H, Mortz CG, et al. Omalizumab prevents anaphylaxis and improves symptoms in systemic mastocytosis: efficacy and safety observations. Allergy 2018;73(1):230–8.

77. Kluin-Nelemans HC, Jansen JH, Breukelman H, et al. Response to interferon alfa-2b in a patient with systemic mastocytosis. N Engl J Med 1992;326(9):619–23.

78. Wimazal F, Geissler P, Shnawa P, et al. Severe life-threatening or disabling anaphylaxis in patients with systemic mastocytosis: a single-center experience. Int Arch Allergy Immunol 2012;157(4):399–405.

79. Gotlib J, Kluin-Nelemans HC, George TI, et al. Efficacy and safety of midostaurin in advanced systemic mastocytosis. N Engl J Med 2016;374(26):2530–41.

80. Valent P, Akin C, Hartmann K, et al. Midostaurin: a magic bullet that blocks mast cell expansion and activation. Ann Oncol 2017;28(10):2367–76.

81. Hartmann K, Gotlib J, Akin C, et al. Midostaurin improves quality of life and mediator-related symptoms in advanced systemic mastocytosis. J Allergy Clin Immunol 2020;146(2):356–66.

82. Gilreath JA, Tchertanov L, Deininger MW. Novel approaches to treating advanced systemic mastocytosis. Clin Pharmacol 2019;11:77–92.

83. Akin C, Elberink HO, Gotlib J, et al. PIONEER: a randomized, double-blind, placebo-controlled, phase 2 study of avapritinib in patients with indolent or smoldering systemic mastocytosis (SM) with symptoms inadequately controlled by standard therapy. J Allergy Clin Immunol 2020;145(2):AB336.

84. Kudlaty E, Perez M, Stein BL, et al. Systemic mastocytosis with an associated hematologic neoplasm complicated by recurrent anaphylaxis: prompt resolution of anaphylaxis with the addition of avapritinib. J Allergy Clin Immunol Pract 2021;9(6):2534–6.

85. Gülen T, Teufelberger A, Ekoff M, et al. Distinct plasma biomarkers confirm the diagnosis of mastocytosis and identify increased risk of anaphylaxis. J Allergy Clin Immunol 2021;2.

Management of Anaphylaxis

Aishwarya Navalpakam, MD, Narin Thanaputkaiporn, MD,
Pavadee Poowuttikul, MD*

KEYWORDS

- Anaphylaxis • Anaphylaxis management • Systemic allergic reaction • Epinephrine
- Epinephrine autoinjector

KEY POINTS

- Early recognition and treatment of anaphylaxis is essential to prevent progression to a fatal reaction. Epinephrine administered intramuscularly into the anterior lateral thigh is the drug of choice. Peak epinephrine levels are achieved more rapidly with intramuscular versus subcutaneous administration.
- Patients with anaphylaxis should be evaluated for airway, breathing, and circulation, then immediately placed in the recumbent supine position.
- The recommended dose of epinephrine to treat anaphylaxis is 0.01 mg/kg of 1 mg/mL (1:1000), not to exceed 0.5 mg/kg in a single dose. Epinephrine is commercially available in a 1 mg/mL (1:1000) vial and can be withdrawn into a syringe for administration. For epinephrine autoinjectors, use the following: for infants ≤10 kg, 0.1 mg; for children 10 to 25 kg, 0.15 mg; for subjects ≥25 kg, 0.3 mg.
- Antihistamines and glucocorticosteroids *should not* be used in the place of epinephrine. They are not helpful in the acute management of anaphylaxis. Inhalational β-2 agonists are used to treat bronchospasm associated with anaphylaxis that persists despite epinephrine administration.
- Intravenous fluids and vasopressors can be considered for patients who have refractory hypotension or shock despite optimal doses of epinephrine.

Anaphylaxis is a systemic allergic or nonallergic reaction that can lead to death. Common systemic symptoms include generalized erythema, itching and urticaria, and/or angioedema; nausea, vomiting, diarrhea, a feeling of impending doom, hypotension, and respiratory difficulty. Other symptoms may also include sneezing, rhinorrhea, nasal pruritus, and/or nasal congestion; throat clearing and/or cough; and conjunctival erythema, pruritus, or tearing. Some patients also experience a metallic taste and abdominal or uterine cramps. Acute management of anaphylaxis includes the early use of epinephrine, assessing airway function, and maintaining circulation. Long-

Division of Allergy, Immunology and Rheumatology, Department of Pediatrics, Children's Hospital of Michigan, Central Michigan University College of Medicine, 3950 Beaubien Boulevard, Detroit, MI 48201, USA
* Corresponding author.
E-mail address: ppoowutt@dmc.org

Immunol Allergy Clin N Am 42 (2022) 65–76
https://doi.org/10.1016/j.iac.2021.09.005
0889-8561/22/© 2021 Elsevier Inc. All rights reserved.

term management includes avoidance of triggers; frequent education of patients, parents, and caregivers as to how to use epinephrine autoinjectors; appropriate treatment of the cause of the reaction, for example, Hymenoptera hypersensitivity, food allergy, etc.; and referral to an allergist/immunologist. The acute management of anaphylaxis is discussed in this article.

ACUTE MANAGEMENT OF ANAPHYLAXIS

Anaphylaxis can develop rapidly and be fatal.[1–4] After exposure to a trigger, respiratory distress, cardiovascular collapse, and death may occur within minutes.[1–4] Early recognition and prompt assessment of anaphylaxis and appropriate intervention can reduce its morbidity and mortality. Recognizing and treating mild symptoms in the early phase can prevent progression to a more serious, even fatal reaction, and may prevent recurrence or biphasic anaphylaxis.[1,5]

Generalized pruritis, erythema, and urticaria, and/or angioedema are the most common early manifestations of a systemic allergic reaction that can lead to anaphylaxis. Although these symptoms and signs are the most common presentation, they do not occur in approximately 10% of patients, that is, severe anaphylaxis may initially present without skin manifestations. It may also initially present with mild symptoms and signs, such as nausea, vomiting, without hypotension.[1,5,6] Patients who do not have skin manifestations of anaphylaxis are at increased risk of fatality.[7] Due to the difficulty in predicting the severity and progression of anaphylaxis, epinephrine should promptly be administered at its onset.[8]

Potential triggers should be identified and discontinued, where possible, and the patient's clinical status assessed at the earliest onset of anaphylaxis. The patient should be placed in a recumbent position and airway, breathing, and circulation should be assessed. Epinephrine is the first and most important medication and it is administered via intramuscular (IM) route into the anterior lateral mid-thigh.[1,5,7,9–13]

Vasodilation and the increased vascular permeability associated with anaphylaxis can cause hypotension and shock. When the patient is supine, there is usually adequate blood volume to reach the heart and maintain circulation. If the patient is in the upright position, blood flow to the heart can decrease significantly, causing the "empty ventricle syndrome"[1,11,14] or "empty heart syndrome,"[15] which can lead to cardiac arrest and death.[1,12,14]

Therefore, patients with anaphylaxis should be placed in a supine position and infants held horizontally, instead of upright or over the shoulder.[16] Pregnant patients should be placed in the semirecumbent position on their left side to avoid compression of the inferior vena cava by the gravid uterus. Hemodynamic normality after anaphylaxis can take up to an hour to stabilize after a single dose of epinephrine and up to 4 hours if multiple doses of epinephrine are administered.[1,5,9,12,14,16]

Individuals who experience respiratory distress may need to optimize their respiratory effort by remaining in the upright position. They should be closely monitored for any signs and symptoms of circulatory collapse. If there is any change in their consciousness or decrease in blood pressure, they must immediately be repositioned, as possible, into a supine position. If they become unconscious or vomit, they should be placed in the lateral recumbent position.[5,10–12]

The Trendelenburg position is proposed in some guidelines to treat anaphylaxis to help prevent hypotension and shock by increasing blood flow to the heart.[17] However, evidence for this position is limited and contradictory.[1,5,12] The Trendelenburg position may result in decreased lung compliance, vital capacity, and tidal volume and increased respiratory effort which could be detrimental in treating anaphylaxis.[12]

Epinephrine is an alpha- and beta-adrenergic agonist and the first-line treatment of anaphylaxis. It is also administered to patients who have clinical symptoms, such as sneezing, itchy nose, runny nose, itchy eyes, and generalized erythema, pruritus, and urticaria associated with the administration of an allergen to which they may be allergic. Such reactions can evolve into anaphylaxis.[2,8,10] Epinephrine is a life-saving drug and should be given intramuscularly into the anterior lateral mid-thigh as soon as signs and symptoms of a systemic allergic reaction are recognized.[5,8,9,12]

It is difficult to predict which patients are at risk for progression to severe anaphylaxis when they present with signs and symptoms of a systemic allergic reaction. Therefore, epinephrine should not be withheld for these patients.[6,8,18] Delayed epinephrine administration is associated with hospitalization and poor outcomes, that is, hypoxemia, ischemia, encephalopathy, and death.[1,8,9,12,18,19] There is no absolute contraindication to the use of epinephrine when anaphylaxis is suspected, for the potential benefits outweigh risks, even for those at highest risk. These include elderly patients, even those with preexisting cardiovascular diseases.[6,8,10,19,20]

The dose of epinephrine for anaphylaxis is 0.01 mg/kg of the 1 mg/mL (1:1000) concentration. It is given IM into the vastus lateralis muscle or anterior lateral mid-thigh.[1,5,8–12] The initial dose for infants ≤10 kg is 0.1 mg; for those between 10 and 25 kg, 0.15 mg; and ≥25 kg, 0.3 mg, with a maximum of 0.5 mg for children and adults ≥25 kg.[8,21] The 0.15 mg autoinjector is recommended for infants who weigh 7.5 to 10 kg when the 0.1 mg device is not available.[8,18]

The dose can be repeated every 5 to 15 minutes, as needed, if symptoms persist.[20] Additional doses may be necessary for patients who have biphasic anaphylaxis, that is, anaphylaxis reoccurring 1 hour after the initial episode, for severe anaphylaxis, or protracted anaphylaxis, the latter of which persists for hours after onset.[20]

Table 1 lists the recommended dose of epinephrine in health care settings where epinephrine autoinjectors are available.[8,19,21] Epinephrine autoinjectors are preferred for self-administration in many health care settings due to the ease of administration. The use of autoinjectors can prevent dosing errors associated with using a syringe to withdraw epinephrine from vials or ampules.

Peak plasma epinephrine levels are achieved faster when epinephrine is given intramuscularly (8 ± 2 minutes) than subcutaneously (34 ± 14 minutes).[1,11,18,22,23] When injected into the muscle, it causes vasodilation and increased absorption.[24] Locally injected epinephrine, at the site of allergen administration suspected of causing the reaction, may reduce the absorption of the allergen. An example would be a reaction caused by an injection of an allergen during allergen immunotherapy. This concept has not yet been evaluated in high-quality studies.[25]

Intravenous (IV) epinephrine should be considered when a patient does not respond to IM epinephrine, especially with hypotension or shock.[1,5,7,8,10,11,18,19,24] In dire circumstances, epinephrine can be administered by drawing up 1/10 of an mL of epinephrine, 1:1000, into a 1 mL tuberculin syringe, inserting it into the vein, drawing

Table 1 Dosing of epinephrine autoinjectors	
Patient	**Epinephrine Autoinjectors Dosing Recommendation**
Infants (≤10 kg)	0.1 mg (If 0.1 mg dose is not available, use 0.15 mg)
Children (10–25 kg)	0.15 mg
Adolescents and Adults (≥25 kg)	0.3 mg

back 9/10 mL of blood, and slowly administering it intravenously.[13] This is a 1:10,000 dilution. An example is where the patient has a rapid onset of cardiovascular collapse, not responding to IM epinephrine.

A continuous drip of IV epinephrine also can be used by mixing 1 mg (1 mL of 1:1000) of epinephrine and 1000 mL of normal saline (concentration of 1 μg/mL) and infusing it at a rate of 2 μg/min. A starting dose of 0.1 μg/kg per minute is recommended for children. The infusion is titrated to the clinical response. The rate can be increased to a maximum of 10 μg/min in adults and adolescents.[1,12,18] Patients who are receiving IV epinephrine ultimately require continuous hemodynamic monitoring in an intensive care unit (ICU).

Alternate routes of epinephrine administration include IV bolus, epinephrine via metered-dose inhaler, and oral epinephrine. An IV bolus is not recommended as a first-line treatment due to an increased risk of arrhythmia. However, if a patient has cardiac arrest, 1 mg of IV epinephrine can be administered every 2 to 3 minutes per advanced cardiovascular life support guidelines.[1,9,18] Epinephrine can also be administered through a metered-dose inhaler for respiratory symptoms.[23] However, this takes up to 20 to 30 inhalations over 4 minutes to be effective and does not replace IM epinephrine in treating systemic reactions.[23] Epinephrine is metabolized in the gastrointestinal tract by catechol-o-methyltransferase or monoamine oxidase, limiting its oral use for treatment.[24]

Epinephrine acts on α-1 adrenergic receptors increasing vasoconstriction and peripheral vascular resistance. This helps reverse hypotension and decrease upper airway edema.[8,10,11] It also acts on β-1 adrenergic receptors, increasing both cardiac inotropic and chronotropic effects and β-2 adrenergic receptors, increasing bronchodilation and reducing the release of inflammatory mediators.[8,10,11]

Epinephrine, in recommended doses, can cause pharmacologic adverse effects including pallor, tremor, nausea, vomiting, anxiety, and palpitations.[8,11] Severe adverse effects include ventricular arrhythmias, myocardial infarction, hypertensive crisis, and pulmonary edema. Side effects usually occur with an excessive amount of epinephrine administered by any route, in particular, by inadvertent IV administration.[9,11] The effects of epinephrine are prolonged in patients on monoamine oxidase inhibitors, which block epinephrine metabolism. Likewise, those on tricyclic antidepressants can have prolonged action of epinephrine.[23]

Airway management and oxygen supplementation are necessary for patients with severe anaphylaxis, that is, those experiencing respiratory and cardiovascular collapse despite treatment with IM epinephrine. Oxygen saturation should be maintained at 94% to 96% with high-flow oxygen administered via nasal prongs[26] or a face mask.[5,9–12] An oropharyngeal airway can be used if needed.[5,9–12]

Advanced airway management should be considered when patients develop stridor or respiratory distress consistent with upper or lower airway compromise and obstruction.[1,7,12] Nebulized epinephrine (2–5 mL, 1 mg/mL) can be used for patients with stridor.[5,10,15]

Patients with anaphylaxis who require intubation are frequently hemodynamically unstable. Therefore, when selecting medications for facilitating tracheal intubation, ones that lower blood pressure should be avoided, that is, fentanyl or midazolam.[1,27] Intubation, especially in the presence of laryngeal edema or swelling of the tongue, is difficult.[1,7,12]

IV fluids are sometimes necessary for patients with severe anaphylaxis because of a massive fluid leak and loss of intravascular volume.[25,28] In such patients, IV normal saline or lactated Ringers via a large-bore catheter (14 or 16 gauge for adults) should be administered.[1,5,10,12] Adults can receive a rapid infusion of 1 to 2 L of either (20 mL/kg bolus). Likewise, children can receive IV fluid boluses of 20 mL/kg over 5 to 10 minutes and up to 30 mL/kg for the first hour.[1,5,12] Intraosseous access is necessary if an IV route is not accessible.[7,18]

Antihistamines have a slow onset of action and are not a first- or even second-line treatment. They reach peak plasma levels in 60 to 120 minutes when administered orally.[18] Intravenously, antihistamines can take up to an hour for maximal therapeutic effect.[25] More often than not, clinicians administer antihistamines for cutaneous signs and symptoms of anaphylaxis, inappropriately delaying the use of epinephrine.[12,18] Likewise, patients often are willing to take an oral antihistamine but are reluctant to self-administer epinephrine, even when they are experiencing the signs and symptoms of anaphylaxis.[18] Therefore, antihistamines should only be considered when epinephrine has been appropriately used to stabilize a patient with anaphylaxis. Antihistamines can relieve generalized pruritus, flushing, and urticaria as well as angioedema. However, they do not prevent or treat cardiovascular and respiratory symptoms associated with anaphylaxis. In summary, antihistamines should not be substituted for the use of epinephrine.[1,10–12,18] Most commonly, they may be considered following the resolution of anaphylaxis to treat persistent cutaneous symptoms, in particular, generalized pruritus and urticaria. Caution must always be used with IV administration of first-generation H1 antihistamines as they can cause hypotension.[29]

First-generation H1 antihistamines include chlorpheniramine, dimenhydrinate, diphenhydramine, and hydroxyzine. Nonsedating second-generation H1 antihistamines include cetirizine, desloratadine, fexofenadine, levocetirizine, and loratadine.[12] The recommended dose for diphenhydramine is 25 to 50 mg in adults and 1 mg/kg to a maximum of 50 mg in children. It can be administered intravenously over 10 to 15 minutes.[1,9,11,12] When administered orally, nonsedating second generation are preferred to sedating first-generation H1 antihistamines.[1,12]

H2 antihistamines, cimetidine, and famotidine are often given with H1 antihistamines.[12] The recommended dose of famotidine is 20 mg by mouth or IV for adults and 0.5 mg/kg/dose in children. IV cimetidine is dosed at 4 mg/kg for adults but a pediatric dose is not established.[1,12,30]

The role of H2 antihistamines to treat anaphylaxis is controversial. H2 and H1 receptors play a minor role in the pathophysiology of allergic reactions. H2 receptors are predominantly located in the gastrointestinal tract and less so in the vascular smooth muscle cells commonly involved in anaphylaxis.[18] To the contrary, H1 receptors are widely distributed in cutaneous sensory nerves, bronchial smooth muscles, and endothelial cells. Stimulation of H1 receptors can lead to bronchoconstriction, increased vascular permeability, generalized urticaria and pruritus, and a burning sensation.[31] Some authors suggest that the combination of H1 and H2 antihistamines may provide additional benefits over the use of just H1 antihistamines in alleviating the cutaneous symptoms of a generalized allergic reaction.[10,11]

Inhaled short-acting bronchodilators are indicated in patients who develop bronchospasm despite epinephrine treatment. β-2 adrenergic agents, such as albuterol, can supplement the use of IM epinephrine to treat this problem. However, it should not be used in the place of epinephrine as it cannot prevent or relieve upper airway obstruction nor treat hypotension associated with anaphylaxis. Albuterol can be administered via metered-dose inhaler (2–6 inhalations) or nebulizer (2.5–5 mg in 3 mL of normal saline) and be repeated as necessary.[1,9,10]

Glucocorticoids are inhibitors of inflammation. They bind to the glucocorticoid receptors on cell membranes and inhibit the expression of genes responsible for the synthesis of inflammatory mediators.[18] They are often inappropriately used as an adjunctive treatment of systemic allergic reactions or anaphylaxis. These medications have little effect on the symptoms or signs of anaphylaxis because of their slow onset of action, that is, 4 to 6 hours. There is minimal evidence for their use in the acute management of anaphylaxis.[1,5,9,18] Moreover, glucocorticoids do not prevent protracted and biphasic reactions.[1,5,6,9,18] They can be considered for use in patients with concomitant asthma or for an individual who has recently received glucocorticoid treatment and may have suppression of the hypophyseal–pituitary–adrenal axis.[25]

Norepinephrine, vasopressin, dopamine, and other vasopressors can be used in patients who are hypotensive despite receiving optimal doses of epinephrine and volume resuscitation.[9,11,12] These medications are used as needed but are best administered in an ICU setting with continuous hemodynamic monitoring.[9] An epinephrine infusion can be started for individuals with unresponsive anaphylaxis. However, for persistent hypotension, dopamine or another vasopressor can be used.[12] Dopamine is an inotropic medication that has dose-dependent effects on alpha and beta-adrenergic and dopamine receptors. Dopamine is a drug of choice and also should be considered in hypotensive shock associated with low cardiac output.[32] The recommended dose of dopamine is 400 mg in 500 mL of 5% dextrose; it is administered at 2 to 20 µg/kg/min and titrated to maintain optimal blood pressure.[33] When administered at a lower dose (2–5 µg/kg/min or more), dopamine's β-adrenergic effects increases cardiac output, stroke volume, and heart rate.[32] When administered at a higher dose (5–10 µg/kg/min), dopamine acts on the α adrenergic receptors and results in vasoconstriction and increased systemic vascular resistance while maintaining renal blood flow.[32] Norepinephrine and vasopressin also have been used along with epinephrine to manage anaphylaxis-induced hypotension and shock.[34] Norepinephrine is an α- and β-adrenergic agonist that results in increased cardiac output and vasoconstriction. It is administered at 0.05 to 0.4 µg/kg/min.[34] Vasopressin is ordinarily produced in the posterior pituitary gland, causes vasoconstriction, and promotes water retention.[34] It is dosed at 0.02 to 0.04 units/min.[34]

The first-line treatment for patients who are on β-blockers and experiencing anaphylaxis is epinephrine. Glucagon is used in patients on β-blockers unresponsive to epinephrine and with refractory bronchospasm and hypotension.[1,5,9,11] Patients on β-blockers seem to be at greater risk for increased severity of anaphylaxis due to β-blockade and decreased response to epinephrine.[9,35] Epinephrine, when administered to such patients, acts unopposed on α-adrenergic receptors sometimes leading to vasoconstriction and a reflex vagotonic response.[9] Patients who are on nonselective β-blockers also are at a higher risk for bronchospasm.[11] Glucagon, by increasing intracellular cAMP, directly bypasses the β-adrenergic receptors, and creates a positive chronotropic and inotropic effect on cardiac and bronchial smooth muscles.[36] This can counteract refractory hypotension and bronchospasm.[1,11,12] It is dosed at 1 to 5 mg in adults (20–30 µg/kg in children, maximum 1 mg) and administered intravenously slowly over 5 minutes and followed by an infusion of 5 to 15 µg/min titrated to clinical response.[1,30,33] Glucagon can induce emesis and increase the risk of aspiration. It is important to place drowsy or obtunded patients in the lateral recumbent position to maintain airway patency before glucagon administration.[1,11,12]

PROTRACTED, BIPHASIC, AND REFRACTORY ANAPHYLAXIS

Protracted anaphylaxis is the persistence of signs and symptoms of anaphylaxis for at least 4 hours.[37] Treatments, such as vasopressors and ventilatory support, for more than 24 hours, may be required.[38] Refractory anaphylaxis is characterized by the persistence of anaphylaxis symptoms despite 3 or more doses of epinephrine and other symptom-directed treatment such as the use of IV fluids for hypotension.[37] IV fluids and vasopressors may be used in refractory anaphylaxis to control and reverse hypotension.[39] In patients unresponsive to traditional resuscitative measures, extra-corporeal membrane oxygenation may be necessary.[1,19]

Biphasic reactions are defined by the recurrence of anaphylaxis symptoms despite no further exposure to the causative trigger beginning after $\geq$1 hour of an asymptom-atic period.[40] Biphasic reactions occur in up to 20% of adults and 11% of children with anaphylaxis.[6,18] Biphasic reactions can occur anywhere from 1 to 78 hours following the resolution of the initial reaction.[17] However, most of the biphasic reactions occur 6 to 12 hours following the initial reaction.[17] Epinephrine is the treatment of choice in both uniphasic and biphasic anaphylaxis.[17] Biphasic and protracted reactions are 2.8 times more likely to occur if the initial onset of the reaction was more than 30 mi-nutes after exposure to the causative allergen.[41]

The duration of observation in medical settings should be individualized depending on the patient characteristics and the severity of anaphylaxis, as illustrated in **Table 2**, because it is difficult to accurately predict the onset of a biphasic reaction.[17] When in doubt, the patient should be admitted and observed in the hospital for up to 24 hours.[5,9,17] **Fig. 1** is the 2021 severity grading classification for acute allergic reac-tions.[42] Signs and symptoms of anaphylaxis are listed under various grades. This anaphylaxis grading system is to be used to classify patients, to help determine the duration of observation, and to communicate with other health care professionals.[42] However, it should not be used solely to determine patient management. Regardless of the severity of anaphylaxis, epinephrine is always the drug of choice.

All patients who experience anaphylaxis should be educated about the signs and symptoms of anaphylaxis, risks of recurrence, and allergen avoidance. They should be provided with a personalized anaphylaxis emergency action plan and epinephrine autoinjectors with appropriate instructions on their use. All patients with anaphylaxis should be referred to an allergist/immunologist for further evaluation and long-term management.[1,5,12,17]

Long-term management is essential to prevent the recurrence of the event and to prevent more serious reactions and fatality. Such management includes avoidance of allergens; identification and elimination, where possible, of cofactors which may in-crease susceptibility to such a reaction; interventions to reduce sensitivity, for

Table 2 Recommended observation time for anaphylaxis	
Duration of Observation	**Clinical Features**
1 h	Patients who remain asymptomatic *and* have resolved mild anaphylaxis with the following characteristics: • Have low risk for anaphylaxis • Have no significant comorbidities or limitations such as severe asthma, cardiovascular disease, lack of access to epinephrine, lack of access to medical care, and poor self-management skills • Have a favorable response to a single dose of epinephrine
Up to 6 h or longer (including hospital admission)	Patients who have severe clinical features or have other comorbidities/risk factors such as: • Hypotension and/or respiratory distress • Coexisting medical comorbidities • Inability to access medical care • Required more than 1 dose of epinephrine

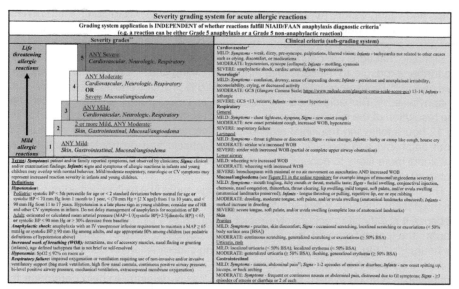

Fig. 1. Severity grading system for acute allergic reactions. This system can be used for both anaphylactic and nonanaphylactic allergic reactions. The clinical criteria determine the severity grading and in patients with multiple signs/symptoms, the most severe symptom determines their grade. This consensus-based severity system is intended to improve communication with providers, provide education to patients regarding their allergic reaction severity, and be used for research purposes. However, this is not intended to determine patient care and management decisions. Epinephrine is the drug of choice for anaphylaxis regardless of the severity. (*From* Dribin TE, Schnadower D, Spergel JM, Campbell RL, Shaker M, Neuman MI, Michelson KA, Capucilli PS, Camargo CA Jr, Brousseau DC, Rudders SA, Assa'ad AH, Risma KA, Castells M, Schneider LC, Wang J, Lee J, Mistry RD, Vyles D, Pistiner M, Witry JK, Zhang Y, Sampson HA. Severity grading system for acute allergic reactions: A multidisciplinary Delphi study. J Allergy Clin Immunol. 2021 Jul;148(1):173-181.)

example, to Hymenoptera insects, via venom immunotherapy; management of comorbidities; and when necessary, patient, parent, and caregiver education. Patient, parent, and caregiver education includes providing an anaphylaxis action plan, use of epinephrine autoinjector instructions, and discussion of how to avoid the causative allergen. Long-term management of anaphylaxis is discussed in other chapters of this textbook.

Medical Identification Jewelry

Medical identification jewelry has been available since 1950s and such information should be provided to subjects at risk for anaphylaxis.[43] They are designed to identify medical conditions, including anaphylaxis, and provide a way of communicating information if and when the patient is unable to do so. A staff of Aesculapius in red is present as a symbol of medicine differentiating it from other jewelry.[43] The jewelry was first designed as a bracelet or necklace worn on pulse points to allow for quick recognition.[43] Now there are anklets, shoe tags, and watches available. Other forms of medical identification include body art, smartphone technology, near field communication alert devices, and wallet cards.[43] Anaphylaxis wallet cards provide inexpensive medical identification for those who cannot afford jewelry and includes a proposed anaphylaxis action plan.[44]

Although medical identification may be important to identify and treat anaphylaxis, the wording on the jewelry is not reviewed by experts who treat it.[43] Patients are responsible for what is contained on their medical identification which possibly decreases the accuracy and relevance of the data included.[43] Physicians and other health care professionals should discuss the information that should be indicated on medical identification jewelry and/or products.

SUMMARY

Early recognition, assessment, and management of anaphylaxis are essential to reduce associated morbidity and mortality. Epinephrine is the treatment of choice. It is administered at a dose of 0.01 mg/kg of 1 mg/mL (1:1000) concentration intramuscularly into the anterior lateral thigh. For infants ≤10 kg, clinicians should consider a 0.1 mg epinephrine autoinjector, if available; for those between 10 and 25 kg, 0.15 mg; and for individuals who weigh ≥25 kg, 0.3 mg. Delayed epinephrine injection is associated with increased risk for fatality. Patients with mild anaphylaxis should be observed for at least an hour and those with more severe features should be observed for up to 6 hours or more. For patients who develop refractory hypotension or bronchospasm, despite adequate and optimal epinephrine treatment, other measures should be considered including IV fluid resuscitation, inhalation β-2 agonist administration, glucagon infusion if on a β-blocker, and a vasopressor for hypotension. Ideally, the latter, when possible, should be performed in an ICU setting with continuous hemodynamic monitoring under the care of a critical care specialist.

All patients with anaphylaxis should be referred to an allergist/immunologist for further evaluation and long-term management. On discharge, instructions on allergen/trigger avoidance, an anaphylaxis emergency treatment plan, and education on the use of an epinephrine autoinjector should be provided.

CLINICS CARE POINTS

- For individuals with anaphylaxis, first-line treatment is epinephrine. Consider the following appropriate doses based on weight and autoinjector availability.
  - Epinephrine dosing is 0.01 mg/kg of the 1 mg/mL (1:1000) concentration and is given intramuscularly to the lateral mid-thigh.
  - For infants less than or equal to 10 kg, consider 0.1mg by autoinjector if available or 0.15mg by autoinjector
  - For children between 10 to 25 kg, 0.15 mg
  - For adolescents and adults greater than or equal to 25 kg, 0.3 mg

- Glucocorticoids have not been shown to prevent protracted and biphasic anaphylactic reactions.

- Antihistamines and glucocorticoids should not replace epinephrine. They are not helpful in the acute management of anaphylaxis.

- Inhaled short-acting β-2 adrenergic agonists are used to treat bronchospasm associated with anaphylaxis that persists despite epinephrine administration.
  - β-2 adrenergic agonists cannot prevent or relieve upper airway obstruction.

- Patients on β-blockers with anaphylaxis should be treated first with epinephrine. Glucagon is used in patients on B-blockers unresponsive to epinephrine and with refractory bronchospasm and hypotension.

- Patients with mild anaphylaxis should be observed for an hour and those with severe features should be observed for 6 or more hours.

- Referral to allergist should be provided when necessary.
- Patients should be provided with information regarding medical identification and clinicians should discuss appropriate wording to communicate relevant and important information.

DISCLOSURE

The authors have nothing to disclose.

REFERENCES

1. Campbell RL, Li JT, Nicklas RA, et al. Emergency department diagnosis and treatment of anaphylaxis: a practice parameter. Ann Allergy Asthma Immunol 2014;113:599–608.
2. Pumphrey RS. Lessons for management of anaphylaxis from a study of fatal reactions. Clin Exp Allergy 2000;30:1144–50.
3. Pumphrey R. Anaphylaxis: can we tell who is at risk of a fatal reaction? Curr Opin Allergy Clin Immunol 2004;4:285–90.
4. Greenberger PA, Rotskoff BD, Lifschultz B. Fatal anaphylaxis: postmortem findings and associated comorbid diseases. Ann Allergy Asthma Immunol 2007; 98:252–7.
5. Cardona V, Ansotegui IJ, Ebisawa M, et al. World allergy organization anaphylaxis guidance 2020. World Allergy Organ J 2020;13:100472.
6. Anagnostou K, Turner PJ. Myths, facts and controversies in the diagnosis and management of anaphylaxis. Arch Dis Child 2019;104:83–90.
7. Poowuttikul P, Seth D. Anaphylaxis in children and adolescents. Pediatr Clin North Am 2019;66:995–1005.
8. Sicherer SH, Simons FER, Section On, A. & Immunology. Epinephrine for first-aid management of anaphylaxis. Pediatrics 2017;139:e20164006.
9. Simons FE, Ardusso LRF, Bilo MB, et al. World allergy organization guidelines for the assessment and management of anaphylaxis. World Allergy Organ J 2011;4: 13–37.
10. Muraro A, Roberts G, Worm M, et al. Anaphylaxis: guidelines from the European Academy of Allergy and Clinical Immunology. Allergy 2014;69:1026–45.
11. Mali S, Jambure R. Anaphyllaxis management: current concepts. Anesth Essays Res 2012;6:115–23.
12. Lieberman P, Nicklas RA, Randolph C, et al. Anaphylaxis–a practice parameter update 2015. Ann Allergy Asthma Immunol 2015;115:341–84.
13. Kemp SF, Lockey RF. Anaphylaxis: a review of causes and mechanisms. J Allergy Clin Immunol 2002;110:341–8.
14. Pumphrey RS. Fatal posture in anaphylactic shock. J Allergy Clin Immunol 2003; 112:451–2.
15. Anthony S, Larry Jameson FJ, Kasper DL, et al, editors. Harrison's Manual of medicine. New York: McGraw Hill Professional Publishing; 2019. Chapter 28.
16. ASCIA Guidelines Acute management of anaphylaxis. Available at: https://www.allergy.org.au/hp/papers/acute-management-of-anaphylaxis-guidelines. Accessed May 15, 2021.
17. Brown SG. Cardiovascular aspects of anaphylaxis: implications for treatment and diagnosis. Curr Opin Allergy Clin Immunol 2005;5:359–64.
18. Shaker MS, Wallas DV, Golden DBK, et al. Anaphylaxis-a 2020 practice parameter update, systematic review, and Grading of Recommendations, Assessment,

Development and Evaluation (GRADE) analysis. J Allergy Clin Immunol 2020;145: 1082–123.

19. Simons FE, Ebisawa M, Sanchez-Borges M, et al. 2015 update of the evidence base: World Allergy Organization anaphylaxis guidelines. World Allergy Organ J 2015;8:32.

20. Simons KJ, Simons FE. Epinephrine and its use in anaphylaxis: current issues. Curr Opin Allergy Clin Immunol 2010;10:354–61.

21. Halbrich M, Mack DP, Carr S, et al. CSACI position statement: epinephrine auto-injectors and children < 15 kg. Allergy Asthma Clin Immunol 2015;11:20.

22. Prince BT, Mikhail I, Stukus DR. Underuse of epinephrine for the treatment of anaphylaxis: missed opportunities. J Asthma Allergy 2018;11:143–51.

23. Simons FE. First-aid treatment of anaphylaxis to food: focus on epinephrine. J Allergy Clin Immunol 2004;113:837–44.

24. Simons FE, Gu X, Silver NA, et al. EpiPen Jr versus EpiPen in young children weighing 15 to 30 kg at risk for anaphylaxis. J Allergy Clin Immunol 2002;109: 171–5.

25. Moore LE, Kemp AM, Kemp SF. Recognition, treatment, and prevention of anaphylaxis. Immunol Allergy Clin North Am 2015;35:363–74.

26. Kemp SF. Navigating the updated anaphylaxis parameters. Allergy Asthma Clin Immunol 2007;3:40–9.

27. Allen P, Desai NM, Lawrence VN. Tracheal Intubation Medications. In: StatPearls [Internet]. Treasure Island (FL): StatPearls Publishing; 2021. [cited 2021 Aug 30]. Available at: https://www.ncbi.nlm.nih.gov/books/NBK507812/.

28. Brown SG, Blackman KE, Stenlake V, et al. Insect sting anaphylaxis; prospective evaluation of treatment with intravenous adrenaline and volume resuscitation. Emerg Med J 2004;21:149–54.

29. Ellis BC, Brown SG. Parenteral antihistamines cause hypotension in anaphylaxis. Emerg Med Australas 2013;25:92–3.

30. Lieberman P, Kemp SF, Oppenheimer J, et al. The diagnosis and management of anaphylaxis. an updated practice parameter. J Allergy Clin Immunol 2005;115: S483–523.

31. White MV. The role of histamine in allergic diseases. J Allergy Clin Immunol 1990; 86:599–605.

32. Lollgen H, Drexler H. Use of inotropes in the critical care setting. Crit Care Med 1990;18:S56–60.

33. Simon GA, Brown SFK, Lieberman PL. In: Bruce SB, Adkinson NF, Burks A, et al, editors. Middleton's allergy: principles and practice, Vol 2. 8th edition. Philadelphia, PA: Elsevier/Saunders; 2014. p.1237–59.

34. van Diepen S, Katz JN, Albert NM, et al. Contemporary management of cardiogenic shock: a scientific statement from the American Heart Association. Circulation 2017;136:e232–68.

35. Krishnaswamy G. Critical care management of the patient with anaphylaxis: a concise definitive review. Crit Care Med 2021;49:838–57.

36. Sherman MS, Lazar EJ, Eichacker P. A bronchodilator action of glucagon. J Allergy Clin Immunol 1988;81:908–11.

37. Dribin TE, Sampson HA, Camargo Jr CA, et al. Persistent, refractory, and biphasic anaphylaxis: a multidisciplinary Delphi study. J Allergy Clin Immunol 2020;146:1089–96.

38. Sampson HA, Mendelson L, Rosen JP. Fatal and near-fatal anaphylactic reactions to food in children and adolescents. N Engl J Med 1992;327:380–4.

39. Francuzik W, Dolle-Bierke S, Knop M, et al. Refractory anaphylaxis: data from the European Anaphylaxis Registry. Front Immunol 2019;10:2482.
40. Lieberman P. Biphasic anaphylactic reactions. Ann Allergy Asthma Immunol 2005;95:217–26 [quiz 226, 258].
41. Stark BJ, Sullivan TJ. Biphasic and protracted anaphylaxis. J Allergy Clin Immunol 1986;78:76–83.
42. Dribin TE, Schnadower D, Spergel JM, et al. Severity grading system for acute allergic reactions: a multidisciplinary Delphi study. J Allergy Clin Immunol 2021; 148:173–81.
43. Rahman S, Walker D, Sultan P. Medical identification or alert jewellery: an opportunity to save lives or an unreliable hindrance? Anaesthesia 2017;72:1139–45.
44. Hernandez-Trujillo V, Simons FE. Prospective evaluation of an anaphylaxis education mini-handout: the AAAAI Anaphylaxis Wallet Card. J Allergy Clin Immunol Pract 2013;1:181–5.

Management of Anaphylaxis in Infants and Toddlers

Nicole Ramsey, MD, PhD, Julie Wang, MD*

KEYWORDS

- Infant • Toddler • Anaphylaxis • Food allergy • Prevention • Management

KEY POINTS

- Anaphylaxis in infants typically has good outcomes and lower severity than other age groups.
- The mainstay of treatment of anaphylaxis is intramuscular epinephrine. In the community setting, a weight-appropriate autoinjector should be used when available.
- Long-term management of anaphylaxis in infants and toddlers includes allergy testing and routine follow-up, epinephrine autoinjector prescription, and maintenance of an age-appropriate allergy emergency plan.

INTRODUCTION

Anaphylaxis is a potentially serious, systemic reaction, either immunologic or nonimmunologic, that is usually rapid in the onset, of variable severity, and may cause death.[1] Anaphylaxis is estimated to affect 1.5 to 757 per 100,000 persons/year worldwide.[2–4] The global prevalence of anaphylaxis over a lifetime has been rising according to studies reported in the United States (US), Europe, Australia, and Asia In recent years, by 1.89- to 3.3-fold.[5–7] One systematic review of fatal anaphylaxis cited fewer cases in France and Canada when compared with increased rates in Finland and Australia, and stable rates in the United Kingdom, the US, and Brazil.[8] Recent studies have also found that anaphylaxis rates are rising in the infant and toddler age group, specifically.[3] In a large US database, from 2006 to 2015, emergency department (ED) visits for infants and toddlers with anaphylaxis increased, whereas hospitalizations remained stable or decreased.[3,9]

Epidemiologic studies on anaphylaxis are based on different parameters, including diagnosis codes from ED visits and hospitalizations, epinephrine use, and voluntary registries of physicians. Unfortunately, these estimators are limited by a 60% to 64% positive predictive value for diagnosis code-based estimates,[10] and

Jaffe Food Allergy Institute, Icahn School of Medicine at Mount Sinai, One Gustave L. Levy Place, Box 1198, New York, NY 10029, USA
* Corresponding author.
E-mail address: Julie.wang@mssm.edu

Immunol Allergy Clin N Am 42 (2022) 77–90
https://doi.org/10.1016/j.iac.2021.09.006
0889-8561/22/© 2021 Elsevier Inc. All rights reserved.

documentation of epinephrine use does not equate to an anaphylaxis diagnosis.[11–14] Limitations of using epinephrine as a surrogate marker for anaphylaxis include that epinephrine may not always be available for an initial allergic reaction, it may sometimes be used preemptively before criteria are met, and underutilization of epinephrine by both providers and caregivers to treat anaphylaxis is common.[15]

Allergic reactions in infants and toddlers are most often triggered by foods, and less often by drugs or insect stings. Food allergens are associated with 91% to 93% of infant anaphylaxis cases presenting in the hospital setting, including ED visits, inpatient, and outpatient encounters, according to 2 studies.[16,17] Egg and milk are the most common triggers of allergic reactions in infants, though the frequency may vary based on geographic locations and feeding practices.[8,15–18] In 2 European studies and a Korean study, milk was the most common food trigger in infants (44%–61%).[8,16,17] Another 2 studies in the US reported that egg was the most common food trigger in infants (33% and 38%).[15,18] In toddlers, peanut is the most common triggering food for allergic reactions in the US[15,18] and tree nuts were noted as the most common trigger in toddlers in a European study.[19]

Infants and toddlers also present with a distinct pattern of allergic symptoms and severity of reactions. Evidence suggests decreased severity of allergic reactions among infants when compared with other pediatric age groups.[8,15,16,18,20,21] Among 512 infants from 3 to 15 months old with milk or egg allergy, Fleischer and colleagues reported that 70% of reactions were mild, 18% were moderate, and 11% were severe.[22] In addition to lower rates of systemic involvement, death and biphasic reactions were also less frequently reported.[8,21,23–27]

CLINICAL PRESENTATION IN INFANTS AND TODDLERS
Context of reactions

In infants and toddlers who have been diagnosed with food allergy, allergic reactions are mainly due to accidental exposures.[22] This age group is more likely to have accidental exposure to allergens due to crawling on the ground and mouthing of hands, fingers, and objects. However, in some cases, caregivers have reported intentional exposures causing reactions. Reasons cited by caregivers include determining whether the child has outgrown the allergy or giving a larger amount of an allergen than previously tolerated, in particular to milk, egg, and peanut.[22] Limited studies have identified that cofactors may increase the likelihood of an allergic reaction in infants and toddlers including upper respiratory infection at the time of reaction.[8,28]

The greatest number of new food exposures occurs during the infant and toddler ages. As such, allergic reactions due to first-time exposures are more likely in infants and toddlers than in older children.[15] As an example of one solid food introduction practice that is recommended, infant peanut introduction guidelines may affect the rate and timing of first-time exposures and therefore reactions. The Learning Early About Peanut (LEAP) clinical trial, a landmark study published in 2015, showed that the early introduction of peanut between 4 and 11 months was linked to a decrease in the development of peanut allergy in high risk infants.[29] The 2017 National Institute of Allergy and Infectious Diseases (NIAID) Addendum Guidelines to Prevent Peanut Allergy which followed, recommends that high-risk infants (with egg allergy or severe eczema) be evaluated for peanut and introduced to peanut between 4 and 6 months of age and that infants with mild to moderate eczema start peanut around 6 months.[30] A retrospective cohort study of 561 patients in California found an increase in the rate of ED visits and epinephrine prescriptions in infants between 2016 and 2018, from 2.2 to 5.7 per 1000, which may represent an impact of these published guidelines in the short term.[31]

Assessing allergic reactions in infants and toddlers

Allergic reactions consist of a constellation of symptoms that present on a continuum from mild reactions (grade 1-cutaneous or upper respiratory without cutaneous) to cardiovascular collapse and/or respiratory distress (grade 4 or 5 – anaphylaxis, **Fig. 1, Table 1**).[32] Studies have shown that infants present most commonly with skin and/or gastrointestinal (GI) symptoms, and cardiovascular, and respiratory symptoms are less frequent.[15–18,20,33,34]

Some differences in anaphylaxis presentation are also noted when comparing infants and toddlers. One study of 374 caregivers reported that infants more frequently experience skin reactions, mottling, ear pulling/scratching, or putting fingers in ears, whereas toddlers experienced throat itching and coughing/wheezing more frequently.[34] Also, GI symptoms are more common in infants than in all other age groups and respiratory symptoms were more common in toddlers than in infants, according to a retrospective study of 357 ED visits.[18] A similar pattern of symptoms was noted in a retrospective European study, with cutaneous and neurologic symptoms also increased in infants of this group of 314 anaphylaxis cases.[19]

Assessments of infants and toddlers can be challenging. Blood pressure measurement in an acutely reacting child can be especially difficult as this requires an appropriate cuff size to be available and behaviors such as fussiness or crying can present barriers to obtaining an accurate measure. The lack of this data point in many cases precludes the use of hypotension as a parameter for assessing the severity of anaphylaxis.[16,35,36] As a surrogate measure, signs and symptoms of hypotension can be assessed by examining for mottled or pale skin, delayed capillary refill, or lethargy. Two other complicating factors related to the assessment of allergic reactions in infants and toddlers include their inability to communicate subjective symptoms and challenges in recognizing nonspecific signs and symptoms as potential markers of

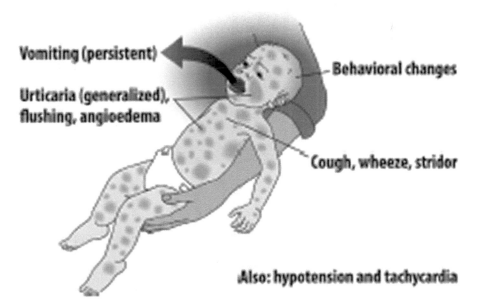

Fig. 1. Potential signs and symptoms of anaphylaxis in infants. (*From* Simons FE, Sampson HA. Anaphylaxis: Unique aspects of clinical diagnosis and management in infants (birth to age 2 years). J Allergy Clin Immunol. 2015 May;135(5):1125 to 31.)

Table 1
Modified WAO grading system

| | Grading System for SARs | | | |
| | | | Anaphylaxis | |
Grade 1	Grade 2	Grade 3	Grade 4	Grade 5
Symptom (sign(s) from l organ system present Cutaneous • Urticaria and/or erythema-warmth and/or pruritus, other than localized at the injection site And/or • Tingling, or itching of the lips* or • Angioedema (not laryngeal)* Or Upper respiratory • Nasal symptoms (eg, sneezing, rhinorrhea nasal pruritus, and/or nasal congestion) And/or • Throat-clearing (itchy throat)* And/or • Cough not related to bronchospasm Or Conjunctival • Erythema, pruritus, or tearing Or Other • Nausea • Metallic taste	Symptom(s)/sign(s) from ≥2 organ symptoms listed in grade 1	Lower airway • Mild bronchospasm. for example, cough, wheezing, shortness of breath which responds to treatment And/or Gastrointestinal • Abdominal cramps* and/or vomiting/diarrhea Other • Uterine cramps • Any symptom(s)/sign(s) from grade 1 would be included	Lower airway • Severe bronchospasm, for example, not responding or worsening in spite of treatment And/or Upper airway • Laryngeal edema with stridor • Any symptom(s)/sign(s) from grades 1 or 3 would be included	Lower or upper airway • Respiratory failure and/or Cardiovascular • Collapse/hypotension* And/or Loss of consciousness (vasovagal excluded) • Any symptom(s)/sign(s) from grades 1, 3, or 4 would be included

From Cox LS, Sanchez-Borges M, Lockey RF. World Allergy Organization Systemic Allergic Reaction Grading System: Is a Modification Needed? J Allergy Clin Immunol Pract. 2017 Jan-Feb;5(1):58 to 62.e5.

anaphylaxis.[37] Infants and toddlers cannot clearly express symptoms such as anxiety, itchiness, congestion, nausea, or dizziness. Some signs that may be difficult to attribute to an allergic reaction in this age group include behavioral changes (fussiness and fear are common in a health care setting), flushing (may occur with fever or crying), drooling (common in infants), and drowsiness (common after feeds or around naptime). Therefore, additional descriptors for anaphylaxis signs and symptoms may help caregivers identify reactions in infants and toddlers (**Table 2**).[34,38]

Differential diagnosis

Although the differential diagnosis of anaphylaxis is addressed in detail in Section 2, an expanded differential needs to be considered in this young age group. For an infant or toddler, infectious, respiratory, GI, and toxicology-related etiologies should also be considered during assessment. Infectious conditions causing septic shock may be considered given the shared symptoms of hypotension, flushing, and coughing symptoms. For infants and toddlers presenting with respiratory symptoms of wheezing and cough, obstruction, congenital abnormalities, and aspiration of a foreign body may be considered. Notably, aspiration of peanuts and tree nuts make up one-third of foreign body aspirations in toddlers.[39] In the GI system, syndromes such as pyloric stenosis, malrotation, and intussusception could cause symptoms of vomiting, abdominal pain, or diarrhea which could be misattributed to an allergic reaction. Non–IgE-mediated food allergies such as food protein-induced enterocolitis syndrome may need to be considered if delayed GI symptoms are observed.[40]

Discernment of anaphylaxis with testing of the mast cell enzyme, tryptase, may be used to support the diagnosis. This enzyme can be measured within a 2 to 4-hour window of allergic reaction onset, but may not always be elevated in food-induced anaphylaxis.[41–43] Blood sampling for tryptase levels may be challenging to obtain in an ill infant, and results should be interpreted with caution as younger patients have higher tryptase levels at baseline.[44]

ACUTE MANAGEMENT

The World Allergy Organization, Joint Task Force of Practice Parameters (US), and European Academy of Allergy and Clinical Immunology have all published guidelines on the acute management of anaphylaxis.[41,43,45] These guidelines are similar across ages and are based on studies performed in older children and adults.[46–48] Epinephrine is the mainstay of treatment in anaphylaxis and should be administered without delay.

Initial treatment in the medical setting

Once there is a concern for anaphylaxis, standard procedures should be followed, including the removal of allergen trigger and administration of intramuscular (IM) epinephrine to the anterolateral thigh (0.01 mg/kg of a 1:1000 [1 mg/mL] solution[49]). The benefits of using epinephrine in anaphylaxis outweigh the risks. In infants and toddlers, epinephrine underuse can be attributed to factors such as lack of access in patients without a previous diagnosis, difficulty with identifying symptoms in this age group, and caregiver or provider hesitancy.

In the clinical setting, after epinephrine administration, the provider should call for help, and position the patient in a supine or semi-reclining manner.[36,50] Next, the patient should be assessed for any disturbances in the airway, breathing, or circulation. If cardiopulmonary arrest is identified, resuscitation should be initiated without delay. Adjunctive medications, such as antihistamines, steroids, beta-agonists, intravenous

Table 2 Alternative, age-specific symptoms/signs used in this study to help identify anaphylaxis in infants/toddlers	
Language Used in Current Diagnostic Criteria*	**Language Used in AAFA Infant Toddler Anaphylaxis Study**
Pruritis	Tongue thrusting, tongue pulling, repetitive lip licking, or licking of hands or objects. Throat itching ear pulling, scratching, or putting fingers in the ears. Eye rubbing, eye itching
Dyspnea	Belly breathing, fast breathing, nasal flaring, chest or, neck "tugging"
Stridor	Hoarse voice, hoarse cry. Barky/croup-like cough
Reduced PEF	*(Currently, no appropriate and practical way to get FEV₁ in this population in an acute setting)*
Reduced BP (low systolic BP [age specific] or >30% decrease in systolic BP)	*(Blood pressure in this population can be challenging to acquire and interpret. Hypotension is also t late phase cardiovascular symptom in this age group. Tachycardia may be an earlier vital sign change)* Wobbly appearance, lethargic, floppy, poor head control, difficult to wake up. Crankiness, withdrawn or clingy, inconsolable crying, subdued or less active, limp. Mottling of the skin or blue/gray skit (cyanosis) around mouth/lips or hands/feet
Hypotonia (collapse), syncope	Wobbly appearance, lethargic, floppy, poor head control, difficult to wake up. Crankiness, withdrawn or clingy, inconsolable crying, subdued or less active, limp
Incontinence	*(Can be challenging to differentiate in diaper wearing population)*
Persistent gastrointestinal symptoms	Abdominal pain, diarrhea, hiccups, spitting up, back arching, vomiting

Abbreviations: AAFA, asthma and allergy foundation of America; *BP,* blood pressure; *PEF,* peak expiratory flow.
From Pistiner M, Mendez-Reyes JE, Eftekhari S, Carver M, Lieberman J, Wang J, Camargo CA Jr. Caregiver-Reported Presentation of Severe Food-Induced Allergic Reactions in Infants and Toddlers. J Allergy Clin Immunol Pract. 2021 Jan;9(1):311 to 320.e2.

fluids, or oxygen supplementation may be considered, but only after epinephrine is administered.

Management in the community setting

In the community setting, a weight-appropriate epinephrine autoinjector (EAI) should be used, if available. Some patients may need more than one EAI administration if symptoms do not resolve soon after the first dose. For caregivers, a patient-specific emergency action plan can help guide management during an acute reaction as it reminds caregivers of signs and symptoms that can occur and provides instructions for additional steps after epinephrine has been administered (aap.org/anaphylaxis).

Epinephrine autoinjectors

In the US, EAIs are currently available in 3 doses, 0.1 mg, 0.15 mg, and 0.3 mg. A summary of the differences between these devices in terms of indication and other parameters can be found in **Table 3**. The 0.1 mg device is not as widely available due to insurance coverage and regulatory approval in many countries. If it is available, the

Table 3
Attributes of FDA-approved epinephrine devices in the United States

Attribute	Auvi-Q	EpiPen	Adrenaclick	Generic EAI	SYMJEPI (Prefilled Syringe)
Manufacturer	Kaleo	Mylan	Amedra	Teva	Adamis
Dosages (mg)	0.10, 0.15, 0.30	0.15, 0.30	0.15, 0.30	0.15, 0.30	0.15, 0.30
Trainer	Yes	Yes	No	Yes	No
Supplied	2-pack	2-pack	2-pack	2-pack	2-pack
Exposed needle length for pediatric EAIs	0.29″ for 0.1 mg 0.50″ for 0.15 mg	0.51″ for 0.15 mg	0.51″ for 0.15 mg	0.63″ for 0.15 mg [a]	0.63″ for 0.15 mg [a]
Injection hold time	2-s hold, no massage	3-s hold, 10-s massage	10-s hold, 10-s massage	3-s hold, 10-s massage	2-s hold, 10-s massage
Needle guard	Yes	Yes	No	Yes	Yes (manual)
Retractable needle	Yes	No	No	No	No
Vocalized audio prompts	Yes	No	No	No	No

Abbreviations: FDA, food and drug administration.

[a] As reported by the company on inquiry.

From Tsuang A, Chan ES, Wang J. Food-Induced Anaphylaxis in Infants: Can New Evidence Assist with Implementation of Food Allergy Prevention and Treatment? J Allergy Clin Immunol Pract. 2021 Jan;9(1):57-69.

package insert states that dosing is 0.1 mg for children between 7.5 kg and 15 kg, whereas the 0.15 mg is for children weighing 15 kg and 25 kg, and 0.3 mg for anyone more than 25 kg. Expert consensus recommends the 0.1 mg dose of EAI for children under 7.5 kg, given the benefits of treatment over delay in treatment or lack of treatment.[35] Based on the same perspective, if the 0.1 mg is unavailable, the 0.15 mg is recommended for young children weighing 7.5 to 15 kg.[41,49]

Another element of EAIs for consideration is the needle length. In smaller infants, there is a theoretical concern of accidentally injecting beyond the muscle to the bone, based on the applied pressure.[51,52] The ideal IM injection needle length, based on studies measuring the distance between skin, muscle, and bone, using ultrasound, is 7 to 8 mm (0.28–0.31 inches) in children 7.5 to 15 kg.[51] Considering the currently available EAIs, only the 0.1 mg EAI fits this range. However, a follow-up study reported the increased risk of subcutaneous injection when any age patient wears winter clothes.[53] These considerations are noteworthy for optimal treatment; according to a randomized, double-blind, placebo-controlled, prospective study in adult males, peak plasma concentrations are highest when epinephrine is injected intramuscularly in comparison with subcutaneous injection.[54]

LONG-TERM MANAGEMENT
Allergy referral and education

In the acute setting, before discharge from the hospital or ED, education and counseling should be provided regarding allergen avoidance and management of future allergic reactions. If the trigger is identifiable, the family should be instructed about the identification and avoidance of specific foods, medications, or insects.[41] Also, a weight-appropriate EAI should be prescribed and a demonstration of how to use the EAI using a device trainer or training video can be beneficial. A referral to an allergist is advisable to evaluate and confirm potential triggers and receive additional education and management guidance. In terms of allergic reaction management, an allergy emergency plan should be provided to the family with guidance on what medications should be administered based on the patient's symptoms.[55,56] An allergy and anaphylaxis emergency plans are available from the American Academy of Pediatrics (both English and Spanish).[56] Emergency plans should also be updated and reviewed with the family at each follow-up visit to reinforce the management of allergic reactions and ensure appropriate medication dosing for the growing child. Annual follow-up is advised for any child with food allergy to ensure that the family has updated medications and emergency plans.[56]

In the allergist's office, a detailed history of reactions to foods, insects, and medications will be taken to help guide targeted testing for possible allergen triggers.[35] In the case of food allergic responses, the history can help distinguish between IgE and non–IgE-mediated reactions. To help confirm a diagnosis, the allergist may perform skin prick testing, allergen-specific IgE measurement, and/or oral food challenge (OFC). These tests provide information about sensitization and support an IgE-mediated allergy diagnosis. If there is a high suspicion and negative test, repeat skin prick testing could be considered at least 4 to 6 weeks after the initial reaction, to avoid the depletion of mast cell mediators after a severe reaction.[35] There is no minimum age for allergy evaluation and testing according to recommendations from a recent consensus panel of experts.[35] Allergy testing panels are strongly discouraged as they often lead to unnecessary avoidance of foods, or EAI prescription, due to the common occurrence of sensitization in the absence of clinically relevant allergy, especially in atopic individuals.[57] If a low level of sensitization is noted in the absence of ever eating the food, home introduction or, physician-supervised OFCs may be considered. An infant peanut OFC guide is available from Bird and colleagues.[50] Annual follow-up is typical in the course of food, drug, and venom allergy management.

Preventing recurrence

Allergen avoidance is the standard of care for the management of most allergic triggers in infants and toddlers. Even in the setting of allergen avoidance, accidental exposures can occur and can trigger symptoms that may require epinephrine.[22,58] Fleischer and colleagues noted that among 512 preschool-aged children, the annualized reaction rate was 0.81 per year, with 87.4% due to accidental reactions, 11.4% of cases classified as severe, and 29.9% requiring treatment with epinephrine.[22] Therefore, caregivers should always be prepared to recognize and manage unexpected allergic reactions.

Emerging therapies for food allergy

Allergen avoidance can be effective, but has been associated with increased stress and anxiety and decreased quality of life in some patients[59] Therefore, there have been ongoing efforts to develop treatments for food allergies. Treatment approaches focus on incremental trigger desensitization or immune dampening using a biologic medication. Oral (OIT) and epicutaneous immunotherapy (EPIT) are both promising approaches to food allergy treatment in infants and toddlers. Currently, there is one FDA-approved product available for peanut OIT, Palforzia that may help prevent or minimize reactions to accidental peanut exposures, by increasing peanut thresholds for patients 4 to 17 years of age.[60] OIT has shown to be efficacious in infants in 2 early studies, and there is an ongoing phase 3 study underway (NCT03736447).[61–63] Another mode of treatment, EPIT, is also being studied in this age group. One study in 1 to 3-year-old children with peanut allergy (EPITOPE) is currently underway (NCT03211247),[64] and another in 2 to 11-year-old children with IgE-mediated milk allergy (MILES) was recently completed (NCT02223182).[65,66] The MILES study showed an increase in milk tolerated, after 1 year of treatment.[65] Biologic medications, such as omalizumab (anti-IgE monoclonal antibody), are also being studied. Currently, an NIH-sponsored Consortium of Food Allergy trial is investigating omalizumab as monotherapy and as adjunctive to OIT for food allergy (NCT03881696)[67] and includes children 1 year and older.

SUMMARY/DISCUSSION

Lifetime anaphylaxis cases are increasing over time and infant and toddler cases are no exception, particularly regarding ED visits. Notably, this increase in ED visits was documented before the NIAID Addendum Guidelines to Prevent Peanut Allergy in 2017.[5]

Anaphylaxis in infants and toddlers should be treated according to established guidelines, and epinephrine is the mainstay of treatment. Epinephrine is a safe and life-saving medication, and its use should never be hesitated. Long-term management of anaphylaxis includes trigger avoidance and follow-up testing and evaluation with an allergy/immunology specialist.

Recent studies have demonstrated that infant and toddler anaphylaxis has good outcomes, is less severe than other age groups, and primarily presents with cutaneous and GI symptoms. This evidence could allay concerns and support the implementation of food allergy prevention guidelines and emerging treatments.

CLINICS CARE POINTS

- Pearls
  - In infants and toddlers, food is the most common trigger of anaphylaxis. In infants, the most common trigger is milk or egg, whereas, in toddlers, the most common trigger is peanuts.
  - Infants and toddlers have favorable outcomes in anaphylaxis.
- Pitfalls
  - Infants and toddlers should be treated with epinephrine without delay; epinephrine is underutilized and this may be due to the lack of access, difficulty identifying symptoms, or caregiver/provider hesitancy.
  - Due to challenges in recognizing signs and symptoms of anaphylaxis in infants and toddlers, age-specific descriptors may be considered to aid caregivers in recognizing anaphylaxis.

DISCLOSURE

N. Ramsey – Nothing to disclose, J. Wang receives research support from the NIAID, Aimmune, DBV Technologies, and Regeneron, and has received consultancy fees from ALK Abello, DBV Technologies, and Genentech.

REFERENCES

1. Turner PJ, Worm M, Ansotegui IJ, et al. Time to revisit the definition and clinical criteria for anaphylaxis? World Allergy Organ J 2019;12(10):100066. https://doi.org/10.1016/j.waojou.2019.100066.
2. Wood RA, Camargo CA, Lieberman P, et al. Anaphylaxis in America: the prevalence and characteristics of anaphylaxis in the United States. J Allergy Clin Immunol 2014;133(2):461–7. https://doi.org/10.1016/j.jaci.2013.08.016.
3. Robinson LB, Arroyo AC, Faridi MK, et al. Trends in US emergency department visits for anaphylaxis among infants and toddlers: 2006-2015. J Allergy Clin Immunol Pract 2021;9(5):1931–8.e2. https://doi.org/10.1016/j.jaip.2021.01.010.
4. Panesar SS, Javad S, de Silva D, et al. The epidemiology of anaphylaxis in Europe: a systematic review. Allergy 2013;68(11):1353–61. https://doi.org/10.1111/all.12272.
5. Wang Y, Allen KJ, Suaini NHA, et al. The global incidence and prevalence of anaphylaxis in children in the general population: a systematic review. Allergy 2019;74(6):1063–80. https://doi.org/10.1111/all.13732.
6. Tejedor-Alonso MA, Moro-Moro M, Mosquera González M, et al. Increased incidence of admissions for anaphylaxis in Spain 1998-2011. Allergy 2015;70(7):880–3. https://doi.org/10.1111/all.12613.
7. Andrew E, Nehme Z, Bernard S, et al. Pediatric anaphylaxis in the prehospital setting: incidence, characteristics, and management. Prehosp Emerg Care 2018;22(4):445–51. https://doi.org/10.1080/10903127.2017.1402110.
8. Pouessel G, Jean-Bart C, Deschildre A, et al. Food-induced anaphylaxis in infancy compared to preschool age: a retrospective analysis. Clin Exp Allergy 2020;50(1):74–81.
9. Robinson LB, Arroyo AC, Faridi MK, et al. Trends in US hospitalizations for anaphylaxis among infants and toddlers: 2006 to 2015. Ann Allergy Asthma Immunol 2021;126(2):168–74.e3. https://doi.org/10.1016/j.anai.2020.09.003.

10. Bann MA, Carrell DS, Gruber S, et al. Identification and validation of anaphylaxis using electronic health data in a population-based setting. Epidemiology 2021; 32(3):439–43. https://doi.org/10.1097/EDE.0000000000001330.

11. Lee S, Hess EP, Lohse C, et al. Epinephrine autoinjector prescribing trends: an outpatient population-based study in Olmsted County, Minnesota. J Allergy Clin Immunol Pract 2016;4(6):1182–6.e1. https://doi.org/10.1016/j.jaip.2016.05.006.

12. Cho H, Kwon J-W. Prevalence of anaphylaxis and prescription rates of epinephrine auto-injectors in urban and rural areas of Korea. Korean J Intern Med 2019; 34(3):643–50. https://doi.org/10.3904/kjim.2018.094.

13. Simons FER, Peterson S, Black CD. Epinephrine dispensing patterns for an out-of-hospital population: a novel approach to studying the epidemiology of anaphylaxis. J Allergy Clin Immunol 2002;110(4):647–51. https://doi.org/10.1067/mai. 2002.127860.

14. Lieberman P, Camargo CA, Bohlke K, et al. Epidemiology of anaphylaxis: findings of the American College of Allergy, Asthma and Immunology Epidemiology of Anaphylaxis Working Group. Ann Allergy Asthma Immunol 2006;97(5):596–602. https://doi.org/10.1016/S1081-1206(10)61086-1.

15. Ko J, Zhu S, Alabaster A, et al. Prehospital treatment and emergency department outcomes in young children with food allergy. J Allergy Clin Immunol In Pract 2020;8(7):2302–9.e2. https://doi.org/10.1016/j.jaip.2020.03.047.

16. Topal E, Bakirtas A, Yilmaz O, et al. Anaphylaxis in infancy compared with older children. Allergy Asthma Proc 2013;34(3):233–8. https://doi.org/10.2500/aap. 2013.34.3658.

17. Jeon YH, Lee S, Ahn K, et al. Infantile anaphylaxis in Korea: a multicenter retrospective case study. J Korean Med Sci 2019;34(13):e106. https://doi.org/10. 3346/jkms.2019.34.e106.

18. Samady W, Trainor J, Smith B, et al. Food-induced anaphylaxis in infants and children. Ann Allergy Asthma Immunol 2018;121(3):360–5. https://doi.org/10.1016/j. anai.2018.05.025.

19. Kahveci M, Akarsu A, Koken G, et al. Food-induced anaphylaxis in infants, as compared to toddlers and preschool children in Turkey. Pediatr Allergy Immunol 2020;31(8):954–61. https://doi.org/10.1111/pai.13320.

20. Rudders SA, Banerji A, Clark S, et al. Age-related differences in the clinical presentation of food-induced anaphylaxis. J Pediatr 2011;158(2):326–8. https://doi. org/10.1016/j.jpeds.2010.10.017.

21. Koplin JJ, Peters RL, Dharmage SC, et al. Understanding the feasibility and implications of implementing early peanut introduction for prevention of peanut allergy. J Allergy Clin Immunol 2016;138(4):1131–41.e2. https://doi.org/10.1016/j. jaci.2016.04.011.

22. Fleischer DM, Perry TT, Atkins D, et al. Allergic reactions to foods in preschool-aged children in a prospective observational food allergy study. Pediatrics 2012;130(1):e25–32. https://doi.org/10.1542/peds.2011-1762.

23. Umasunthar T, Leonardi-Bee J, Hodes M, et al. Incidence of fatal food anaphylaxis in people with food allergy: a systematic review and meta-analysis. Clin Exp Allergy 2013;43(12):1333–41.

24. Pumphrey RSH, Gowland MH. Further fatal allergic reactions to food in the United Kingdom, 1999-2006. J Allergy Clin Immunol 2007;119(4):1018–9. https://doi.org/ 10.1016/j.jaci.2007.01.021.

25. Poirot E, He F, Gould LH, et al. Deaths, hospitalizations, and emergency department visits from food-related anaphylaxis, New York City, 2000-2014: implications

for fatality prevention. J Public Health Manag Pract 2020;26(6):548–56. https:// doi.org/10.1097/PHH.0000000000001137.

26. Osborne NJ, Koplin JJ, Martin PE, et al. The HealthNuts population-based study of paediatric food allergy: validity, safety and acceptability. Clin Exp Allergy 2010; 40(10):1516–22.

27. Koplin JJ, Tang MLK, Martin PE, et al. Predetermined challenge eligibility and cessation criteria for oral food challenges in the HealthNuts population-based study of infants. J Allergy Clin Immunol 2012;129(4):1145–7. https://doi.org/10. 1016/j.jaci.2011.09.044.

28. Vega MG, Alonso SB, España AP, et al. Treatment with proton pump inhibitors as a cofactor in adverse reactions of patients undergoing oral food immunotherapy. Allergol Immunopathol (Madr) 2021;49(3):169–72. https://doi.org/10.15586/aei. v49i3.58.

29. Du Toit G, Roberts G, Sayre PH, et al. Randomized trial of peanut consumption in infants at risk for peanut allergy. N Engl J Med 2015;372(9):803–13. https://doi. org/10.1056/NEJMoa1414850.

30. Togias A, Cooper SF, Acebal ML, et al. Addendum guidelines for the prevention of peanut allergy in the United States: report of the National Institute of Allergy and Infectious Diseases–sponsored expert panel. J Allergy Clin Immunol 2017; 139(1):29–44. https://doi.org/10.1016/j.jaci.2016.10.010.

31. Ko J, Zhu S, Alabaster A, et al. Health care utilization outcomes after implementation of early peanut introduction guidelines. J Allergy Clin Immunol In Pract 2021;9(1):531–3.e1. https://doi.org/10.1016/j.jaip.2020.08.054.

32. Cox LS, Sanchez-Borges M, Lockey RF. World allergy organization systemic allergic reaction grading system: is a modification needed? J Allergy Clin Immunol Pract 2017;5(1):58–62.e5. https://doi.org/10.1016/j.jaip.2016.11.009.

33. Pouessel G, Lejeune S, Dupond M-P, et al. Individual healthcare plan for allergic children at school: lessons from a 2015-2016 school year survey. Pediatr Allergy Immunol 2017;28(7):655–60. https://doi.org/10.1111/pai.12795.

34. Pistiner M, Mendez-Reyes JE, Eftekhari S, et al. Caregiver-reported presentation of severe food-induced allergic reactions in infants and toddlers. J Allergy Clin Immunol In Pract 2021;9(1):311–20.e2. https://doi.org/10.1016/j.jaip.2020. 11.005.

35. Greenhawt M, Gupta RS, Meadows JA, et al. Guiding principles for the recognition, diagnosis, and management of infants with anaphylaxis: an expert panel consensus. J Allergy Clin Immunol In Pract 2019;7(4):1148–56.e5. https://doi. org/10.1016/j.jaip.2018.10.052.

36. Simons FER, Sampson HA. Anaphylaxis: unique aspects of clinical diagnosis and management in infants (birth to age 2 years). J Allergy Clin Immunol 2015;135(5): 1125–31. https://doi.org/10.1016/j.jaci.2014.09.014.

37. Tsuang A, Chan ES, Wang J. Food-induced anaphylaxis in infants: can new evidence assist with implementation of food allergy prevention and treatment? J Allergy Clin Immunol Pract 2021;9(1):57–69. https://doi.org/10.1016/j.jaip. 2020.09.018.

38. Sampson HA, Muñoz-Furlong A, Campbell RL, et al. Second symposium on the definition and management of anaphylaxis: summary report—Second National Institute of Allergy and Infectious Disease/Food Allergy and Anaphylaxis Network symposium. J Allergy Clin Immunol 2006;117(2):391–7. https://doi.org/10.1016/j. jaci.2005.12.1303.

39. Simons FER. Anaphylaxis in infants: can recognition and management be improved? J Allergy Clin Immunol 2007;120(3):537–40. https://doi.org/10.1016/j.jaci.2007.06.025.

40. Nowak-Węgrzyn A, Chehade M, Groetch ME, et al. International consensus guidelines for the diagnosis and management of food protein–induced enterocolitis syndrome: Executive summary—Workgroup Report of the Adverse Reactions to Foods Committee, American Academy of Allergy, Asthma & Immunology. J Allergy Clin Immunol 2017;139(4):1111–26.e4. https://doi.org/10.1016/j.jaci.2016.12.966.

41. Shaker MS, Wallace DV, Golden DBK, et al. Anaphylaxis—a 2020 practice parameter update, systematic review, and Grading of Recommendations, Assessment, Development and Evaluation (GRADE) analysis. J Allergy Clin Immunol 2020;145(4):1082–123. https://doi.org/10.1016/j.jaci.2020.01.017.

42. De Schryver S, Halbrich M, Clarke A, et al. Tryptase levels in children presenting with anaphylaxis: temporal trends and associated factors. J Allergy Clin Immunol 2016;137(4):1138–42. https://doi.org/10.1016/j.jaci.2015.09.001.

43. Simons FER, Ebisawa M, Sanchez-Borges M, et al. 2015 update of the evidence base: World Allergy Organization anaphylaxis guidelines. World Allergy Organ J 2015;8(1):32. https://doi.org/10.1186/s40413-015-0080-1.

44. Belhocine W, Ibrahim Z, Grandné V, et al. Total serum tryptase levels are higher in young infants. Pediatr Allergy Immunol 2011;22(6):600–7.

45. Muraro A, Agache I, Clark A, et al. EAACI food allergy and anaphylaxis guidelines: managing patients with food allergy in the community. Allergy 2014;69(8):1046–57. https://doi.org/10.1111/all.12441.

46. Lee S, Peterson A, Lohse CM, et al. Further evaluation of factors that may predict biphasic reactions in emergency department anaphylaxis patients. J Allergy Clin Immunol Pract 2017;5(5):1295–301. https://doi.org/10.1016/j.jaip.2017.07.020.

47. Campbell RL, Bellolio MF, Knutson BD, et al. Epinephrine in anaphylaxis: higher risk of cardiovascular complications and overdose after administration of intravenous bolus epinephrine compared with intramuscular epinephrine. J Allergy Clin Immunol Pract 2015;3(1):76–80. https://doi.org/10.1016/j.jaip.2014.06.007.

48. Fleming JT, Clark S, Camargo CA, et al. Early treatment of food-induced anaphylaxis with epinephrine is associated with a lower risk of hospitalization. J Allergy Clin Immunol In Pract 2015;3(1):57–62. https://doi.org/10.1016/j.jaip.2014.07.004.

49. Sicherer SH, Simons FER, Section on Allergy and Immunology. Epinephrine for first-aid management of anaphylaxis. Pediatrics 2017;139(3):e20164006. https://doi.org/10.1542/peds.2016-4006.

50. Bird JA, Groetch M, Allen KJ, et al. Conducting an oral food challenge to peanut in an infant. J Allergy Clin Immunol Pract 2017;5(2):301–11.e1. https://doi.org/10.1016/j.jaip.2016.07.019.

51. Kim H, Dinakar C, McInnis P, et al. Inadequacy of current pediatric epinephrine autoinjector needle length for use in infants and toddlers. Ann Allergy Asthma Immunol 2017;118(6):719–25.e1. https://doi.org/10.1016/j.anai.2017.03.017.

52. Kim L, Nevis IF, Tsai G, et al. Children under 15 kg with food allergy may be at risk of having epinephrine auto-injectors administered into bone. Allergy Asthma Clin Immunol 2014;10(1):40. https://doi.org/10.1186/1710-1492-10-40.

53. Dreborg S, Tsai G, Kim H. Epinephrine auto-injector needle length: the impact of winter clothing. Allergy Asthma Clin Immunol 2020;16:24. https://doi.org/10.1186/s13223-020-00422-4.

54. Simons FER, Gu X, Simons KJ. Epinephrine absorption in adults: Intramuscular versus subcutaneous injection. J Allergy Clin Immunol 2001;108(5):871–3. https://doi.org/10.1067/mai.2001.119409.

55. Casale TB, Wang J, Nowak-Wegrzyn A. Acute at home management of anaphylaxis during the Covid-19 pandemic. J Allergy Clin Immunol In Pract 2020;8(6): 1795–7. https://doi.org/10.1016/j.jaip.2020.04.022.

56. Wang J, Sicherer SH, Section on Allergy and Immunology. Guidance on completing a written allergy and anaphylaxis emergency plan. Pediatrics 2017; 139(3):e20164005. https://doi.org/10.1542/peds.2016-4005.

57. NIAID-Sponsored Expert Panel, Boyce JA, Assa'ad A, Burks AW, Jones SM, Sampson HA, Wood RA, et al. Guidelines for the diagnosis and management of food allergy in the United States: report of the NIAID-sponsored expert panel. J Allergy Clin Immunol 2010 Dec;126(6 Suppl):S1–58. https://doi.org/10.1016/j.jaci.2010.10.007. PMID: 21134576.

58. Huang F, Chawla K, Järvinen KM, et al. Anaphylaxis in a New York City pediatric emergency department: triggers, treatments, and outcomes. J Allergy Clin Immunol 2012;129(1):162–8. https://doi.org/10.1016/j.jaci.2011.09.018, e1–3.

59. Rubeiz CJ, Ernst MM. Psychosocial Aspects of Food Allergy: Resiliency, Challenges and Opportunities. Immunol Allergy Clin North Am 2021 May;41(2): 177–88. https://doi.org/10.1016/j.iac.2021.01.006. Epub 2021 Mar 24. PMID: 33863478.

60. Peanut allergen powder (Palforzia). Med Lett Drugs Ther 2020;62(1593):33–4.

61. Vickery BP, Berglund JP, Burk CM, et al. Early oral immunotherapy in peanut-allergic preschool children is safe and highly effective. J Allergy Clin Immunol 2017;139(1):173–81.e8. https://doi.org/10.1016/j.jaci.2016.05.027.

62. Aimmune Therapeutics, Inc. Peanut Oral Immunotherapy Study of Early Intervention for Desensitization (POSEIDON). clinicaltrials.gov. 2021. Available at: https://clinicaltrials.gov/ct2/show/NCT03736447. Accessed June 3, 2021.

63. Soller L, Abrams EM, Carr S, et al. First Real-World Safety Analysis of Preschool Peanut Oral Immunotherapy. J Allergy Clin Immunol Pract 2019;7(8):2759–67.e5. https://doi.org/10.1016/j.jaip.2019.04.010.

64. DBV Technologies. A double-blind, placebo-controlled, randomized phase III trial to assess the safety and efficacy of viaskin peanut in peanut-allergic young children 1-3 years of age. clinicaltrials.gov. 2021. Available at: https://clinicaltrials.gov/ct2/show/NCT03211247. Accessed June 3, 2021.

65. DBV Technologies. Phase II Study of Viaskin Milk in MilkAllergic Patients. DBV technologies announces results from phase II study of Viaskin Milk in MilkAllergic patients. 2018. Available at: https://www.dbv-technologies.com/wp-content/uploads/2018/02/4511-pr-miles-final_eng-pdf.pdf. Accessed June 6, 2021.

66. DBV Technologies. A double-blind, placebo-controlled randomized trial to study the Viaskin milk efficacy and safety for treating IgE-mediated Cow's milk allergy in children. clinicaltrials.gov; 2019. Available at: https://clinicaltrials.gov/ct2/show/NCT02223182. Accessed July 22, 2020.

67. National Institute of Allergy and Infectious Diseases (NIAID). Omalizumab as Monotherapy and as Adjunct Therapy to Multi-Allergen Oral Immunotherapy (OIT) in Food Allergic Children and Adults (CoFAR-11). clinicaltrials.gov. 2021. Available at: https://clinicaltrials.gov/ct2/show/NCT03881696. Accessed June 3, 2021.

Recognition and Management of Food Allergy and Anaphylaxis in the School and Community Setting

Susan Waserman, MSc, MDCM, FRCPC, Anita Shah, HBSc,
Heather Cruikshank, BA, Ernie Avilla, MBA*

KEYWORDS

- Anaphylaxis • Food allergy • Epinephrine • Food allergy training • Food bans
- Stock epinephrine • School • Community

KEY POINTS

- Current evidence supports food allergy management training in schools and food service establishments as a means to improve knowledge and skills, but more research is needed.
- Although there are challenges involved in implementing unassigned stock epinephrine programs, they have potential life-saving benefits in school and community settings.
- Food bans in schools were previously regarded as an important component of allergy management; however, these measures may not be as effective as once thought, according to more recent evidence.

INTRODUCTION

Immunoglobulin E-mediated food allergy (FA) is a response to food protein that can lead to anaphylaxis, a life-threatening reaction that can cause breathing difficulty, drop in blood pressure, and loss of consciousness.[1,2] In the United States, it is estimated that 10.8% of adults have FA.[3] The condition is also prevalent among children, affecting approximately 1% to 10% of infants and preschool-aged children and 1% to 2.5% of children older than 5 years of age.[4]

FA has a considerable impact on quality of life, often affecting social and psychological domains.[5–7] This is due to the persistent need for vigilance and often-restricted ability to engage in social activities involving food.[5,7] Among children with FA, the negative impact on quality of life often extends to parents and/or caregivers.[6]

Department of Medicine, Clinical Immunology and Allergy, McMaster University, Hamilton, Ontario, Canada
* Corresponding author. Department of Medicine, Clinical Immunology and Allergy, McMaster University, 1280 Main Street West, HSC 3V49, Hamilton, Ontario L8S 4K1, Canada.
E-mail address: avillae@mcmaster.ca

Immunol Allergy Clin N Am 42 (2022) 91–103
https://doi.org/10.1016/j.iac.2021.09.008
0889-8561/22/© 2021 Elsevier Inc. All rights reserved.

Given the public health burden of FA—including the need for caution in workplaces, schools, restaurants, other public areas—shared community responsibility is necessary to accommodate those with the condition. However, there are documented gaps in FA knowledge among children, parents, teachers, food service personnel, and others.[8] Two particularly important community entities and potential sites of allergic reaction from accidental exposure are schools and food services.[9,10] There are many potential strategies and interventions for managing FA, one of which is staff training. Staff education has been shown to significantly improve FA knowledge and confidence in managing an allergic reaction.[11] Another important consideration is whether to stock unassigned epinephrine autoinjectors (EAIs) for use in allergy emergencies.[12] Extensive evidence has shown that epinephrine is generally underused in the treatment of anaphylaxis, sometimes because of lack of availability.[12,13] Finally, there has been much discussion as to whether food bans on common allergens in schools are beneficial and warranted for preventing accidental allergen exposure.[14] The objective of this review is to highlight recent evidence on FA management in school and community settings, with a focus on staff training, stocking EAIs, and food bans/restrictions.

Training Staff in School and Community Settings

Although emphasis is often placed on training patients and parents on FA management, training is also important for workers in school and other community settings. Experts recommend that such training should focus on reducing the risk of accidental exposure to food allergens, developing communication protocols, recognizing symptoms of acute allergic reaction, and administering emergency treatment.[15]

Schools

Training on recognition and management of allergic reaction is especially important in the school setting, given the prevalence of FA among children. Children with FA may not have a mature understanding of the strategies necessary to keep themselves safe. One study showed that children, regardless of their FA status, have a similar level of knowledge on the topic.[16] In addition, FA bullying is not uncommon. In one survey, approximately 24% of children with FA in the United States reported having been bullied about their allergy.[17] Surprisingly, more than one-fifth of reported cases were perpetrated by teachers.[17] Evidence has also demonstrated deficits in the knowledge and attitudes of school personnel regarding FA. A study in US school nurses found deficiencies in both FA knowledge and attitudes.[18] Knowledge scores were highest for symptom recognition and lowest for treatment.[18] In addition, more than half of nurses (55%) held negative perceptions of parents of children with FA, feeling that they were "overprotective."[18]

In many jurisdictions, there are no standardized FA training requirements, and little research has been conducted on the impact that training has on the risk of allergic reactions in schools. However, research has linked FA training to improved test scores and self-reported knowledge, confidence, and attitudes among teachers, childcare workers, and cafeteria staff—including significant improvements in their capacity to recognize symptoms and identify appropriate treatment of allergic reactions.[19–22] The educational interventions in most of these studies incorporated topics such as common allergens, routes of exposure, symptom recognition, and treatment of anaphylaxis. In one study of childcare workers, allergy training was linked to improved knowledge and confidence, even among participants who had prior training and self-reported proficiency in allergy management.[21] Another study found that FA training may improve allergy management preparedness at the school level.[20] In the 2 years following training for school nurses, the availability of EAIs increased and the number of allergic reactions decreased at participating schools.[23]

Recent practice guidelines by Waserman and colleagues[14] recommend that schools and childcare centers implement expert-designed training for teachers and other personnel to facilitate the prevention, recognition, and treatment of allergic reactions. Moreover, the guidelines recommend that parents of children with FA be required to provide an allergy action plan (AAP), outlining the recommended emergency response to a suspected reaction.[14] Limited low-quality evidence suggests that implementing AAPs along with FA training may decrease the frequency of allergic reactions.[14,24–30] Finally, the guidelines recommend that schools and childcare centers implement protocols for managing suspected food allergic reactions in students and personnel with no existing AAP.[14]

Community

More research is needed to evaluate the effects of FA training for workers in other community settings, including restaurants. FA training is especially important in this setting, given that dining out accounts for the second most commonly reported location of food allergic reactions.[9] Allergic reactions have occurred even when allergens have been identified on the menu and customers have shared their FA status with restaurant staff.[9] There are known deficits in the FA knowledge and attitudes of restaurant personnel. For example, a study of 295 restaurant staff in Germany found that only 30% were able to correctly identify 3 food allergens, and many expressed unfavorable attitudes toward customers with FA.[31] Another study of 278 restaurants in the United States identified important knowledge gaps and misconceptions among managers and staff, including the belief that people with FA can safely consume a small amount of allergen.[32]

As with the school setting, limited research over the past 10 years has demonstrated benefits of FA training for improving the knowledge and attitudes of restaurant staff. Generally, training in these studies has focused on knowledge of common allergens, methods to reduce the risk of allergic reactions, symptoms of allergic reactions, the emergency response required in the case of an allergic reaction, and effective communication techniques to use with customers with FA. A systematic review and meta-analysis of FA training for restaurant personnel showed that most participants had not received prior training, and very few studies have examined the benefit of training through an interventional approach.[33] Although there was significant variability between studies, one common theme that emerged was the presence of important deficits in knowledge regarding in the emergency response to an allergic reaction.[33] A pilot evaluation of restaurant staff in the United Kingdom showed considerable improvements in knowledge posttraining (91% accuracy score vs 82% pretraining) in topics such as common allergens, the severity of FA, and cross-contamination.[34] Likewise, a study of 121 food service workers in Romania showed that trained employees exhibited higher levels of knowledge, which translated to safer practices for customers with FA.[35] Moreover, allergy training has also been associated with more positive attitudes among restaurant managers.[32]

An American Academy of Allergy, Asthma and Immunology Work Group Report published in 2020 presented several recommendations for restaurants to safely serve those with FA, emphasizing communication, knowledge, and safe practices as 3 main themes.[36] With respect to communication, the report recommends that restaurant staff establish clear communication with customers and chefs and ask all customers about their FA status.[36] Regarding knowledge, the report suggests using appropriate cleaning techniques to remove allergens and implementing regular training for all restaurant staff that incorporates education on cross-contamination and symptoms of anaphylaxis.[36] Finally, the investigators suggest several possible safe practices, including allergy-designated spaces in the kitchen, menus with clearly labeled allergens, and computer technology that automatically identifies the safety of certain menu items for food allergic customers.[36]

Stocking Epinephrine Autoinjectors

Intramuscular epinephrine is the first-line recommended treatment for suspected systemic allergic reaction and anaphylaxis.[37] It may be administered using an EAI, a self-injectable device that contains a premeasured dose of epinephrine. In some countries, multiple brands of EAI are available in a variety of doses for patients of different weights.

To ensure that epinephrine is available to treat anaphylaxis, people with FA should always keep an EAI accessible. Those who are mature enough to do so should carry one or more personal EAIs with them. Some schools and other community sites also stock unassigned EAIs to treat suspected cases of anaphylaxis in individuals experiencing a first-time reaction or those with a known history of FA who do not have a personal EAI available. Stock EAIs have also been used after a personal EAI has malfunctioned or the patient requires additional doses of epinephrine after receiving treatment with their personal EAI.[38–42]

Schools

Schools often ask each student at risk of anaphylaxis to have one or more personal EAIs available on site. Depending on school policies, at-risk students who are mature enough to do so may carry their personal EAIs with them to, from, and at school—or be asked to submit personal EAIs to be stored on site (eg, in their classroom or a nurse's office).[43,44] Some schools also stock unassigned EAIs to treat anaphylaxis when a personal EAI is not available. In schools where stock EAIs are available, they have been used in 20% to 77% (median: 49%) of reported cases of epinephrine use.[38–41,45–50]

Studies have found that delays in epinephrine use are associated with increased risks of hospitalization and increased risk of death from anaphylaxis.[51–57] Administering a stock EAI when a personal EAI is not available could potentially prevent severe outcomes from anaphylaxis. Stocking EAI may also improve epinephrine access for students who face socioeconomic barriers to obtaining personal EAIs.[58–67] However, socioeconomic disparities have also been reported in the implementation of stock EAI programs.[68,69] In the United States, researchers have found that schools in wealthier counties and urban or suburban areas are more likely than schools in poorer and rural areas to have stock EAIs.[68,69]

The feasibility of stocking EAIs varies from one jurisdiction to another. EAIs remain unavailable in many countries, and the unsubsidized price per unit in countries where they are available varies widely.[70] Reported barriers to stocking EAIs include cost, lack of funding, lack of prescribing physicians, lack of school nursing support, gaps in knowledge among school personnel, and legal concerns.[43,68,71–74] In some districts, EAI manufacturers offer a limited number of free stock EAIs to schools that fulfill certain criteria. However, in jurisdictions where schools require a prescription to obtain stock EAIs, legal concerns among physicians may contribute to a reluctance to prescribe.[68,71,74]

A computer simulation study in the United States found that when schools required each at-risk student to have 2 personal EAIs available, it was only cost-effective to stock EAIs when the annual cost did not exceed $339 per school.[75] It was more cost-effective for schools to stock EAIs without requiring at-risk students to have multiple personal EAIs on site.[75] In the more cost-effective approach, each at-risk student still had one personal EAI that they could carry with them to and from school. Regardless of whether stock EAIs are available, promoting self-carriage among at-risk students helps to ensure that epinephrine is available in any setting where anaphylaxis may occur, including when students are traveling to or from school or participating in other off-site activities. Importantly, it promotes self-management and earlier treatment.

Studies suggest that school nurses and parents of at-risk children generally support stock EAI programs,[43,69,72,76,77] although some parents have concerns about the adequacy of stock EAI coverage on large school campuses.[77] Among school administrators, teachers, and other personnel, concerns about increased responsibility, legal liability, or other issues may reduce support for stock EAI programs.[43,71,77,78] According to one survey of school nurses, packing stock EAIs on field trips and other off-site activities is more costly and less acceptable to personnel than stocking EAIs on site alone.[43] In order to pack stock EAIs on field trips while maintaining an adequate supply on site, schools must stock a larger number of EAIs. They must also invest administrative labor in ensuring that stock EAIs are appropriately distributed, returned, and replaced if lost on field trips. Thus, for many schools, packing stock EAIs on field trips and other off-site activities may not be feasible or cost-effective. In fact, this precautionary measure was not supported in recent guidelines published by Waserman and colleagues.[14]

If schools decide to stock EAIs, guidelines from Waserman and colleagues[14] advise them to implement formalized procedures for obtaining, storing, administering, and replacing those devices as needed. More research is needed to learn how many stock EAIs are required to provide adequate coverage, based on school size, layout, and population. Sometimes, more than 1 dose of epinephrine is needed to treat anaphylaxis.[79] Thus, schools should stock at least 2 EAIs of each dose required to provide a weight-appropriate option for all students. They should also promptly replace stock EAIs after they have been used or expired. One survey in the United States found that arrangements to replace used stock EAIs were made in only 84% of cases.[39]

Schools should store stock EAIs at an appropriate temperature (20°C–25°C/68°F–77°F) in a location that is known and easily accessible to all school personnel. If stock EAIs will not be available on field trips or other off-site activities, it is recommended that school personnel inform at-risk students and their parents beforehand; require at-risk students to have personal EAIs with them; and ensure that their personal EAIs are always easily accessible during the activity.[14]

Community
Our search yielded only 2 studies that describe stock EAIs in community settings outside of schools and childcare centers. First, Waserman and colleagues[80] implemented a stock epinephrine program between September 2014 and March 2016 to better understand FA management in food service establishments, specifically in a shopping mall setting. Security guards and food service staff participated in a 3-hour training session. Posttraining, security personnel carried 2 doses of stock EAIs (0.15 mg and 0.3 mg) and had additional access to secured first-aid kits located in the central administration offices within the mall.[80] In stand-alone owner-operated restaurants at the mall, trained staff had access to 2 doses of stock EAIs in a central location (eg, behind the counter), with emergency backup in secured first-aid kit located in a central office.[80] Overall, these findings suggest that it is feasible to use stock epinephrine programs in malls with personnel who are trained to administer it.[80] However, more research is needed to learn if it is cost-effective to do so.

Previous studies have shown that anaphylaxis can occur even in those with no prior history of anaphylaxis, thus underscoring the benefits of stock epinephrine in protecting all individuals at risk of anaphylaxis, not just those with a previous diagnosis. The study revealed that the provision of stock EAIs was widely accepted by food-allergic individuals as well as food service establishments who continued to stock EAIs beyond the study and integrated the processes into their emergency response procedures and new employee training policies.[80]

The second study evaluated the cost-effectiveness of stock EAIs on commercial aircraft.[68] The study demonstrated that the provision of supplemental stock EAIs is cost-effective, with an incremental cost-effectiveness ratio less than $20,000 per cost of quality-adjusted life-year—under the accepted cost-thresholds for medical interventions in the United States, which are generally $50,000 to $100,000.[81] Although emergency medical kits on US flights must include epinephrine solutions of both 1:1000 and 1:10,000, the complexities of selecting the correct ampule and appropriately using the syringe may cause confusion and delay administration during emergency response.[81] Providing access to supplemental stock EAIs on all flights may potentially improve epinephrine delivery by nonmedical personnel.[81]

Food Bans

Some schools have implemented school-wide, lunchroom-wide, or classroom-wide bans on foods that contain peanut, tree nuts, or in some cases, other allergens.[82–85] The presumed purpose of these bans is to prevent allergic reactions by preventing accidental exposure to banned allergens. However, researchers have not found strong or consistent evidence that food bans actually reduce the risk of allergic reactions in schools.[86–88]

In one observational study, peanut-allergic children were less likely to experience an allergic reaction at school if they attended a school where peanut was restricted (1%, n = 12/1230 students vs 3%, n = 5/181 students).[87] Another observational study found that a greater proportion of reported reactions occurred in schools that prohibited peanut versus schools that allowed peanut (5% vs 3%).[86] In both studies, most of the reported reactions were classified as mild or moderate.[86,87] A third observational study compared the use of EAIs to treat allergic reactions in schools with different peanut policies.[88] No difference was found between schools with site-wide peanut bans versus schools that allowed peanut on site (3 epinephrine administrations per 100,000 student-years).[88] Overall, peanut-free classrooms had no significant effect on epinephrine use either.[88]

Support for food bans is variable among school personnel and parents,[76,82,89–95] and effectively monitoring and promoting adherence to food bans can be challenging.[43,96,97] In a survey of school nurses in the United States, resistance from staff or parents was the most frequently reported barrier to implementing food bans.[43] When researchers in Quebec, Canada inspected lunches in classrooms with peanut-free policies, they found that most but not all lunches were actually free of peanut.[37] A study of food allergens in floor dust and table wipe samples found that peanut allergen was detectable in elementary school environments, but not at levels higher than in peanut-allergic students' own homes.[98] Peanut-restricted policies did not consistently lower environmental exposure to peanut in schools.[98]

Compared with school-wide or classroom-wide bans, allergen-restricted tables affect the autonomy and food choices of fewer students, and they might be easier to monitor and enforce. Some limited evidence suggests they may also be more effective. In the study on epinephrine use, researchers found that schools with peanut-free tables had lower rates of epinephrine use than those without (2 vs 6 epinephrine administrations per 100,000 student-years).[88] However, the absolute difference was small, and the rate of epinephrine use was low regardless.[88] The implementation of allergen-restricted tables may negatively affect the autonomy of at-risk students if they are compelled to eat there against their wishes. These tables may also limit the social development of at-risk students by isolating them from peers.

Whether they implement food bans or allergen-restricted tables, schools may implement other risk-reduction strategies to help prevent accidental exposure to food allergens. For example, common-sense strategies include promoting handwashing before and after eating, discouraging students from sharing food or utensils, helping at-risk students check ingredient lists for allergens, and proactively addressing incidents of "food fights" or FA-related bullying. Active adult supervision during snacks and meals and proper cleaning of surfaces where food is prepared and eaten are also important. In addition, teachers and other school personnel can promote inclusion and manage the risk of allergic reactions by taking steps to avoid students' allergens when planning field-trip and classroom activities, such as home economics projects, science experiments, and crafts.

SUMMARY

FA is a common cause of anaphylaxis, a life-threatening condition that should be treated with epinephrine. Given the public health burden of FA, community entities, such as schools and food service establishments, have a shared responsibility to accommodate those with the condition. Although more research is needed to standardize anaphylaxis management in school and community settings, allergy training has been shown to improve knowledge and skills and should be strongly considered. Stocking unassigned EAIs in schools and other community settings also provides benefits, including quick access to potentially life-saving treatment; however, challenges remain regarding the maintenance of successful stock epinephrine programs. Conversely, food bans as a means of allergy management in schools are not consistently supported by currently available evidence. Other risk mitigation measures may be more effective for preventing allergic reactions in schools and require further study.

CLINICS CARE POINTS

- Remind patients at risk of anaphylaxis to always carry an epinephrine autoinjector and practice other strategies to mitigate the risk of an allergic reaction in community settings (eg, communicate with others about their allergy, wash hands before and after eating, read ingredient lists).

- Advise patients to clearly communicate information about their food allergy to food service staff, including the fact that trace amounts of allergen may trigger a reaction.

- Encourage patients to pack their own safe food from home, when they are not certain of the safety of food at their childcare center, school, or other community settings.

- Help children with food allergy and their caregivers to complete allergy action plans for their childcare centers and schools.

- Support families in advocating for evidence-based interventions to manage food allergy in childcare centers and schools, including allergy training for childcare and school personnel and implementation of stock epinephrine programs. Advise them of the lack of evidence supporting food bans and help them advocate for other common-sense strategies to reduce the risk of accidental exposure. For example, these could include adult supervision during eating, washing of surfaces where food is prepared and eaten, rules against sharing foods, and avoidance of allergens in classroom activities, such as crafts and science experiments.

CONFLICT OF INTEREST DISCLOSURES

S. Waserman reports the following financial relationships: Aimmune Therapeutics, Medexus Pharma, AstraZeneca Canada, CSL Behring, GSK, kaléo, Merck, Mylan, Novartis, Pediapharm, Pfizer Canada, Sanofi Canada, Takeda Canada, Trudell, Avir Pharma, Food Allergy Canada Healthcare Advisory Board, Canadian Hereditary Angioedema Network, and Health Canada Consultant. E. Avilla reports the following financial relationships: Pfizer Canada, AllerGen NCE, Canadian Hereditary Angioedema Network, Aimmune Therapeutics outside the submitted work. A. Shah has nothing to disclose. H. Cruikshank has nothing to disclose.

REFERENCES

1. Food Allergy Canada. Food allergy FAQs. Available at: https://foodallergycanada.ca/food-allergy-basics/food-allergies-101/food-allergy-faqs/. Accessed on July 18 2021.
2. National Health Service. Available at: https://www.nhs.uk/conditions/anaphylaxis/. Accessed on July 18 2021.
3. Gupta RS, Warren CM, Smith BM, et al. Prevalence and severity of food allergies among US adults. JAMA Netw Open 2019;2(1):e185630.
4. Prescott SL, Pawankar R, Allen KJ, et al. A global survey of changing patterns of food allergy burden in children. World Allergy Organ J 2013;6(1):21.
5. DunnGalvin A, Dubois AE, Flokstra-de Blok BM, et al. The effects of food allergy on quality of life. Chem Immunol Allergy 2015;101:235–52.
6. Nowak-Wegrzyn A, Hass SL, Donelson SM, et al. The Peanut Allergy Burden Study: impact on the quality of life of patients and caregivers. World Allergy Organ J 2021;14(2):100512.
7. Antolín-Amérigo D, Manso L, Caminati M, et al. Quality of life in patients with food allergy. Clin Mol Allergy 2016;14:4.
8. Gupta RS, Kim JS, Barnathan JA, et al. Food allergy knowledge, attitudes and beliefs: focus groups of parents, physicians and the general public. BMC Pediatr 2008;8:36.
9. Oriel RC, Waqar O, Sharma HP, et al. Characteristics of food allergic reactions in United States restaurants. J Allergy Clin Immunol Pract 2021;9(4):1675–82.
10. Nowak-Wegrzyn A, Conover-Walker MK, Wood RA. Food-allergic reactions in schools and preschools. Arch Pediatr Adolesc Med 2001;155(7):790–5.
11. Karim J, Gabrielli S, Torabi B, et al. Bridging knowledge gaps in anaphylaxis management through a video-based educational tool. J Allergy Clin Immunol 2021;147(2):AB159.
12. Posner LS, Camargo CA Jr. Update on the usage and safety of epinephrine auto-injectors, 2017. Drug Healthc Patient Saf 2017;9:9–18.
13. Prince BT, Mikhail I, Stukus DR. Underuse of epinephrine for the treatment of anaphylaxis: missed opportunities. J Asthma Allergy 2018;11:143–51.
14. Waserman S, Cruickshank H, Hildebrand KJ, et al. Prevention and management of allergic reactions to food in child care centers and schools: practice guidelines. J Allergy Clin Immunol 2021;147(5):1561–78.

15. Food Allergy Canada. Training for foodservice. Available at: https://foodallergycanada.ca/food-allergy-basics/food-allergies-101/what-are-food-allergies/. Accessed on July 18 2021.

16. Choi Y, Ju S, Chang H. Food allergy knowledge, perception of food allergy labeling, and level of dietary practice: a comparison between children with and without food allergy experience. Nutr Res Pract 2015;9(1):92–8.

17. Oppenheimer J, Bender B. The impact of food allergy and bullying. Ann Asthma, Allergy Immunol 2010;105(6):P410–1.

18. Twichell S, Wang K, Robinson H, et al. Food allergy knowledge and attitudes among school nurses in an urban public school district. Children (Basel) 2015; 2(3):330–41.

19. Canon N, Gharfeh M, Guffey D, et al. Role of food allergy education: measuring teacher knowledge, attitudes, and beliefs. Allergy Rhinol (Providence) 2019;10. 2152656719856324.

20. Shah SS, Parker CL, Davis CM. Improvement of teacher food allergy knowledge in socioeconomically diverse schools after educational intervention. Clin Pediatr (Phila) 2013;52(9):812–20.

21. Lanser BJ, Covar R, Bird JA. Food allergy needs assessment, training curriculum, and knowledge assessment for child care. Ann Allergy Asthma Immunol 2016 Jun;116(6):533–7.e4.

22. Gonzalez-Mancebo E, Gandolfo-Cano MM, Trujillo-Trujillo MJ, et al. Analysis of the effectiveness of training school personnel in the management of food allergy and anaphylaxis. Allergol Immunopathol (Madr) 2019;47(1):60–3.

23. Chokshi NY, Patel D, Davis CM. Long-term increase in epinephrine availability associated with school nurse training in food allergy. J Allergy Clin Immunol Pract 2015;3(1):128–30.

24. Clark AT, Ewan PW. Good prognosis, clinical features, and circumstances of peanut and tree nut reactions in children treated by a specialist allergy center. J Allergy Clin Immunol 2008;122:286–9.

25. Patel D, Johnson G, Guffey D, et al. Longitudinal effect of food allergy education on epinephrine availability in public schools. J Allergy Clin Immunol 2014;133: AB288.

26. Tsuang A, Atal Z, Demain H, et al. Benefits of school nurse training sessions for food allergy and anaphylaxis management. J Allergy Clin Immunol Pract 2019;7: 309–11.e2.

27. Ewan PW, Clark AT. Long-term prospective observational study of patients with peanut and nut allergy after participation in a management plan. Lancet 2001; 357:111–5.

28. Ewan PW, Clark AT. Efficacy of a management plan based on severity assessment in longitudinal and case-controlled studies of 747 children with nut allergy: proposal for good practice. Clin Exp Allergy 2005;35:751–6.

29. Moneret-Vautrin DA, Kanny G, Guenard L, et al. Food anaphylaxis in schools: evaluation of the management plan and the efficiency of the emergency kit. Allergy 2001;56:1071–6.

30. Kourosh A, Davis CM. School staff food allergy (FA) education increases epinephrine coverage and recognition of allergic reactions. J Allergy Clin Immunol 2015;135:AB211.

31. Loerbroks A, Tolksdorf SJ, Wagenmann M, et al. Food allergy knowledge, attitudes and their determinants among restaurant staff: A cross-sectional study. PLoS One 2019;14(4):e0214625.

32. Radke TJ, Brown LG, Hoover ER, et al. Food allergy knowledge and attitudes of restaurant managers and staff: an EHS-Net Study. J Food Prot 2016;79(9): 1588–98.

33. Young I, Thaivalappil A. A systematic review and meta-regression of the knowledge, practices, and training of restaurant and food service personnel toward food allergies and celiac disease. PLoS One 2018;13(9):e0203496.

34. Bailey S, Billmeier Kindratt T, Smith H, et al. Food allergy training event for restaurant staff: a pilot evaluation. Clin Transl Allergy 2014;4:26.

35. Jianu C, Goleţ I. Food allergies: knowledge and practice among food service workers operating in western Romania. J Food Prot 2019;82(2):207–16.

36. Carter CA, Pistiner M, Wang J, et al. Food Allergy in Restaurants Work Group Report. J Allergy Clin Immunol Pract 2020;8(1):70–4.

37. Banerjee DK, Kagan RS, Turnbull E, et al. Peanut-free guidelines reduce school lunch peanut contents. Arch Dis Child 2007;92:980–2.

38. Feuille E, Lawrence C, Volel C, et al. Time trends in food allergy diagnoses, epinephrine orders, and epinephrine administrations in New York City schools. J Pediatr 2017;190:93–9.

39. Hogue SL, Muniz R, Herrem C, et al. Barriers to the administration of epinephrine in schools. J Sch Health 2018;88:396–404.

40. Tyquin B, Ford L, Hollinshead K, et al. Review of the use of adrenaline EAIs (AAI) in NSW Department of Education schools in terms 1 and 2 2017. Intern Med J 2017;47(Suppl 5):20.

41. Vale S, Netting MJ, Ford LS, et al. Anaphylaxis management in Australian schools: review of guidelines and adrenaline EAI use. J Paediatr Child Health 2019;55:143–51.

42. Vokits K, Pumphrey I, Baker D, et al. Implementation of a stock epinephrine protocol. NASN Sch Nurse 2014;29:287–91.

43. Kao LM, Wang J, Kagan O, et al. School nurse perspectives on school policies for food allergy and anaphylaxis. Ann Allergy Asthma Immunol 2018;120:304–9.

44. Ben-Shoshan M, Kagan R, Primeau MN, et al. Availability of the epinephrine EAI at school in children with peanut allergy. Ann Allergy Asthma Immunol 2008;100: 570–5.

45. Dickson MA, Ng CW, Neupert K, et al. Epinephrine administration trends in a large urban school district after implementing unassigned epinephrine. J Allergy Clin Immunol 2019;143:AB147.

46. Leo HL, McCormack KL, Patel PH, et al. Characterization of epinephrine utilization in Michigan public schools 2014-17. J Allergy Clin Immunol 2019;143:AB84.

47. Neupert K, Cherian S, Varshney P. Epinephrine use in Austin Independent School District after implementation of unassigned epinephrine. J Allergy Clin Immunol Pract 2019;7:1650–2.e4.

48. White MV, Hogue SL, Odom D, et al. Anaphylaxis in schools: results of the EPIPEN4SCHOOLS survey combined analysis. Pediatr Allergy Immunol Pulmonol 2016;29:149–54.

49. Wright BL, Fogg M, Sparks C, et al. Availability and utilization of epinephrine in Utah schools for the management of anaphylaxis. J Allergy Clin Immunol 2014; 1:AB25.

50. Aktas ON, Kao LM, Hoyt A, et al. Development and implementation of an allergic reaction reporting tool for school health personnel: a pilot study of three Chicago schools. J Sch Nurs 2019;35:316–24.

51. Fleming JT, Clark S, Camargo CA Jr, et al. Early treatment of food-induced anaphylaxis with epinephrine is associated with a lower risk of hospitalization. J Allergy Clin Immunol Pract 2015;3:57–62.
52. Hochstadter E, Clarke A, De Schryver S, et al. Increasing visits for anaphylaxis and the benefits of early epinephrine administration: a 4-year study at a pediatric emergency department in Montreal, Canada. J Allergy Clin Immunol 2016;137: 1888–90.
53. Robinson M, Greenhawt M, Stukus DR. Factors associated with epinephrine administration for anaphylaxis in children before arrival to the emergency department. Ann Allergy Asthma Immunol 2017;119(2):164–9.
54. Bock SA, Munoz-Furlong A, Sampson HA. Fatalities due to anaphylactic reactions to foods. J Allergy Clin Immunol 2001;107:191–3.
55. Pumphrey RS. Lessons for management of anaphylaxis from a study of fatal reactions. Clin Exp Allergy 2000;30:1144–50.
56. Pumphrey RS, Gowland MH. Further fatal allergic reactions to food in the United Kingdom, 1999-2006. J Allergy Clin Immunol 2007;119:1018–9.
57. Sampson HA, Mendelson L, Rosen JP. Fatal and near-fatal anaphylactic reactions to food in children and adolescents. N Engl J Med 1992;327:380–4.
58. Bilaver LA, Kester K, Smith B, et al. Socioeconomic disparities in the economic impact of childhood food allergy. J Allergy Clin Immunol 2016;137:AB283.
59. Coombs R, Simons E, Foty RG, et al. Socioeconomic factors and epinephrine prescription in children with peanut allergy. Paediatr Child Health 2011;16:341–4.
60. Davis CM, Parker CL, Shah SS. Under-recognition of food allergies in lower socioeconomic status (SES) schools in a large urban school district. J Allergy Clin Immunol 2011;127:AB266.
61. Frost DW, Chalin CG. The effect of income on anaphylaxis preparation and management plans in Toronto primary schools. Can J Public Health 2005;96:250–3.
62. Minaker LM, Elliot SJ, Clarke A. Exploring low-income families' financial barriers to food allergy management and treatment. J Allergy 2014;2014:1–7.
63. Mullins RJ, Clark S, Camargo CA Jr. Socio-economic status, geographic remoteness and childhood food allergy and anaphylaxis in Australia. Clin Exp Allergy 2010;40:1523–32.
64. Neuport K, Uderngba C, Huntwork M, et al. Improving access to stock epinephrine in a de-centralized school district: the New Orleans experience. J Allergy Clin Immunol 2020;145:AB183.
65. Shah SS, Parker CL, Davis CM. The power of education: food allergy intervention and prevention in Houston Independent School District (HISD). J Allergy Clin Immunol 2011;127:AB139.
66. Wang E, Plunk A, Morales M. Attitudes and beliefs toward epinephrine autoinjector price increase. Ann Allergy Asthma Immunol 2018;121:S58.
67. Shah SS, Parker CL, O'Brian Smith E, et al. Disparity in the availability of injectable epinephrine in a large, diverse US school district. J Allergy Clin Immunol Pract 2014;2:288–93e1.
68. Love MA, Breeden M, Dack K, et al. A law is not enough: geographical disparities in stock epinephrine access in Kansas. J Allergy Clin Immunol 2016;137:AB56.
69. Szychlinski C, Schmeissing KA, Fuleihan Z, et al. Food allergy emergency preparedness in Illinois schools: rural disparity in guideline implementation. J Allergy Clin Immunol Pract 2015;3:805–7.e8.
70. Waserman S, Avilla E, Harada L, et al. Decades of poor availability of epinephrine EAIs: global problems in need of global solutions. Ann Allergy Asthma Immunol 2020;124:205–7.

71. Denny SA, Merryweather A, Kline JM, et al. Stock epinephrine in schools: a survey of implementation, use, and barriers. J Allergy Clin Immunol Pract 2020;8: 380–2.

72. Odhav A, Ciaccio CE, Serota M, et al. Barriers to treatment with epinephrine for anaphylaxis by school nurses. J Allergy Clin Immunol 2015;135:AB211.

73. Morris P, Baker D, Belot C, et al. Preparedness for students and staff with anaphylaxis. J Sch Health 2011;81:471–6.

74. Yeh CY, Wheeler A, Schwind K, et al. Identifying barriers to implementation of stock epinephrine bills: the Texas experience. J Allergy Clin Immunol 2018;141: AB88.

75. Shaker MS, Greenhawt MJ. Analysis of value-based costs of undesignated school stock epinephrine policies for peanut anaphylaxis. JAMA Pediatr 2019; 173:169–75.

76. Mustafa SS, Russell AF, Kagan O, et al. Parent perspectives on school food allergy policy. BMC Pediatr 2018;18:e11.

77. Norton L, Dunn Galvin A, Hourihane JO. Allergy rescue medication in schools: modeling a new approach. J Allergy Clin Immunol 2008;122:209–10.

78. Tran D, Minard CG, Staggers KA, et al. School personnel apprehension related to stock epinephrine in Greater Houston Area. J Allergy Clin Immunol 2019;143: AB76.

79. Tsuang A, Menon NR, Bahri N, et al. Risk factors for multiple epinephrine doses in food-triggered anaphylaxis in children. Ann Allergy Asthma Immunol 2018;121: 469–73.

80. Waserman S, Avilla E, Harada L, et al. To stock or not to stock? Implementation of epinephrine autoinjectors in food establishments. J Allergy Clin Immunol Pract 2019;7(2):678–80.e5.

81. Shaker M, Greenhawt M. Cost-effectiveness of stock epinephrine autoinjectors on commercial aircraft. J Allergy Clin Immunol Pract 2019;7(7):2270–6.

82. C.S. Mott Children's Hospital. Are schools doing enough for food allergic-kids? C.S. Mott Children's Hospital National Poll of Children's Health 2009;6. Available at: https://mottpoll.org/reports-surveys/are-schools-doing-enough-food-allergic-kids. Accessed November 5, 2020.

83. Eldredge C, Patterson L, White B, et al. Assessing the readiness of a school system to adopt food allergy management guidelines. WMJ 2014;113:155–61.

84. Field MJ, Sasaki M, Koplin JJ, et al. Are schools banning nuts? Results from a population-based survey of Australian schools. Allergy 2019;74(Suppl 106):304.

85. Pham MN, Pistiner M, Wang J. National School Nurse Survey of food allergy and anaphylaxis policies and education. J Allergy Clin Immunol Pract 2019;7: 2440–2.e7.

86. Cherkaoui S, Ben-Shoshan M, Alizadehfar R, et al. Accidental exposures to peanut in a large cohort of Canadian children with peanut allergy. Clin Transl Allergy 2015;5:e6.

87. Nguyen-Luu NU, Ben-Shoshan M, Alizadehfar R, et al. Inadvertent exposures in children with peanut allergy. Pediatr Allergy Immunol 2012;23:133–9.

88. Bartnikas LM, Huffaker MF, Sheehan WJ, et al. Impact of school peanut-free policies on epinephrine administration. J Allergy Clin Immunol 2017;140:465–73.

89. C.S. Mott Children's Hospital. Nut-free lunch? Parents speak out. C.S. Mott Children's Hospital National Poll of Children's Health 2014;20. Available at: https://mottpoll.org/reports-surveys/nut-free-lunch-parents-speak-out.   Accessed November 5, 2020.

90. Gupta RS, Springston EE, Smith B, et al. Food allergy knowledge, attitudes, and beliefs of parents with food-allergic children in the United States. Pediatr Allergy Immunol 2010;21:927–34.

91. Gupta RS, Kim JS, Springston EE, et al. Food allergy knowledge, attitudes, and beliefs in the United States. Ann Allergy Asthma Immunol 2009;103:43–50.

92. Sharma HP, Robinson H, Twichell SA, et al. Food allergy attitudes and beliefs among school nurses in an urban public school district. J Allergy Clin Immunol 2012;129:AB133.

93. Ross NL, Filuk S, Kulbaba B, et al. Impact of food allergy on school-age students: perceptions of Winnipeg parents, teachers and school staff. J Allergy Clin Immunol 2019;143:AB215.

94. Sampson MA, Munoz-Furlong A, Sicherer SH. Risk-taking and coping strategies of adolescents and young adults with food allergy. J Allergy Clin Immunol 2006; 117:1440–5.

95. Watson W, Woodrow AM, Bruce A, et al. Are teachers knowledgeable and confident about dealing with allergy emergencies? Allergy Asthma Clin Immunol 2010; 6:P10.

96. Munoz VL. 'Everybody has to think – do I have any peanuts and nuts in my lunch?' School nurses, collective adherence, and children's food allergies. Sociol Health Illn 2018;40:603–22.

97. Ozen A, Boran P, Torlak F, et al. School board policies on prevention and management of anaphylaxis in Istanbul: Where do we stand? Balkan Med J 2016;33: 539–42.

98. Maciag MC, Sheehan WJ, Bartnikas LM, et al. Detection of food allergens in school and home environments of elementary students. J Allergy Clin Immunol 2021;9(10):P3735–43.

Systemic Allergic Reactions and Anaphylaxis Associated with Allergen Immunotherapy

Yashu Dhamija, MD[a],*, Tolly E.G. Epstein, MD, MS[a,b],
David I. Bernstein, MD[a]

KEYWORDS

- Allergen immunotherapy • Subcutaneous immunotherapy
- Sublingual immunotherapy • Systemic reactions • Anaphylaxis

KEY POINTS

- Fatal reactions (FRs) are uncommon but still occur at a rate of 1 in every 7,000,000 injection visits.
- Risk factors for FRs include uncontrolled asthma, a prior systemic reaction (SR), and allergen immunotherapy (AIT) during the peak pollen season.
- Suggested interventions to reduce SR rates in patients undergoing AIT are reviewed.

INTRODUCTION

Subcutaneous allergen immunotherapy (SCIT) is used to treat allergic rhinitis, asthma, atopic dermatitis, and prevent Hymenoptera sting-induced anaphylaxis.[1,2] The known benefit of SCIT, however, must be considered in each patient relative to the potential risk of a systemic allergic reaction (SR). The lifetime prevalence of anaphylaxis from any cause is estimated to be 0.05% to 2%.[3] Limitations, such as recognition, varying definitions, underreporting, miscoding, and attributable causes, may confound population-based estimates. In 1987, known cases of fatalities due to immunotherapy and skin testing dating back to 1945 were reviewed, leading to the first survey of fatal reactions (FRs).[4,5] Data regarding SRs from allergen immunotherapy (AIT) have been systematically gathered in the North American Immunotherapy Surveillance Study since 2008 and from annual retrospective surveys conducted among members of the American Academy of Allergy, Asthma, & Immunology (AAAAI) and American College of Allergy, Asthma, & Immunology (ACAAI). Although physicians and other health

[a] Division of Immunology, Allergy and Rheumatology, University of Cincinnati College of Medicine, 231 Albert Sabin Way, ML 0563, Medical Science Bldg. (MSB), Rm 7409, Cincinnati, OH 45267-0563, USA; [b] Allergy Partners of Central Indiana, 7430 N Shadeland Ave, Suite 150, Indianapolis, IN 46250, USA
* Corresponding author.
E-mail address: dhamijyu@ucmail.uc.edu

Immunol Allergy Clin N Am 42 (2022) 105–119
https://doi.org/10.1016/j.iac.2021.09.012
0889-8561/22/© 2021 Elsevier Inc. All rights reserved.
immunology.theclinics.com

care professionals' participation rates in these surveys vary from year to year, these annual data evaluate millions of injections administered to more than 200,000 patients by hundreds of allergists/immunologists and their associates.[6] These data result in estimates of the annual incidence of SRs, their severity, and possible risk factors for susceptibility to SRs and anaphylaxis from AIT.[6] Data, collected between 2013 and 2017, indicate that SRs of varying severity occurred in up to 85% of clinical allergy/immunology practices. A mean of 1 SR per 1000 injection visits (0.1%) is estimated to have occurred between 2008 and 2018.[6] Life-threatening or near-fatal anaphylactic events, that is, Grade 4, based on World Allergy Organization (WAO) grading criteria for SRs to SCIT, are relatively uncommon and estimated to occur in 0.005% of patients receiving SCIT injections and in 1/160,000 injection visits.[7] Evidence identifying factors that contribute to SRs and FRs are reviewed in this article. Risk management strategies are proposed to prevent or decrease future SCIT, SRs, anaphylaxis, and FRs.

FATAL REACTIONS AND CONTRIBUTING FACTORS

Fatal anaphylactic reactions from SCIT are rare. Since 1972, 92 confirmed FRs due to SCIT have been reported by physicians in North America.[4–6] From 1990 to 2001, 41 FRs were reported, for an estimated rate of 1 in every 2.5 million injections or 3.4 FR per year.[8] Although the number of reported FRs has decreased, 10 confirmed FR have been reported in the North American Surveillance Study between 2008 and 2019 (1 in every 7.2 million injection visits) in patients receiving care from allergists/immunologists.[6] This includes 5 new confirmed FRs since 2017. The data from the European surveillance study, prospectively obtained in 3 countries from 2012 to 2014, did not report any FR.[9] A lack of reports on FR from European studies is likely limited by geographic reporting and brief, periodic data collection.[9,10]

Details were provided of 273 near-FRs to SCIT injections in the 1990 to 2001 North American Immunotherapy Surveillance Study.[8,11] This survey identified differences between clinical manifestations during FRs and near-fatal anaphylactic reactions manifested by acute respiratory insufficiency and/or hypotension. As illustrated in **Fig. 1**, SRs versus near-FRs were characterized by a more frequent occurrence of

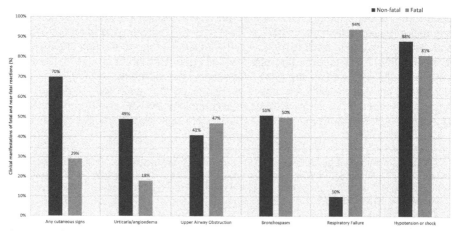

Fig. 1. Fatal reactions: low occurrence of skin manifestations. (*Adapted from* Amin HS, Liss GM, Bernstein DI. Evaluation of near-fatal reactions to allergen immunotherapy injections. J Allergy Clin Immunol. 2006 Jan;117(1):169-75.)

respiratory failure in the absence of cutaneous signs and symptoms. The absence of cutaneous manifestations in these FRs could have delayed recognition and the timely initiation of treatment in some of these cases. **Fig. 2** compares baseline asthma severity characteristics, demonstrating that patients with FRs had higher frequencies of poor asthma control, acute emergency room visits, and hospitalization for asthma, preceding the FR. These data are consistent with other reports, indicating that asthma is a major contributing factor for FRs.

A review of 34 FRs to SCIT from 1985 to 2001 identified contributing risk factors.[7,8,12] After uncontrolled asthma, prior SRs, administration of injections during the peak pollen seasons, sub-optimal treatment of anaphylaxis, and dosing errors were recognized by treating physicians as possible factors contributing to these FRs in at least 35% of reported cases (**Table 1**). Less frequent factors cited include inadequate postinjection observation periods, administration in a medically unsupervised setting, delayed onset of reactions following the 30-min wait, and coadministration of β-blockers or angiotensin-converting enzyme (ACE) inhibitors.[8] No contributing factors were reported in 17% of cases.

FATAL REACTIONS SINCE 2008

Details regarding 10 fatalities that have occurred since 2008 are presented in **Table 1**.[6,13–15] One of the most important findings is that at least 6 of the FRs occurred in patients with asthma; it was unknown whether the other 4 had asthma. At least 2 of the FRs occurred in patients with severe persistent asthma. Another important risk factor in at least 3 FRs was the lack of immediate treatment at the onset of the SRs, in 2 because the patients left the clinic facility before the recommended waiting time, and in the third, because of a lack of recognition of the signs and symptoms of anaphylaxis by health care personnel. At least 2 fatalities occurred in obese individuals. Morbid obesity is suspected to have played a role in lack of response to epinephrine in at least one FR. Two FRs occurred in teenagers and one in a 19-year-old

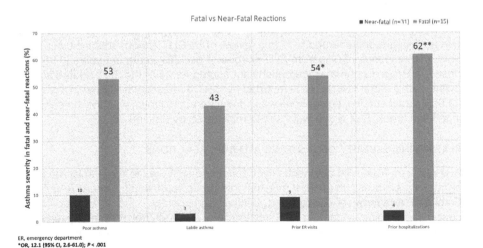

ER, emergency department
*OR, 12.1 (95% CI, 2.6-61.0); *P* < .001
**OR, 34.7 (95% CI, 5.7-251.1); *P* < .001

Fig. 2. Comparison of asthma characteristics: fatal versus near-fatal reactions.[a]OR, 12.2 (95% CI, 2.6-61.0); P < .001. [b]OR, 34.7 (95% CI, 5.7-251.1); P < .001. (*Adapted from* Amin HS, Liss GM, Bernstein DI. Evaluation of near-fatal reactions to allergen immunotherapy injections. J Allergy Clin Immunol. 2006 Jan;117(1):169-75.)

Table 1
Risk factors for SCIT fatal systemic reactions

Risk Factor	Prevalence 1985–2001 (n = 34)
Uncontrolled asthma	62%
Prior systemic reaction	53%
Pollen season	47%
Suboptimal treatment of anaphylaxis (epinephrine)	43%
Dosing error	35%
< 3' observation	12%
Unsupervised setting (home)	9%
Delayed reaction? (onset after 30' observation)	9%
None	17%
β-blocker/ACEI	2%/2%

Abbreviations: ACEI, angiotensin-converting enzyme inhibitor.
Data from Refs [6,10]

woman. More FRs occurred in men, if the information on gender was provided, although the sample size was too small to know whether these data are significant. FRs occurred in both the buildup and maintenance phase of SCIT. At least one FR was associated with an accelerated cluster schedule, that is, the FR occurred at maintenance dose, 2 weeks after cluster buildup.

SYSTEMIC ALLERGIC REACTIONS ASSOCIATED WITH SUBLINGUAL IMMUNOTHERAPY

Patients commonly experience local oral reactions (80% of all treatment-related adverse events) to FDA-approved sublingual immunotherapy (SLIT) products. Six SRs occurred among 8000 patients treated with SLIT.[16] There are rare case reports of anaphylaxis with SLIT, either as drop as or approved sublingual tablet formulations, and no FRs are documented.[17–21] In a review of 66 SLIT studies that included safety data, the incidence of SRs from SLIT is about 1 per 384 treatment years (0.056% of doses).[22] Severe asthma exacerbations accounted for 14 of the SLIT-related adverse events in this same review. None reported hypotension-associated SRs. In a review of 29 SLIT tablet studies, epinephrine was administered 16 times, with the majority given in the first week, 5 of which were self-administered by patients.[23]

CLASSIFYING SEVERITY OF SYSTEMIC ALLERGIC REACTIONS

SRs can vary from mild cutaneous symptoms and signs to life-threatening near-fatal or fatal anaphylaxis.[1] In 2010, a multinational group representing the AAAAI, ACAAI, European Academy of Allergy and Clinical Immunology, and WAO published a consensus grading system for SCIT-related SRs. Although not adapted by regulatory agencies for use in clinical trials, the WAO grading criteria have been used for SCIT reactions in the annual North American Immunotherapy Surveillance Study conducted among practicing allergists/immunologists, since their introduction in 2010. This has enabled the estimation of the annual incidence rate of SCIT-related SRs based on SR severity and identification of factors possibly contributing to Grades 3 and 4 anaphylactic events versus milder Grades 1 and 2. Before the introduction of the

WAO grading system for SCIT-related SRs, the AAAAI/ACAAI North American Immunotherapy Surveillance Study used mild, moderate, and severe reactions to guide responders on grading systemic SRs, retrospectively.[24,25] Before the implementation of the North American Immunotherapy Surveillance Study, studies evaluating SRs categorized reactions simply as mild or severe.[26]

CLINICAL AND OTHER FACTORS THAT ENHANCE THE RISK FOR SYSTEMIC ALLERGIC REACTIONS TO SUBCUTANEOUS ALLERGEN IMMUNOTHERAPY
Asthma

Uncontrolled asthma is a risk factor for SCIT-related SRs. The National Immunotherapy Surveillance Study confirms that uncontrolled asthma is a significant risk factor for nonfatal SRs and severe and fatal SRs. Data consistently show practices treating patients with asthma have higher rates of severe and fatal SRs.[6,14] Two-thirds of all severe Grade 3 or 4 nonfatal SRs occurred in patients with asthma and 50% of Grades 3 and 4 SRs in individuals with severe asthma.[6,13] Clinical practices that did not prescribe SCIT for individuals with uncontrolled asthma reported fewer severe Grade 3 SRs and those who did prescribe SCIT to such individuals reported significantly more Grades 1 and 2 SRs.[6] Other studies also show a higher rate of SRs in patients with asthma.[27–29] Seventy percent of patients with an FEV1 less than 80% predicted versus 12% with an FEV1 $\geq$ 80% of predicted receiving rush SCIT experienced an SR in a prospective trial of 125 patients.[30]

Therefore, routine clinical screening of patients with asthma and, where necessary, measurement of lung function (peak flow spirometry) is recommended prior to SCIT administration.[2] Such screening has resulted in significantly fewer Grades 3 and 4 SRs.[14]

Clinical trial data from Phase 3 allergic rhinitis studies of grass and ragweed pollen and house dust mite (HDM) SLIT indicate no increased risk of SRs for subjects with concomitant asthma.[31–33] However, FDA-approved SLIT tablets are not recommended in patients with uncontrolled asthma.[34] No SRs were reported in a 2016 placebo-controlled trial evaluating efficacy and safety of HDM SLIT tablet therapy for asthma in 834 adult patients not well controlled by inhaled corticosteroids.[35] The safety of commercial therapeutic extract drops used off label for SLIT has not been systematically evaluated in patients with asthma.

Pollen Seasons

Severe and fatal SRs have previously been associated with the administration of SCIT during peak pollen seasons, particularly among highly sensitized individuals.[4,12,15] North American Immunotherapy Surveillance Study data of 34 FRs before 2005 demonstrate that 47% of cases occurred during the pollen season to which the patient was sensitive.[8,12] A similar review of 68 near-fatal SRs between 1990 and 2001 found that 46% of cases occurred during peak allergy seasons, the most commonly cited possible contributing factor for these reactions.[11] The initiation of SCIT during the pollen season was a risk factor for SRs in a 2020 retrospective study of 12,284 injections in 261 children.[36] The results show that most SRs occurred, in decreasing frequency, during the grass, ragweed, and tree pollen seasons.[14,37]

Data from the National Immunotherapy Surveillance Study indicate that clinical practices that do not increase SCIT doses during pollen seasons were less likely to report Grade 2 (moderate) or 3 (severe) SRs.[37] This was most significant for SRs of all severity grades in practices that did not increase SCIT doses in highly sensitized individuals during their peak pollen seasons.[14]

No significant differences in SR rates occurred during versus not during the mountain cedar season in a 2017 retrospective study of patients receiving SCIT for mountain cedar.[38] However, interpretation of this study was limited by the low number of severe SRs. Albuhairi and colleagues also reviewed SCIT injections in 2 groups of 246 pediatric patients, one in which doses were not increased during peak pollen seasons and the other in which they were increased.[39] There was no significant difference in the rate of SRs. In conclusion, because of these differences, more prospective studies are necessary to determine whether and when adjustments of doses during peak pollen seasons are necessary.

Waiting Times, Delayed Systemic Allergic Reactions, Epinephrine Auto-Injectors, and Home Immunotherapy

Most SRs and FRs associated with SCIT occur within the first 30 min of the injection.[2] Inadequate waiting times following SCIT injections and delays in treatment have also been associated with such reactions.[4,6,13] Therefore, the third update of the Immunotherapy Practice Parameter recommends a 30-min postinjection waiting period.[2] Extract manufacturers' product labeling recommend waiting periods of 20 to 30 min.[40,41] Data from the North American Immunotherapy Surveillance Study do not show a difference in SRs for severity based on a 20- or 30-min postinjection waiting time; however, these data may have been skewed by under-reporting of SRs in clinical practices with shorter observation times.[6,13] The 2021 North American Immunotherapy Surveillance Study shows a statistically significant difference in total Grades 3 and 4 SRs versus less severe grades based on the enforcement of postinjection waiting periods, that is, monitoring patient waiting times and requiring check-out with office personnel before leaving postinjection.[6]

A 2019 study indicates that around 15% of SRs may begin after 30 min postinjection, although some studies report up to 50% of SCIT-related SRs after 30 min.[13,42] Most SRs after 30 min are mild or moderate, but severely delayed SRs including anaphylaxis are reported.[42] Therefore, epinephrine autoinjectors should be considered for patients on SCIT, or at least those who are considered to be at higher risk or have had an SR after 30 min. This recommendation is still debated.[43] When last assessed in 2016, almost 30% of practitioners reported that they routinely prescribe epinephrine autoinjectors for all patients on SCIT. However, this did not lower the risk of severe SRs, possibly because of low rates of adherence with the self-administration of autoinjectors among patients experiencing delayed SRs.[13] In fact, surveillance data show that only 8% to 30% of patients used prescribed autoinjectors for severe Grades 3 or 4 SRs that began after departing the outpatient injection facility.[13] Based on these data, it is estimated that 8,261 patients would have to be prescribed epinephrine auto-injectors for one delayed SR.[44]

Home administration of SCIT is not recommended due to risks associated with delays in the recognition and administration of epinephrine. These concerns arise from previous rare reports of FRs associated with home administration.[2,8,36] The only possible exception, whereby the benefit of home administration could outweigh the risk, is for patients with a history of Hymenoptera sting-induced anaphylaxis, with no access to a medical facility, requiring venom immunotherapy (VIT).[2] Informed consent is necessary and the patient must be educated on recognizing the signs and symptoms of an SR and its treatment.

Accelerated Buildup

Accelerated regimens refer to "cluster" and "rush" buildup protocols for AIT. Cluster AIT involves administering 2 or more SCIT injections per day that are subsequently increased every 2 to 7 days with the goal of achieving maintenance therapy more rapidly.[45] Rush schedules are used to increase doses every 15 to 60 min over 1–3 consecutive days until the target dose is achieved.[46] North American Immunotherapy Surveillance Study data from 270 practices show that 27% use cluster and 12% rush protocols; however, 93% of patients are initiated on standard buildup protocols.[15] Cluster and rush buildups were associated with a higher incidence of SR per injection, than slow buildup, in a 5-year review of a large, multicenter practice. A higher incidence of SRs (11.9%) occurred for cluster versus standard or rush protocols, 2.8% and 2.5, respectively.[47] The North American Immunotherapy Surveillance Study data show a significant increase in the risk of Grades 1 to 4 SRs in practices using cluster therapy.[14,37]

Practices that require a lower final cluster dose before transitioning to maintenance had a lower SR rate.[7,15] This suggests that practices that switch from accelerated buildup to conventional SCIT before reaching maintenance have a lower SR rate (689 SRs) than those which continue an accelerated buildup until maintenance (1,023 SRs).

Doses of Allergen

The National Surveillance Study assessed the relationship between allergen doses and SRs. Practices with Grade 3 versus those with Grade 1 SRs used higher doses of standardized doses of standard HDM allergen products, 1,000 and 1,999 allergy units ($P = .025$). No similar significant dose–response relationship was found with grass pollen or cat allergen products.[48] SR rates identified in small studies indicate that higher target doses for maintenance are linked with higher rates of SRs.[49–51]

Previous Systemic Allergic Reactions to Subcutaneous Allergen Immunotherapy

In Year 2 of the North American Immunotherapy Surveillance Study among 630 participating practices, approximately 25% of patients with an SR had a history of a previous SR.[7] In a review of 177 SRs occurring in a practice of 459 patients receiving 74,183 SCIT injections, a history of SR was not identified as a risk for subsequent SRs.[52] Smaller studies show approximately one-third to two-thirds of patients with an SR typically had Grade 1 SRs.[29,53]

It is unclear whether the severity of a subsequent SR is related to the previous SR. For example, among patients in a study from 2010 to 2011 who experienced severe delayed SRs, none had prior SRs.[24] There is also no consensus about dose adjustment strategies following SRs; however, stopping SCIT should be considered with repeated SRs.[2] In summary, prior SRs are considered the second most common risk factor for FRs.

Large Local Reactions

There is conflicting evidence about the risk of SRs following prior large local reactions. This could be due to how such reactions are defined, that is, size and duration.[54] Two retrospective studies show no difference in the incidence of SRs between dose-adjustments and no-dose-adjustment protocols in patients with large SCIT local reactions. Other retrospective studies found that among patients with SRs, the rate of large local reactions preceding SR events was up to fourfold greater.[55–58] In summary, large local reactions are poor predictors for future local reactions as well as SRs.[52,58,59] Also, appropriate intervention for these reactions remains unknown.[60]

Morbid Obesity

Morbid obesity is not a risk factor for severe SRs.[15] North American Immunotherapy Surveillance Study data collected from 2016 to 2018 also did not show an increased rate of severe SRs from SCIT in patients with morbid obesity when adjusting for its prevalence in the general population.[6] Body mass index was identified as a risk factor in China tor local reactions but not SRs in a study of 91 children receiving HDM SCIT.[61]

Risks of Concomitant Medications

A theoretic concern about the use of β-blockers in patients on SCIT exists because of the theoretically increased risk of mast cell mediators and inadequate response to injectable epinephrine associated with β-receptor blockade.[62] However, the use of β-blockers has not been associated with an increased frequency of SRs to SCIT. The AIT Practice Parameter recommends avoiding SCIT in patients requiring β-blockers even though there is little evidence to support this recommendation.[2] Hepner and colleagues evaluated more than 3,000 patients over 1 year and identified one with an SR who was on a β-blocker.[63] Future randomized controlled trials (RCTs) to evaluate the safety of β-blockers in AIT are unlikely due to ethical considerations and the need for large sample sizes.[64]

The use of β-blockers in patients receiving VIT for anaphylaxis to Hymenoptera stings is justified when considering the risk versus the benefit of VIT.[62] β-blocker use concern arose from a single case report of an FR in a patient receiving VIT while on a β-blocker.[65] Retrospective studies, however, support the use of β-blockers in patients receiving VIT.[66]

Cases of severe anaphylaxis in patients receiving ACE inhibitors have been anecdotally reported in patients on VIT. However, the assessment of large patient databases did not find an association between their use and SRs to SCIT.[13,67,68]

MITIGATING RISK FOR SYSTEMIC ALLERGIC REACTIONS: WHAT HAVE WE LEARNED?

There is no precise approach to predict the relative risk of SCIT. It is incumbent on the practicing allergist/immunologist to gauge the risk–benefit for each patient for prescribing SCIT or SLIT. For example, in general, SCIT should not be used in patients with uncontrolled asthma and those with compromised baseline lung function, that is, pretreatment FEV1 $\leq$ 70%. Practices avoiding SCIT in patients with uncontrolled asthma versus those that provide such therapy report 70% fewer life-threatening Grade 4 SRs.[14] Alternative therapies, whereby necessary, should be considered in such patients in lieu of SCIT, for example, biological agents.

Patients with asthma are at highest risk for any SR including severe SRs and strategies to mitigate risk are outlined in **Box 1**. Preinjection asthma screening is recommended, that is, assessing asthma symptoms at the injection visit. This also provides for the opportunity to assess the patient's clinical status and when necessary, treat exacerbations.[7]

General recommendations to improve the safety of SCIT are listed in **Box 2**. It should be administered only in facilities whereby staff members are trained to recognize and treat SRs.[7] Careful monitoring of SCIT patients for at least 30 min following an injection and requiring checkout with staff members may reduce this risk.[13]

Pharmacotherapy for the Prevention of Systemic Allergic Reactions

Pretreatment can reduce rates of SRs. Treatment with an antihistamine 2 hours before a SCIT injection significantly reduced the rate of severe SRs and shortened the time for

Box 1
Suggested strategies to reduce the risk of anaphylaxis in patients with asthma undergoing AIT.

1. Preinjection screening for asthma symptoms with or without lung function.
2. Do not initiate SCIT or SLIT in patients with uncontrolled asthma.
3. Withhold SCIT and use alternative treatments in patients with severe, treatment-refractory asthma.
4. Consider potentially safer modalities of AIT (eg, SLIT for patients with controlled asthma).
5. Administer SCIT injections only in adequately equipped clinic facilities with medical staff trained to manage anaphylaxis.
6. Adherence to the 30-min postinjection observation period and check out system.

Abbreviations: AIT, allergen immunotherapy; SCIT, subcutaneous immunotherapy; SLIT, sublingual immunotherapy.

Adapted from Bernstein DI, Epstein TEG. Safety of allergen immunotherapy in North America from 2008-2017: Lessons learned from the ACAAI/AAAAI National Surveillance Study of adverse reactions to allergen immunotherapy. Allergy Asthma Proc. 2020 Mar 1;41(2):108-111.

the target dose for cedar pollen and dust mite in an open-label prospective study of 134 patients.[69] Pretreatment with a combination of H-1 and H-2 antihistamines and prednisone likewise reduced the occurrence of SRs to rush therapy for mixed allergens.[70] A prospective RCT of omalizumab in patients with persistent asthma showed significantly fewer SRs to SCIT with perennial allergens.[71] Omalizumab also significantly reduced the rate of SRs to rush immunotherapy.[72,73] However, cost-effectiveness using omalizumab remains a major concern.[74] Pretreatment with second-generation antihistamines also reduced the rates of SRs and large local reactions for accelerated buildup schedules.[75,76] However, in spite of this evidence, there is no definitive evidence to support routine pretreatment with antihistamines to prevent SRs with a routine SCIT buildup schedule.

Box 2
General recommendations for improving SCIT tolerability in all treated patients

1. Modify doses or discontinue SCIT after grade 3 or 4 SRs.
2. Adapt clinic protocols to prevent dosing errors.
3. Administer SCIT injections only in clinics with adequate facilities, and personnel to manage anaphylaxis, and adhere to a 30-min observation period.
4. Modify allergen doses in highly sensitized patients during peak aeroallergen periods.
5. Consider reducing target doses for an accelerated cluster buildup.
6. Prescribe self-injectable epinephrine in SCIT patients at heightened risk for SRs.

Abbreviation: SCIT, subcutaneous immunotherapy.

Adapted from Bernstein DI, Epstein TEG. Safety of allergen immunotherapy in North America from 2008-2017: Lessons learned from the ACAAI/AAAAI National Surveillance Study of adverse reactions to allergen immunotherapy. Allergy Asthma Proc. 2020 Mar 1;41(2):108-111.

LESSONS LEARNED FROM COVID-19

The COVID-19 pandemic, beginning in 2020, resulted in interruptions in SCIT administration worldwide. Close to 30% of patients who suspend their AIT treatment may not resume it.[77] This is in spite of the fact that the total number of patients on AIT has increased during the COVID-19 pandemic. Strategies used to mitigate this decrease include deferring initiation, extending the interval between doses, discontinuing patients at an increased risk of complications from COVID-19, and considering SLIT as an alternative treatment.[78–80] COVID-19-related restrictions also have provided an opportunity to evaluate the impact of lengthening the time interval between doses for aeroallergens and still maintain efficacy and safety. Optimal strategies to restart SCIT following a break are also indicated. Studies designed to help answer these questions are necessary and ongoing.[81]

SUMMARY

Although the rates of SRs have declined to an estimated rate of 1 per 1000 injections, FRs still occur. A risk stratification before the initiation of AIT may be of value to better select patients for such treatment. Risk versus benefit is a consideration for any treatment program, including SCIT. Risk factors for FRs include the following: uncontrolled asthma, a history of SR, and injections administered during a peak pollen season. Suggested interventions to reduce AIT SR rates are outlined in **Boxes 1** and **2**. Unmet needs include the safety of SLIT versus SCIT in high-risk populations and safety of modified recombinant allergens. In addition, the impact of COVID-19 on the use of SCIT and SLIT, as well as SRs, is still unclear.

CLINICS CARE POINTS

- Although rates of systemic reactions to SCIT have declined over the years, FRs continue to be reported.
- The most cited potential contributing factors to FRs to SCIT are uncontrolled asthma, a history of prior systemic reaction, administration during pollen season, suboptimal treatment of systemic reactions, and dosing errors.
- A risk–benefit consideration is recommended before initiation for all patients to identify high-risk individuals.
- Suggestions are presented in **Boxes 1** and **2** of the article to reduce rates of systemic and FRs to SCIT.

DISCLOSURE

No external funding for this article. All authors have no financial relationships relevant to this article to disclose. All authors have indicated they have no potential conflicts of interest to disclose.

REFERENCES

1. Cox L, Larenas-Linnemann D, Lockey RF, et al. Speaking the same language: The World Allergy Organization subcutaneous immunotherapy systemic reaction grading system. J Allergy Clin Immunol 2010;125(3):569–74, 574 e1-574 e7.
2. Cox L, Nelson H, Lockey R, et al. Allergen immunotherapy: a practice parameter third update. J Allergy Clin Immunol 2011;127(1 Suppl):S1–55.
3. Simons FE. Anaphylaxis. J Allergy Clin Immunol 2010;125(2 Suppl 2):S161–81.

4. Lockey R, Benedict L, Turkeltaub P, et al. Fatalities from immunotherapy (IT) and skin testing (ST). J Allergy Clin Immunol 1987;79(4):660–77.

5. Reid M, Lockey R, Turkeltaub P, et al. Survey of fatalities from skin testing and immunotherapy 1985–1989. J Allergy Clin Immunol 1993;92(1):6–15.

6. Epstein TG, Murphy-Berendts K, Liss GM, et al. Risk factors for fatal and nonfatal reactions to immunotherapy (2008-2018): postinjection monitoring and severe asthma. Ann Allergy Asthma Immunol 2021;127(1):64–9.e1.

7. Bernstein DI, Epstein TEG. Safety of allergen immunotherapy in North America from 2008-2017: Lessons learned from the ACAAI/AAAAI National Surveillance Study of adverse reactions to allergen immunotherapy. Allergy Asthma Proc 2020;41(2):108–11.

8. Bernstein DI, Wanner M, Borish L, et al. Twelve-year survey of fatal reactions to allergen injections and skin testing: 1990-2001. J Allergy Clin Immunol 2004; 113(6):1129–36 (Research Support, Non-U.S. Gov't) (In eng).

9. Calderón MA, Vidal C, Rodríguez del Río P, et al. European Survey on Adverse Systemic Reactions in Allergen Immunotherapy (EASSI): a real-life clinical assessment. Allergy 2017;72(3):462–72.

10. Moreno C, Cuesta-Herranz J, Fernandez-Tavora L, et al. Immunotherapy Committee SEdAeIC. Immunotherapy safety: a prospective multi-centric monitoring study of biologically standardized therapeutic vaccines for allergic diseases. Clin Exp Allergy 2004;34(4):527–31.

11. Amin HS, Liss GM, Bernstein DI. Evaluation of near-fatal reactions to allergen immunotherapy injections. J Allergy Clin Immunol 2006;117(1):169–75.

12. Reid MJ, Lockey RF, Turkeltaub PC, et al. Survey of fatalities from skin testing and immunotherapy 1985-1989 (Research Support, U.S. Gov't, P.H.S.) (In eng). J Allergy Clin Immunol 1993;92(1 Pt 1):6–15. Available at: http://www.ncbi.nlm. nih.gov/pubmed/8335856.

13. Epstein TG, Liss GM, Berendts KM, et al. AAAAI/ACAAI subcutaneous immunotherapy surveillance study (2013-2017): fatalities, infections, delayed reactions, and use of epinephrine autoinjectors. J Allergy Clin Immunol Pract 2019;7(6): 1996–2003 e1.

14. Epstein TG, Liss GM, Murphy-Berendts K, et al. Risk factors for fatal and nonfatal reactions to subcutaneous immunotherapy: National surveillance study on allergen immunotherapy (2008-2013). Ann Allergy Asthma Immunol 2016; 116(4):354–9.e2.

15. Epstein TG, Liss GM, Murphy-Berendts K, et al. AAAAI/ACAAI surveillance study of subcutaneous immunotherapy, years 2008-2012: an update on fatal and nonfatal systemic allergic reactions. J Allergy Clin Immunol Pract 2014;2(2): 161–7.e3.

16. Bernstein DI, Bardelas JA Jr, Svanholm Fogh B, et al. A practical guide to the sublingual immunotherapy tablet adverse event profile: implications for clinical practice. Postgrad Med 2017;129(6):590–7.

17. Blazowski L. Anaphylactic shock because of sublingual immunotherapy overdose during third year of maintenance dose. Allergy 2008;63(3):374.

18. de Groot H, Bijl A. Anaphylactic reaction after the first dose of sublingual immunotherapy with grass pollen tablet. Allergy 2009;64(6):963–4.

19. Antico A, Pagani M, Crema A. Anaphylaxis by latex sublingual immunotherapy. Allergy 2006;61(10):1236–7.

20. Eifan AO, Keles S, Bahceciler NN, et al. Anaphylaxis to multiple pollen allergen sublingual immunotherapy. Allergy 2007;62(5):567–8.

21. Cochard MM, Eigenmann PA. Sublingual immunotherapy is not always a safe alternative to subcutaneous immunotherapy. J Allergy Clin Immunol 2009; 124(2):378–9.

22. Cox LS, Linnemann DL, Nolte H, et al. Sublingual immunotherapy: a comprehensive review. J Allergy Clin Immunol 2006;117(5):1021–35.

23. Nolte H, Casale TB, Lockey RF, et al. Epinephrine use in clinical trials of sublingual immunotherapy tablets. J Allergy Clin Immunol Pract 2016;5(1):84–9.e3.

24. Epstein TG, Liss GM, Murphy-Berendts K, et al. Immediate and delayed-onset systemic reactions after subcutaneous immunotherapy injections: ACAAI/AAAAI surveillance study of subcutaneous immunotherapy: year 2. Ann Allergy Asthma Immunol 2011;107(5):426–431 e1 (Research Support, Non-U.S. Gov't) (In eng).

25. Bernstein DI, Epstein T, Murphy-Berendts K, et al. Surveillance of systemic reactions to subcutaneous immunotherapy injections: year 1 outcomes of the ACAAI and AAAAI collaborative study. Ann Allergy Asthma Immunol 2010;104(6):530–5 (Randomized Controlled Trial Research Support, Non-U.S. Gov't) (In eng).

26. Matloff SM, Bailit IW, Parks P, et al. Systemic reactions to immunotherapy (In eng). Allergy Proc 1993;14(5):347–50. Available at:http://www.ncbi.nlm.nih.gov/pubmed/8288117.

27. Liu JL, Ning WX, Li SX, et al. The safety profile of subcutaneous allergen immunotherapy in children with asthma in Hangzhou, East China. Allergol Immunopathol (Madr) 2017;45(6):541–8.

28. González-Diaz SN, De La Rosa-López JH, Arias-Cruz A, et al. Reacciones sistémicas relacionadas a la inmunoterapia con alergenos en Monterrey, México. Rev Alerg Mex 2011;58(2):79–86.

29. Erdem SB, Nacaroglu HT, Karaman S, et al. Risk of systemic allergic reactions to allergen immunotherapy in a pediatric allergy clinic in Turkey. Int J Pediatr Otorhinolaryngol 2016;84:55–60.

30. Bousquet J, Hejjaoui A, Dhivert H, et al. Immunotherapy with a standardized dermatophagoides pteronyssinus extract: III. Systemic reactions during the rush protocol in patients suffering from asthma. J Allergy Clin Immunol 1989;83(4): 797–802.

31. Nolte H, Bernstein DI, Nelson HS, et al. Efficacy of house dust mite sublingual immunotherapy tablet in North American adolescents and adults in a randomized, placebo-controlled trial. J Allergy Clin Immunol 2016;138(6):1631–8.

32. Maloney J, Prenner BM, Bernstein DI, et al. Safety of house dust mite sublingual immunotherapy standardized quality tablet in children allergic to house dust mites. Ann Allergy Asthma Immunol 2016;116(1):59–65.

33. Nolte H, Amar N, Bernstein DI, et al. Safety and tolerability of a short ragweed sublingual immunotherapy tablet. Ann Allergy Asthma Immunol 2014;113(1): 93–100.e3.

34. Greenhawt M, Oppenheimer J, Nelson M, et al. Sublingual immunotherapy: a focused allergen immunotherapy practice parameter update. Ann Allergy Asthma Immunol 2017;118(3):276–82.e2.

35. Virchow JC, Backer V, Kuna P, et al. Efficacy of a house dust mite sublingual allergen immunotherapy tablet in adults with allergic asthma: a randomized clinical trial. JAMA 2016;315(16):1715–25.

36. Gur Cetinkaya P, Kahveci M, Esenboga S, et al. Systemic and large local reactions during subcutaneous grass pollen immunotherapy in children. Pediatr Allergy Immunol 2020;31(6):643–50.

37. Epstein TG, Liss GM, Murphy-Berendts K, et al. AAAAI and ACAAI surveillance study of subcutaneous immunotherapy, Year 3: what practices modify the risk of systemic reactions? Ann Allergy Asthma Immunol 2013;110(4):274–8.e1.

38. Wong PH, Quinn JM, Gomez RA, et al. Systemic reactions to immunotherapy during mountain cedar season: implications for seasonal dose adjustment. J Allergy Clin Immunol Pract 2017;5(5):1438–9.e1.

39. Albuhairi S, Sare T, Lakin P, et al. Systemic reactions in pediatric patients receiving standardized allergen subcutaneous immunotherapy with and without seasonal dose adjustment. J Allergy Clin Immunol Pract (Cambridge, MA) 2018;6(5):1711–6.e4.

40. ALK-Abello, Inc.. Standardized mite, mixed injection, solution [package insert]. U.S. Food and Drug Administration website. 2020. Available at: https://dailymed.nlm.nih.gov/dailymed/fda/fdaDrugXsl.cfm?setid=4a3539da-7f51-401b-8ac2-101b8a4658f4&type=display. Accessed August 15, 2021.

41. Nelco Laboratories, Inc.. Allergenic Exract [package insert]. U.S. Food and Drug Administration website. 2009. Available at: https://dailymed.nlm.nih.gov/dailymed/fda/fdaDrugXsl.cfm?setid=ade1e6ce-57e8-4b25-9a07-636f2df69d36&type=display. Accessed August 15, 2021.

42. Bernstein DI, Epstein T. Systemic reactions to subcutaneous allergen immunotherapy. Immunol Allergy Clin North Am 2011;31(2):241–9, viii-ix. (Review) (In eng).

43. Fitzhugh DJ, Bernstein DI. Should epinephrine autoinjectors be prescribed to all patients on subcutaneous immunotherapy? J Allergy Clin Immunol Pract 2016;4(5):862–7.

44. Bernstein D, Tankersley M, Russell H. Controversies in allergy: injectable epinephrine should be prescribed to all patients on subcutaneous aeroallergen immunotherapy. J Allergy Clin Immunol Pract (Cambridge, MA) 2020;8(4):1211–5.

45. Parmiani S, Fernández Távora L, Moreno C, et al. Clustered schedules in allergen-specific immunotherapy. Allergologia Immunopathol (Madr) 2002;30(5):283–91.

46. Smits WL, Giese JK, Lotz KL, et al. Safety of rush immunotherapy using a modified schedule: a cumulative experience of 893 patients receiving multiple aeroallergens (In eng). Allergy Asthma Proc 2007;28(3):305–12. Available at: http://www.ncbi.nlm.nih.gov/pubmed/17619559.

47. Winslow AW, Turbyville JC, Sublett JW, et al. Comparison of systemic reactions in rush, cluster, and standard-build aeroallergen immunotherapy. Ann Allergy Asthma Immunol 2016;117(5):542–5.

48. Liss GM, Murphy-Berendts K, Epstein T, et al. Factors associated with severe versus mild immunotherapy-related systemic reactions: a case-referent study. J Allergy Clin Immunol 2011;127(5):1298–300 (Letter Research Support, U.S. Gov't, Non-P.H.S.) (In eng).

49. Moreno V, Alvariño M, Rodríguez F, et al. Randomized dose-response study of subcutaneous immunotherapy with a Dermatophagoides pteronyssinus extract in patients with respiratory allergy. Immunotherapy 2016;8(3):265–77 (In English).

50. Holland CL, Samuels KM, Baldwin JL, et al. Systemic reactions to inhalant immunotherapy using 1:1 target dosing. Ann Allergy Asthma Immunol 2014;112(5):453–8.

51. Sola J, Da Silva Ferreira JA, Dionicio Elera J, et al. Timothy grass pollen therapeutic vaccine: optimal dose for subcutaneous immunotherapy. Immunotherapy 2016;8(3):251–63 (In English).

52. Sani S, Gupta R, Fonacier L, et al. Risk stratification of systemic reactions to subcutaneous immunotherapy: a retrospective study. Allergy Asthma Proc 2019; 40(5):338–42.
53. DaVeiga SP, Liu X, Caruso K, et al. Systemic reactions associated with subcutaneous allergen immunotherapy: timing and risk assessment. Ann Allergy Asthma Immunol 2011;106(6):533–7.e2.
54. Lieberman P, Tankersley M. Significance of large local reactions that occur during allergen immunotherapy. J Allergy Clin Immunol Pract 2015;3(2):310–1.
55. Tankersley MS, Butler KK, Butler WK, et al. Local reactions during allergen immunotherapy do not require dose adjustment. J Allergy Clin Immunol 2000;106(5): 840–3.
56. Kelso JM. The rate of systemic reactions to immunotherapy injections is the same whether or not the dose is reduced after a local reaction. Ann Allergy Asthma Immunol 2004;92(2):225–7.
57. Roy SR, Sigmon JR, Olivier J, et al. Increased frequency of large local reactions among systemic reactors during subcutaneous allergen immunotherapy. Ann Allergy Asthma Immunol 2007;99(1):82–6.
58. Calabria CW, Stolfi A, Tankersley MS. The REPEAT study: recognizing and evaluating periodic local reactions in allergen immunotherapy and associated systemic reactions. Ann Allergy Asthma Immunol 2011;106(1):49–53.
59. Calabria CW, Coop CA, Tankersley MS. The LOCAL Study: local reactions do not predict local reactions in allergen immunotherapy. J Allergy Clin Immunol 2009; 124(4):739–44 (In eng).
60. Epstein TE, Tankersley MS. Are allergen immunotherapy dose adjustments needed for local reactions, peaks of season, or gaps in treatment? J Allergy Clin Immunol Pract (Cambridge, MA) 2017;5(5):1227–33.
61. Yang Y, Ma D, Huang N, et al. Safety of house dust mite subcutaneous immunotherapy in preschool children with respiratory allergic diseases. Ital J Pediatr 2021;47(1):101.
62. Nelson HS. Allergy immunotherapy for inhalant allergens: Strategies to minimize adverse reactions. Allergy Asthma Proc 2020;41(1):38–44.
63. Hepner MJ, Ownby DR, Anderson JA, et al. Risk of systemic reactions in patients taking beta-blocker drugs receiving allergen immunotherapy injections. J Allergy Clin Immunol 1990;86(3 Pt 1):407–11. Available at: http://www.ncbi.nlm.nih.gov/entrez/query.fcgi?cmd=Retrieve&db=PubMed&dopt=Citation&list_uids=1976666.
64. Lang DM. Do β-blockers really enhance the risk of anaphylaxis during immunotherapy? Curr Allergy Asthma Rep 2008;8(1):37–44 (In English).
65. Fatal course of Vespula venom immunotherapy: pretreatment withdrawl of the beta blocker may have been involved. Novartis Found Symp 2004;257:226–7. Available at:.
66. Muller UR, Haeberli G. Use of beta-blockers during immunotherapy for Hymenoptera venom allergy. J Allergy Clin Immunol 2005;115(3):606–10 (Research Support, Non-U.S. Gov't) (In eng).
67. White KMMD, England RWMD. Safety of angiotensin-converting enzyme inhibitors while receiving venom immunotherapy. Ann Allergy Asthma Immunol 2008; 101(4):426–30.
68. Stoevesandt J, Hain J, Stolze I, et al. Angiotensin-converting enzyme inhibitors do not impair the safety of Hymenoptera venom immunotherapy build-up phase. Clin Exp Allergy 2014;44(5):747–55.

69. Yoshihiro O, Yoshinori N, Kiyotaka M. Effect of pretreatment with fexofenadine on the safety of immunotherapy in patients with allergic rhinitis. Ann Allergy Asthma Immunol 2006;96(4):600–5.

70. Portnoy J, Bagstad K, Kanarek H, et al. Premedication reduces the incidence of systemic reactions during inhalant rush immunotherapy with mixtures of allergenic extracts. Ann Allergy 1994;73(5):409–18.

71. Massanari M, Nelson H, Casale T, et al. Effect of pretreatment with omalizumab on the tolerability of specific immunotherapy in allergic asthma. J Allergy Clin Immunol 2010;125(2):383–9.

72. Casale TB, Busse WW, Kline JN, et al. Omalizumab pretreatment decreases acute reactions after rush immunotherapy for ragweed-induced seasonal allergic rhinitis. J Allergy Clin Immunol 2006;117(1):134–40.

73. Casale TB, Kline JN, Busse WW, et al. Omalizumab pretreatment prevents allergic reactions due to rush immunotherapy (RIT). J Allergy Clin Immunol 2005;115(2):S65.

74. Rosenberg JL. Lack of pretreatment cost-effectiveness and side effects of omalizumab versus prednisone/montelukast on tolerability of immunotherapy. J Allergy Clin Immunol 2011;127(2):548 (In English).

75. Nielsen L, Johnsen CR, Mosbech H, et al. Antihistamine premedication in specific cluster immunotherapy: a double-blind, placebo-controlled study. J Allergy Clin Immunol 1996;97(6):1207–13.

76. Berchtold E, Maibach R, MÜLler U. Reduction of side effects from rush-immunotherapy with honey bee venom by pretreatment with terfenadine. Clin Exp Allergy 1992;22(1):59–65.

77. Tsao LR, Villanueva SA, Pines DA, et al. Impact of rapid transition to telemedicine-based delivery on allergy/immunology care during COVID-19. J Allergy Clin Immunol Pract 2021;9(7):2672–2679 e2.

78. Shaker MS, Oppenheimer J, Grayson M, et al. COVID-19: Pandemic contingency planning for the allergy and immunology clinic. J Allergy Clin Immunol Pract 2020;8(5):1477–88.e5.

79. Searing DA, Dutmer CM, Fleischer DM, et al. A phased approach to resuming suspended allergy/immunology clinical services. J Allergy Clin Immunol Pract 2020;8(7):2125–34.

80. Compalati E, Erlewyn-Lajeunesse M, Runa Ali F, et al. Allergen immunotherapy in the era of sars-cov-2. J Investig Allergol Clin Immunol 2020;30(6):459–61.

81. Larenas-Linnemann DE, Epstein T, Ponda P, et al. Gaps in allergen immunotherapy administration and subcutaneous allergen immunotherapy dose adjustment schedules: Need for prospective data. Ann Allergy Asthma Immunol 2020;125(5):505–6.e2.

Anaphylaxis to Drugs, Biological Agents, and Vaccines

Ruchi H. Shah, MD, Margaret M. Kuder, MD, MPH, David M. Lang, MD*

KEYWORDS

- Anaphylaxis • Aspirin-exacerbated respiratory disease
- Contrast-induced anaphylaxis • Drug-induced anaphylaxis
- NSAID-Induced anaphylaxis • Vaccine-induced anaphylaxis

KEY POINTS

- -Drug allergy is a common cause of anaphylaxis in adults, most often from antibiotic or analgesic use.
- There are few antibiotics with well-validated skin testing concentrations; however, evaluation by a board-certified allergist/immunologist in cases of antibiotic anaphylaxis is paramount to consider skin testing and graded dose challenge.
- Aspirin and NSAIDs may cause serious adverse reactions, including anaphylaxis; desensitization can be accomplished successfully for patients with aspirin-exacerbated respiratory disease and nonsteroidal anti-inflammatory drug-induced urticaria/angioedema, but not for patients with nonsteroidal anti-inflammatory drug exacerbated cutaneous disease.
- As the use of biological agents is becoming more common, immediate and nonimmediate hypersensitivity reactions are being observed; elucidating the mechanism for these reactions can direct the next steps in diagnosis and management.
- Risk of anaphylaxis after vaccines is rare; when it occurs, typically this is due to an additive rather than the active antigen component.

INTRODUCTION

Anaphylaxis is a life-threatening systemic reaction, defined by a range of clinical characteristics. Definitions for the diagnosis of anaphylaxis generally include acute onset and involvement of multiple organ systems.[1] The reported prevalence of anaphylaxis is 1.6% to 5.1%,[1,2] which is increasing, and is likely an underestimate.[3] Older age and comorbidities (eg, cardiac and lung disease) are associated with greater risk for severe anaphylaxis.[4] The most common inciting agents for anaphylaxis are foods,

Department of Allergy and Clinical Immunology, Respiratory Institute, Cleveland Clinic
* Corresponding author.
E-mail address: LANGD@ccf.org

Immunol Allergy Clin N Am 42 (2022) 121–144
https://doi.org/10.1016/j.iac.2021.10.001
0889-8561/22/© 2021 Elsevier Inc. All rights reserved.

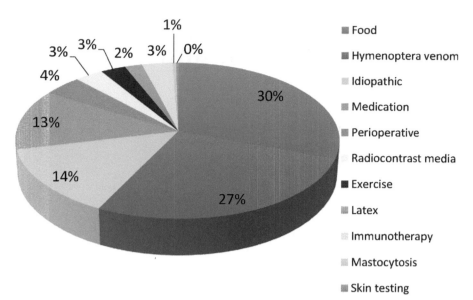

Fig. 1. Causative agents for anaphylaxis. This pie figure displays relative proportions of causes for anaphylaxis in the Department of Allergy and Clinical Immunology at Cleveland Clinic for 730 cases from July 2002 to October 2013. Food allergy was the most common etiology of anaphylaxis, followed by hymenoptera venom, idiopathic anaphylaxis, and medications; 3.6% of cases had more than a single cause for anaphylaxis.

hymenoptera venom, and medications (**Fig. 1**).[5] The frequency of these triggers varies by age: for adults medications and hymenoptera venom are more commonly observed, for children, foods, and hymenoptera venom.[2]

DRUGS

Drugs account for a large proportion of anaphylaxis cases in adults, ranging from 22% to 42%, depending on geographic location. In the United States, 1% of the population experiences at least one episode of drug-induced anaphylaxis (DIA).[6] In an electronic medical record (EMR) review of over 2.7 million patients, 14% of individuals in the United States reported a drug-induced hypersensitivity reaction (HSR), 8% were consistent with anaphylaxis.[6]

The incidence of DIA increases with age. In a Latin American registry, DIA comprised 43.5% of cases in those over 40 years old, 33% of cases in 18 to 40 years old, and 20% of cases in those under 20 years old.[7] These findings have been replicated in other countries.[8,9] Apart from age, female sex is associated with higher rates of DIA and more severe reactions.[9,10] Although older individuals may acquire this risk due to greater medication exposures, chromosomal genetics, or hormonal factors could account for the female predilection for DIA.

DIA is associated with increased reaction severity; for this reason, in evaluating potential etiologies it is paramount to maintain a high index of suspicion for DIA. Among emergency department visits for anaphylaxis, DIA has been associated with more frequent hospitalizations.[9] DIA is more likely to result in fatality, accounting for over half of anaphylaxis fatalities in the United States and Australia.[11,12] Antibiotics, radioiodinated urographic contrast media (RUCM), and other diagnostic agents have been implicated most commonly in fatal anaphylactic events.[11]

The most common causative agents for DIA are antibiotics and analgesics, dependent on geographic location. In the United States, antibiotics account for 66% of DIA cases.[13] Data from the United Kingdom and China report similar rates. Studies from Portugal and Latin America found nonsteroidal anti-inflammatory drugs (NSAIDs) comprised the majority (73%) of DIA cases.[7] The causes of these variations are unknown, but likely are related to drug prescription patterns and genetic predisposition for HSRs.

Antibiotics

Although nearly one-third of patients report allergy to antibiotics, this is still a relatively rare occurrence. Although up to 15% of individuals self-report beta-lactam allergy,[14] fewer individuals have documented cases of anaphylaxis. A review of 1.7 million patients found penicillin anaphylaxis in 45.9 per 10,000 patients, followed by sulfonamides (15.1 per 10,000 patients), cephalosporins (6.1 per 10,000 patients), and macrolides (3.8 per 10,000 patients).[13] Fatal anaphylactic events are rare: one fatal anaphylactic event from oral amoxicillin was found over 35 years, with 100 million treatment courses in the United Kingdom.[15]

The prevalence of antibiotic-induced anaphylaxis is low; nevertheless, the life-threatening nature of this reaction necessitates careful evaluation when drug allergy is listed in the medical record. It is imperative to determine which patients with self-reported allergy are at risk for anaphylaxis and should avoid future exposure to a given medication. Alternatively, it is important to identify which patients can safely reintroduce antibiotics listed as "allergic", as needless avoidance is also associated with untoward outcomes.[16] Thoughtful consideration of drug allergy history, risk factors, and availability of validated testing all play a role in determining appropriate antibiotic allergy evaluation.

DIA can occur through immunologic or nonimmunologic means. Nonimmunologic reactions involve direct stimulation of mast cells or basophils. This occurs more commonly with analgesic medications, but is also reported with RUCM and antibiotics (eg, vancomycin). Comprehensive clinical history, skin testing, and/or serologic testing can aid in identifying IgE-mediated sensitivity.

Anaphylaxis is a clinical diagnosis. When clinical suspicion is warranted, based on symptoms that occur soon after antibiotic exposure, skin testing is often the next step. Drug skin testing involves percutaneous ("prick") and intradermal skin tests at nonirritating concentrations.[17,18] This is a safe procedure, even in individuals with a history of severe anaphylaxis. Validity of these skin tests varies considerably by drug. For example, skin testing for penicillin is well-established, and carries a high negative predictive value of 98%.[19,20] Most other antibiotic skin testing is based on limited data of nonirritating concentrations.

Serum-specific IgE testing to beta-lactams is available, but not recommended due to poor sensitivity. A negative result necessitates skin testing, thus most providers proceed directly to skin testing. Basophil activation testing measures mediator release after in vitro basophil stimulation. This testing is not frequently used, as it has low sensitivity and limited availability.[21]

If skin testing and/or serologic evaluation is negative, observed direct provocation challenge is recommended. This can be conducted as a single dose or a graded-dose challenge, depending on drug reaction history and patient risk factors. Much of the data regarding the safety of oral challenge derives from beta-lactams. After negative penicillin skin testing with major and minor determinants, only 2% to 3% of individuals exhibit clinical reaction—generally mild and limited to the skin—on challenge.[20,22]

If skin testing is positive, continued avoidance with the use of an equally efficacious alternative is recommended. When no equally effective substitute can be used, drug desensitization can be performed. This procedure induces drug tolerance using gradually increasing doses of the medication. Drug desensitization does not "cure" the IgE-mediated sensitivity, but rather induces a temporary state of tolerance to allow for treatment.[23] Anaphylaxis during this procedure is infrequent, but still can occur.

Nonsteroidal Anti-inflammatory Drugs

Aspirin (ASA) and NSAIDs have been implicated in a wide variety of adverse reactions, including cutaneous reactions in patients with NSAID exacerbated cutaneous disease (NECD) and NSAID-induced urticaria angioedema (NIUA), and respiratory reactions in patients with aspirin-exacerbated respiratory disease (AERD)—each occurring via cyclooxygenase (COX)-1 inhibition.[24–26] Although patients and health care providers may label such reactions as an "allergy", it is important to establish the understanding that such reactions are more related to biochemistry than to IgE-mediated pathogenesis. Aspirin and NSAIDs also account for other drug-induced adverse reactions—including anaphylaxis[27,28]; in contrast to the above sensitivity syndromes, patients with single NSAID-induced urticaria, angioedema, or anaphylaxis (SNIUAA) do not cross-react with structurally unrelated NSAIDs. The characteristics of these aspirin sensitivity syndromes are displayed in **Table 1**.

AERD

The initial report of ASA intolerance appeared more than a century ago, only 3 years after aspirin was synthesized.[29] Fatal reactions from aspirin were described in the 1930s.[30,31] However, it was not until 1968 that Samter and Beers described a clinical "triad" of nasal polyposis, bronchial asthma, and "life-threatening reactions to acetylsalicylic acid" as a clinical syndrome.[32]

Table 1 Aspirin sensitivity syndromes			
Aspirin Sensitivity Syndrome	Underlying Condition	Cross-Reaction with Structurally Unrelated COX-1 Inhibitors	Induction of Tolerance Achievable
AERD	Chronic Rhinosinusitis with Nasal Polyposis and Asthma*	Yes	Yes
NECD	Chronic Urticaria	Yes	No
NIUA	N/A	Yes	Yes
SNIUAA	N/A	No	Possibly

Abbreviations: AERD: aspirin-exacerbated respiratory disease; NECD: Nonsteroidal anti-inflammatory drug exacerbated cutaneous disease; NIUA: Nonsteroidal anti-inflammatory drug-induced urticaria/angioedema; SNIUAA: Single nonsteroidal anti-inflammatory drug-induced urticaria, angioedema, and/or anaphylaxis.

* In a small proportion of AERD cases, chronic rhinosinusitis with nasal polyps is present without asthma.[24]

In patients with AERD, respiratory reaction with potentially serious bronchospasm occurs after exposure to ASA or an ASA-like drug; even a subtherapeutic dosage of ASA or NSAID can lead to potentially life-threatening bronchospasm. ASA and NSAIDs, including ibuprofen, naproxen, indomethacin, and so forth, share the action of COX-1 inhibition and are 100% cross-reactive in AERD patients. Cross-reaction may also occur with higher doses of nonacetylated salicylates[33] or acetaminophen,[34] which are poor inhibitors of COX-1 and COX-2. Selective inhibitors of COX-2 (eg, celecoxib) do not cross-react.[35]

AERD affects an estimated 7% of adult asthmatics, and twice as many with severe asthma.[36] AERD generally develops in the 3rd or 4th decade of life.[37] Once AERD develops, it is present lifelong.

The pathogenesis of respiratory reaction provoked by ASA or NSAID in patients with AERD is related to COX-1 inhibition.[24,37] COX-1 blockade leads to loss of inhibition of the enzyme PGE_2, leading in turn to the activation of inflammatory cells—mast cells, basophils, eosinophils, and platelets, and excessive production of histamine, PGD2, tryptase, and sulfidopeptide leukotrienes (LTC_4, LTD_4, LTE_4). Upper and/or lower respiratory reaction occurs in 30 to 180 minutes. These inflammatory cells and mediators also contribute to ongoing airway obstruction and inflammation that persists in AERD despite avoidance of ASA and other COX-1 inhibiting drugs.[24] Although AERD includes several phenotypes,[38] this condition can appropriately be designated as an endotype in terms of being a mechanistically distinct asthma subgroup.

ASA-provoked reaction can be attenuated by administration of antileukotriene drugs; however, the protection is incomplete, and the response is heterogeneous.[39] Antileukotriene drugs shift the dose-response curve to the right, and transfer ASA-provoked reaction to the upper airway. More recently, omalizumab has also been associated with attenuation of ASA-provoked respiratory reaction.[40]

Management of AERD includes avoidance of ASA/NSAIDs, medications as appropriate based on best evidence for chronic rhinosinusitis with nasal polyps (CRSwNP) and asthma, and performance of sinus surgery in properly selected patients.[24]

The term "desensitization" has traditionally been used to describe a procedure that entails modification of IgE-mediated (allergic/anaphylactic) potential to a substance—frequently an antibiotic such as penicillin, via its repetitive administration in a graded-dose fashion. Widal managed a patient in 1922,[41] with gradually increasing doses of ASA, such that instead of reacting when a previously-established provoking dose was administered, ASA re-exposure was tolerated without adverse reaction. Zeiss and Lockey[42] observed the same phenomenon of tolerance induction, and ultimately this procedure was used to allow individuals with AERD who required ASA (eg, for the treatment of cardiovascular conditions) to take ASA safely.

The ASA desensitization procedure, in which a state of "tolerance" can be induced and maintained, entails the administration of incremental oral doses of aspirin until a dosage of 325 mg can be taken without respiratory reaction.[24] Several protocols for ASA desensitization have been published,[43] some including intranasal ketorolac challenge.[44] ASA tolerance can be perpetuated indefinitely if ASA is taken on a daily basis.

Improvement with ASA desensitization treatment has included improved upper and lower airway symptoms, reduced medication reliance, and less morbidity as reflected in fewer annual episodes of infection and fewer sinus surgery procedures over time.[45] ASA desensitization can be considered for patients with AERD who are not well controlled, including those with frequent corticosteroid reliance and/or refractory rhinosinusitis who require repeated sinus surgeries.[24]

Dupilumab, omalizumab, and mepolizumab are efficacious for the treatment of patients with AERD,[46,47] and have been approved by the FDA for refractory asthma and

CRSwNP, respectively. Each has been associated with improved outcome measures of upper and lower airways and quality of life. No head-to-head studies comparing the relative efficacy or safety of these biologic agents have been published to date, nor has there been a study comparing a biological agent vis-à-vis ASA desensitization for treatment outcomes of AERD.

There are 5 randomized controlled trials,[48–52] as shown in **Table 2**, in which the efficacy of ASA desensitization treatment was assessed. All demonstrated benefit, however, several do not provide high-quality evidence in support of ASA desensitization treatment as a therapeutic intervention. Of note is the study by Swierczynska-Krepa, and colleagues—which included subjects who were ASA-tolerant. In contrast to the benefit observed in AERD subjects, those without AERD exhibited no benefit with ASA compared with placebo, underscoring the importance of not encouraging patients who are ASA tolerant to proceed with the daily administration of ASA with the expectation this may have a salutary effect.

NONSTEROIDAL ANTI-INFLAMMATORY DRUG EXACERBATED CUTANEOUS DISEASE

Approximately 20% to 30% of patients with chronic urticaria have NECD—which entails the acute exacerbation of urticaria/angioedema with exposure to ASA/NSAID.[53] This can be viewed as a cutaneous form of ASA sensitivity in which all agents that inhibit COX-1, via release of cysteinyl leukotrienes,[54] provoke the exacerbation of the underlying disease. Similar to AERD, COX-2 inhibitors are tolerated in patients with NECD without untoward reaction. Attempts to induce tolerance via desensitization protocols have been unsuccessful, and in general, these patients should be encouraged to avoid ASA and NSAIDs. When ASA is clearly indicated without an equally effective alternative, such as for cardioprotection,[53] direct challenge should be carried out as the provoking dose for the reaction is frequently less than 81 mg.

NONSTEROIDAL ANTI-INFLAMMATORY DRUGS-INDUCED URTICARIA ANGIOEDEMA

In patients with NIUA, ASA/NSAIDs provoke urticaria or angioedema in the absence of underlying chronic urticaria. The mechanism also entails COX-1 inhibition. These patients will also cross-react with structurally unrelated NSAIDs. If favorable from an individualized risk/benefit standpoint, when aspirin is required for primary or secondary cardioprotection, NIUA patients are candidates for ASA challenge. In contrast to NECD, when a reaction occurs the induction of tolerance in properly selected cases can be achieved.[53]

SINGLE NON-STEROIDAL ANTI-INFLAMMATORY DRUG INDUCED URTICARIA, ANGIOEDEMA, AND/OR ANAPHYLAXIS (SNIUAA)

Although any NSAID can theoretically cause anaphylaxis, this has been most commonly recognized with certain NSAIDs, such as phenylbutazone.[55] Anaphylaxis has also been observed more frequently than expected with tolmetin.[56] Zomepirac,[57] a structurally analogous pyrrole acetic acid differing in structure by only one methyl and one chlorine atom, was voluntarily withdrawn by its manufacturer from the US market, based on more than 1000 suspected "allergic" reactions, including 5 deaths.[58]

Typically, anaphylaxis is provoked by a single NSAID or 2 NSAIDs that are structurally similar.[26] Patients with DIA to one NSAID generally tolerate structurally unrelated NSAIDs, including ASA, without untoward reaction; unlike AERD and NECD, all

Table 2
Randomized controlled trials examining the role of aspirin desensitization in aspirin-exacerbated respiratory disease

	Study Design	Subjects Enrolled	Subjects Completing Participation	Results	Comments
Stevenson et al,[48] 1984	RDBPC Cross-over	38	25	Improved symptoms and reduced medication reliance for rhinosinusitis, 50/50 for asthma. Trend for greater improvement with higher ASA dose	Subjects were treated with 325 mg daily, 325 mg QID, 650 mg QID.
Fruth et al,[49] 2013	RDBPCPG	70	31	Improved rhinosinusitis symptoms and QOL, trends for lower polyp score and polyp relapse.	Subjects enrolled after sinus surgery. ASA desensitization treatment dose 100 mg/d.
Swierczynska-Krepa et al,[52] 2014	RDBPCPG	20	15	Improved symptoms, SNOT-20, ACQ, PNIF, ICS reliance	ASA-tolerant asthmatics also randomized to treatment or placebo – no benefit with ASA
Esmaelizadeh et al,[50] 2015	RDBPCPG	39	31	Improved symptom scores, FEV1, QOL.	Antihistamines, beta-agonists, corticosteroids suspended 48 h before intranasal ketorolac/oral ASA challenge
Mortazavi et al,[51] 2017	RDBPCPG	41	38	Improved symptom and medication scores, FEV1, QOL.	Antihistamines, beta-agonists, corticosteroids suspended 48 h before intranasal ketorolac/oral ASA challenge

Abbreviations: ACQ, asthma control questionnaire; ASA, aspirin; FEV1, forced pexired volume in 1 s; ICS, inhaled corticosteroid; PNIF, peak nasal inspiratory flow; QOL, quality of life; RDBPC, randomized, double-blind, placebo-controlled; RDBPCPG, randomized, double-blind, placebo-controlled, parallel-group.

NSAIDs need not be avoided. Positive skin tests have been reported in cases of anaphylaxis to pyrazolones[29]; however, in most cases, it is prudent to recommend avoidance of the culprit drug and structurally similar NSAIDs, and perform oral challenge under observation to ASA or a structurally dissimilar NSAID. Some reactions may occur via IgE-mediated pathogenesis; however, DIA with initial exposure to the NSAID implies non–IgE-mediated anaphylaxis also accounts for a proportion of these cases.[30] Desensitization is generally not recommended for patients with NSAID-provoked anaphylaxis, as a structurally unrelated NSAID that is, equally efficacious can be tolerated. Should anaphylaxis occur related to ASA, assuming this is IgE-mediated and that ASA is required without an equally effective substitute—for example, for secondary cardioprotection, a desensitization procedure may be entertained. However, IgE-mediated anaphylaxis to aspirin is very rare, if it exists at all.

BLENDED REACTIONS

It should also be noted there are patients who exhibit a "blend" of cutaneous and respiratory reaction, with/without gastrointestinal symptoms, to ASA/NSAIDs,[59] and do not neatly fit into one of the categories displayed in **Table 1**. This subgroup has not been as well characterized, but seems to reflect a combination of AERD and NIUA, which otherwise present as distinct phenotypes.

Radioiodinated Urographic Contrast Media

Anaphylaxis to RUCM is relatively rare, reported in 0.02% to 0.04% of patients.[60] Fatal anaphylaxis is reported in 1 to 3 per 100,000 RUCM administrations. Most reactions begin within 5 minutes of RUCM exposure. These reactions were thought to be primarily nonimmunologic, reflecting mast cell/basophil degranulation leading to anaphylaxis. However, recent data also implicate IgE-mediated sensitization accounting for RUCM HSRs.

These media previously were high-osmolar relative to plasma, consisting of a single benzene ring that ionized in solution. This was associated with a relatively high rate of adverse reactions (including non–IgE-mediated HSRs), with one study identifying a prevalence of 12.66%. In the late 1980s, low-osmolar contrast media were introduced. These monomers dissolved in water, but did not dissociate, thus their "low osmolar" designation. Rates of adverse reactions were much lower. Iso-osmolar agents that do not dissolve in solution have also been developed. These also have a lower rate of adverse reactions. Iso-osmolar agents have been associated with a higher rate of HSRs than low-osmolar agents.[61]

Standard of care for the management of prior reactors who require administration of RUCM involved pretreatment with antihistamines and corticosteroids. Administering these medications at specific time intervals to prior reactors before RUCM re-exposure significantly reduced the rate of HSRs. Because high-osmolality contrast material is rarely used, pretreatment has become more controversial. A 2020 systematic review found no reduction of risk for HSRs in patients receiving glucocorticoid and/or antihistamine pretreatment, with a calculated risk ratio of 1.07 (95% CI 0.67–1.71).[1] Davenport and colleagues found that premedication with a 13-h prednisone regimen was associated with increased length of hospital stay, longer time to obtain imaging, and increased risk of hospital-acquired infections.[62] Based on this evidence, the 2020 anaphylaxis practice parameter issued a conditional recommendation against the use of prophylactic glucocorticoid and/or antihistamine pretreatment for prior reactors who require RUCM.[1]

Skin testing is not routine; however, this may be considered in the evaluation of selected patients with RUCM anaphylaxis. Skin testing may be performed with undiluted RUCM, and if negative completing intradermal testing with a 1:10 dilution.[60,63] If positive, testing to other RUCMs may also be performed. Cross-reactivity between different RUCMs has been defined sufficiently to guide the use of alternative agents.[64]

Gadolinium-based Contrast Media

Gadolinium is a heavy metal with paramagnetic properties that provides contrast for intravascular or intraluminal use in MRI studies. Gadolinium-based contrast media (GBCM) can be categorized based on net charge (ionic or nonionic) and structure (linear or macrocyclic),[65,66] as shown in **Table 3**.

Adverse reactions to GBCM occur at a lower rate than to RUCM. The rate of anaphylaxis ranges from 0.004% to 0.7%; severe reactions occur rarely, in a range of 0.001%–0.01%.[67] Fatal anaphylaxis has been reported.[68]

Similar to RUCM reactions, pathogenesis frequently entails activation of mast cells and basophils due to the hyperosmolar nature of GBCM, with elevation in serum tryptase.[65] Some cases of anaphylaxis occur on first exposure to GBCM, consistent with a non–IgE-mediated mechanism. However, wheal/flare reaction on skin testing has also been reported[69]; positive Prausnitz–Kustner reaction has been observed.[70]

As is the case for RUCM, elevated risk for anaphylaxis exists in prior reactors with re-exposure to GBCM and has been reported in association with female gender, patients with "drug allergy", "food allergy", or patients with a history of "allergies and asthma".[71] It is unclear whether patients who have had non–IgE-mediated anaphylaxis from RUCM are directly at elevated risk from receiving GBCM, as there may be an indirect hazard associated with shared risk factors; however, the overwhelming most of the prior reactors to RUCM tolerate GBCM without adverse reaction.

Skin testing with a panel of GBCM has been recommended to confirm IgE-mediated potential to the GBCM associated with anaphylaxis and to identify a skin test negative alternative GBCM that can be used.[65] When GBCM administration is required despite wheal/flare reactions to all GBCM, desensitization can be performed so that GBCM re-exposure can be tolerated without remarkable untoward reaction.[72]

Management of anaphylaxis to GBCM is similar to anaphylaxis from other causes, with the additional recommendation that patients be immediately removed from the imaging room so that none of the resuscitative equipment becomes a magnetic threat.[67]

BIOLOGICAL AGENTS

Monoclonal antibodies (mAB) are used as targeted therapy in many medical conditions—including allergic/immunologic disorders, chronic inflammatory conditions, and malignancy. As mAB are used more commonly, more frequent HSRs, both immediate and nonimmediate, have been observed.[73] As detailed in **Table 4**, there are 3 categories of immediate reactions associated with mAB; clinical symptoms vary accordingly.[73] Elucidating the likely mechanism of reaction can direct next steps in evaluation and management.[73]

Omalizumab

Omalizumab is a humanized mAB administered subcutaneously for treatment of moderate to severe allergic asthma, chronic idiopathic urticaria, and nasal polyps.[63] Its mechanism of action entails the formation of small immune complexes with free IgE antibodies.[74] Anaphylaxis to omalizumab is rare and has been reported in 0.09% to

Table 3
Gadolinium-based contrast agents

Brand Name	Generic Name	Molecular Structure and Net Charge	Comments
Magnevist	Gadopentetate dimeglumine	Linear, ionic	Oldest agent in use
MultiHance	Gadobenate dimeglumine	Linear, ionic	
Omniscan	Gadodiamide	Linear, nonionic	
Dotarem, Clariscan	Gadoterate meglumine	Macrocyclic, ionic	
ProHance	Gadoteridol	Macrocyclic, nonionic	Lowest osmolality and viscosity
Gadavist	Gadobutrol	Macrocyclic, nonionic	Highest viscosity
Eovist	Gadoxetate disodium	Linear, ionic	Used for hepatic imaging

0.2% of patients.[75,76] A majority occur within 1 hour of administration. Delayed reactions have also been reported. Two hours observation after the first 3 doses of omalizumab, when anaphylaxis is more likely,[76] has been recommended, followed by 30 minutes with subsequent doses.[75] More recently, at-home administration was approved by the FDA for properly selected patients.[77] A recent case-control study found a prior history of anaphylaxis was associated with greater risk of anaphylaxis to omalizumab (odds ratio (OR): 8.1; 95% confidence interval (CI): 2.7–24.3)[78] The mechanism of anaphylaxis to omalizumab is unclear. In the same study, no serum IgE or IgG toward omalizumab was detected in 21 patients with anaphylaxis.[78] Skin testing protocols have been described, using skin prick testing with full strength omalizumab and intradermal testing with a 1:10,000 dilution. In patients with HSR to omalizumab, it is not recommended to rechallenge. Successful desensitization has been reported.[79]

Anti-IL-5/IL-5 Receptor Biologics

Mepolizumab

Mepolizumab, approved for the treatment of persistent asthma, CRSwNP, and eosinophilic granulomatosis polyangiitis is a humanized mAb that exerts its effect by binding to IL-5. The FDA package insert reports no anaphylaxis.[80,81] In several studies of subjects with severe eosinophilic asthma treated with mepolizumab, there were no

Table 4
Mechanisms of immediate HSRs to monoclonal antibodies

Mechanism	Clinical Features	Skin Test
IgE mediated	• May occur on first exposure but onset usually after at least one exposure • Elevated tryptase	Positive
IgG mediated	• Onset usually after several exposures	Negative
Cytokine release syndrome	• Fever and chills • Onset usually on first exposure	Negative

Adapted from Picard M, Galvão VR. Current Knowledge and Management of Hypersensitivity Reactions to Monoclonal Antibodies. J Allergy Clin Immunol Pract. 2017 May-Jun;5(3):600 to 609.

reports of anaphylaxis.[80,82,83] DREAM, a multicenter study done between 2009 and 2011, reported HSRs in $\leq$ 1% of patients who received mepolizumab, than 2% who received placebo. There were no reports of anaphylaxis.[80,84]

Reslizumab
Reslizumab is an IL-5 antagonist mAb used in the treatment of persistent asthma. An RCT reported 2 subjects of 477 randomized to reslizumab had anaphylaxis.[85] A study looking at long-term safety data reported no cases of anaphylaxis.[86] The FDA prescribing information reports anaphylaxis in 3 patients treated with reslizumab[80,85]

Benralizumab
Benralizumab is a humanized mAb that binds to the α-subunit of the IL-5 receptor used for the treatment of severe eosinophilic and allergic asthma.[87] The FDA label describes a 3% incidence of HSRs (anaphylaxis, urticaria, rash, and angioedema) in subjects randomized to benralizumab.[87] A meta-analysis of 8 RCTs did not show an increased risk of HSR with benralizumab than placebo.[80,88]

Dupilumab
Dupilumab, a humanized mAb, binds to the α unit of the IL-4 receptor and modulates signaling of IL-4 and IL-13. It is approved for the treatment of atopic dermatitis, refractory asthma, and CRSwNP.[89] one meta-analysis that analyzed 8 RCTs comparing dupilumab to placebo found dupilumab had a higher incidence of injection-site reactions, conjunctivitis, and headache, but no cases of anaphylaxis.[80,90] In the 2019 EMA report, anaphylactic reaction or angioedema was reported in 3 patients, and anaphylactic shock was reported in one patient.[80,91] The FDA drug report for dupilumab describes no information about anaphylaxis.[80,89]

Lanadelumab
Lanadelumab is a humanized mAb used for the treatment of hereditary angioedema, which inhibits plasma kallikrein.[92] In a 2018 study with 84 subjects, one treated with lanadelumab developed oral tingling and pruritus without need for treatment.[93] There have been no reports of anaphylaxis.[80]

Anti-CD20 biologics
Rituximab is a chimeric mAb against CD20, used in the treatment of B-cell malignancies and certain autoimmune conditions.[73,94] Immediate reactions have been associated with rituximab in 25% to 50% of patients on first exposure, with fewer reported reactions in patients with inflammatory conditions than malignancies.[73,94] Most reactions were likely consistent with cytokine release syndrome; IgE-mediated reactions were also reported. Though TNF-a and IL-6 levels were shown to correlate with the severity of reaction, these reactions may present solely with cutaneous and respiratory symptoms without classic cytokine syndrome symptoms such as fevers, chills, or rigors.[95,96] Some patients will go on to tolerate further exposures, often with premedication; others will initially tolerate rituximab, then develop immediate HSRs on subsequent exposures.[73,97] The latter group should be considered to have IgE-mediated reactions unless proven otherwise.[73] Skin testing protocols have been reported.[97] In patients thought to have IgE-mediated reaction, desensitization can be considered.[98] In patients whose reactions are thought to be consistent with cytokine release syndrome, premedication with acetaminophen, antihistamines, corticosteroids, and alteration of infusion rates have been recommended.[73,94,96] Ofatumumab and obinutuzumab are human and humanized mAbs, respectively, which also target CD20 in the treatment of B cell malignancies. These have not been as well studied as rituximab. Both have been reported to cause immediate

HSRs in more than 50% on first exposure. This has been thought to be caused by cytokine release and may occur even with pretreatment.[99,100] Skin testing has not been described. Severe and fatal reactions to ofatumumab have occurred.[101]

Cetuximab

Cetuximab is a chimeric mAB that binds and targets the epidermal growth factor receptor (EGFR) for the treatment of head and neck, lung, skin, and colorectal cancers.[73] An interesting phenomenon was discovered related to HSRs to cetuximab: the prevalence of immediate HSRs to cetuximab was less than 3%, except in the southeastern United States, whereby the prevalence was 22%.[73,102] Interestingly, Chung and colleagues found that 17/25 (68%) of patients with a severe immediate HSR to cetuximab on first exposure had pre-existing IgE antibodies directed against an oligosaccharide, galactose-alpha-1,3 galactose (alpha-gal), present on the mAB. Alpha-gal antibodies were then associated with delayed-onset IgE-mediated reactions to mammalian meats.[103] With further investigation, the Lone Star tick was identified as the main etiology for sensitization to alpha-gal in the United States.[104] Skin testing protocols and a serum-specific anti-cetuximab IgE test are available for the evaluation of patients who have had immediate HSR to cetuximab; however, preemptive skin testing or blood studies before administration are not currently recommended. In patients with positive skin testing or a detectable anti-cetuximab IgE greater than 0.35, desensitization can be attempted.[73,105–107] Panitumumab, a fully human mAB which also targets EGFR and does not contain alpha-gal, may be used as an alternative.[108,109]

TNF-a inhibitors

Multiple TNF-a inhibitors are used in the treatment of autoimmune conditions— including but not limited to: rheumatoid arthritis, psoriasis, inflammatory bowel disease, and ankylosing spondyloarthritis. Infliximab is a chimeric mAB that is, administered intravenously, while others such as certolizumab (humanized), adalimumab (fully human), golimumab (fully human), and etanercept (fusion protein) are administered subcutaneously.[110–113] IgE-mediated reactions have been implicated as the cause of injection site as well as systemic reactions with TNF-a inhibitors. About 10% of patients treated with infliximab develop immediate HSRs with symptoms ranging from flushing, pruritus, dyspnea, dizziness/hypotension as well as headache, fevers, and chills. Although these reactions can occur with first exposure, they are more commonly present after multiple exposures.[63] Systemic reactions have rarely been reported with subcutaneous TNF-a inhibitors.[63] Skin testing protocols have been published for the evaluation of immediate reactions to infliximab. If skin testing is positive, or patients have severe or recurrent HSRs, desensitization can be attempted.[63] Anti-infliximab antibodies can also be measured. Anti-infliximab antibodies do not cross-react with anti-adalimumab antibodies, but patients who develop anti-infliximab antibodies may be more prone to developing anti-adalimumab antibodies.[114] Switching to adalimumab remains an option for patients who develop an immediate reaction to infliximab.[115] One case series evaluating 12 patients who developed injection site and systemic reactions to adalimumab and etanercept showed that all had a positive skin test to the culprit mAB, implying an IgE-mediated cause of reaction.[116] For patients in whom an IgE-mediated reaction is suspected, desensitization can be performed.[116] Immediate HSRs related to other commonly prescribed biologics are summarized in **Table 5**.[73,98,117–121]

Table 5
Summary of biologics and reported hypersensitivity reactions

Biologic	Type of Biologic	Conditions Treated	Reaction type Reported	Skin Testing Reported?	Successful Desensitization Reported?
Trastuzumab	Humanized mAb targeting HER2	Breast cancer	Immediate hypersensitivity: reactions consistent with cytokine release syndrome and/or IgE mediated[74]	Yes[118]	Yes[118]
Pertuzumab	Humanized mAb targeting HER2	Breast cancer	Immediate hypersensitivity	Yes[119]	Yes[119]
Tocilizumab	Humanized mAb targeting IL-6	RA and polyarticular juvenile arthritis	Immediate hypersensitivity	Yes[120]	Yes[121]
Bevacizumab	Humanized mAb targeting VEGF	Multiple cancers	Immediate hypersensitivity	Yes[74,98]	Yes[74,98]
Brentuximab	Chimeric mAb	CD30+ lymphoma	Immediate hypersensitivity	No[74,122]	Yes[74,122]

Abbreviations: HER2, human epidermal growth factor receptor 2; IL-6, interleukin 6; mAb, monoclonal antibody; RA, rheumatoid arthritis; VEGF, vascular endothelial growth factor.

Table 6
Vaccine additives commonly associated with allergic reaction[a]

Vaccine	Relevant Additives to Consider
MMR	• Gelatin[127,128] • Alpha-gal[127] • Previous concern, no longer clinically relevant: egg[127]
MMRV	• Gelatin[127,128] • Alpha-gal[127]
Varicella	• Gelatin[127,128] • Alpha-gal[127]
Zoster	• Gelatin[127,128] • Alpha-gal[127] • Polysorbate 80[a,132]
Influenza	• Polysorbate 20[a,132] • Polysorbate 80[a,132] • Previous concern, no longer clinically relevant: egg[127]
Intranasal live attenuated influenza vaccine	• Potential concern: alpha-gal[127]
DTaP, TdaP	• Polysorbate 80[a,132] • Potential concern: cow's milk[127]
Yellow Fever	• Gelatin[127,128] • Potential concerns: egg, chicken[127]
Rabies	• Potential concerns: egg[127]
Hepatitis A	• Polysorbate 20[a,132]
Hepatitis B	• Polysorbate 80[a,132] • Potential concern: yeast[127]
Hepatitis A&B	• Polysorbate 20[a,132]
Oral polio vaccine	• Potential concern: cow's milk[127]
Pneumococcal 13-valent	• Polysorbate 80[a,132]
HPV	• Polysorbate 80[a,132]
Japanese encephalitis	• Polysorbate 80[a,132]
Rotavirus	• Polysorbate 80[a,132]
Meningococcal group	• Polysorbate 80[a,132]
Combination vaccines: • DTaP + IPV • DTaP + HepB + IPV • DTaP + IPV • DTap + IPV + HepB + Hib	• Polysorbate 80[a,132]
SARS-CoV-2 (AstraZeneca, Johnson&Johnson)	• Polysorbate 80[a,132]
SARS-CoV2 (Moderna, Pfizer)	• PEG2000[a,132]

Abbreviations: DTaP, diphtheria tetanus acellular pertussis; HepB, hepatitis B; Hib, haemophilus influenzae B; HPV, human papillomavirus; IPV, inactivated polio vaccine; MMR, measles, mumps, rubella; MMRV, measles, mumps, rubella, varicella; TDaP, tetanus, diphtheria, acellular pertussis.
   [a] dose dependent on vaccine manufacturer.

VACCINES

The risk of anaphylaxis after any vaccine is rare: 1.31 per million vaccine doses.[122] To induce an immune response, vaccines must contain an active component (the antigen) and additional components or additives. Rather than the antigen of the vaccine, immediate HSR is caused by additives such as gelatin, latex, yeast, and egg protein (**Table 6**).[123,124] More recently, alpha-gal, polysorbate 80 and polyethylene glycol (PEG) have been implicated as causes of vaccine-associated anaphylaxis.[123–125] An IgE-mediated reaction to a vaccination typically occurs promptly after vaccination. Classic symptoms include urticaria, angioedema, flushing, pruritus, wheezing, dyspnea, and hypotension.[63] Patients who develop IgE-mediated symptoms after vaccination should undergo skin testing to both the vaccine (using an identical dose and manufacturer) as well as potential culprit components that are contained in the vaccine (gelatin, egg, and so forth).[63,126]

Skin testing protocols for vaccine anaphylaxis include skin prick testing with 1:1 concentration, and if negative, proceeding to intradermal testing using a 1:100 dilution. Skin testing to components (eg, egg, latex) should be done in the standard manner.[127] Patients who test positive to the vaccine should be considered allergic; however, in selected cases, patients with positive skin tests have received the vaccine without immediate reaction.[63,127] Patients with a known allergy to a component may warrant further evaluation via skin testing. For example, a patient with a known history of gelatin allergy should be tested before receiving the varicella-zoster, MMR, or rabies vaccine.[63]

If a patient tests positive for a culprit component, the patient may still potentially receive the vaccine in a graded fashion. Kelso and colleagues published a 5 step protocol[127] which is adapted later in discussion in **Table 7**.

Egg allergy was a concern for patients receiving the influenza vaccine. However, the amount of ovalbumin protein in egg-based vaccines is below the threshold for reaction. The most recent practice parameter, published in 2017, indicated that egg-allergic patients who receive any influenza vaccine, even those that are egg-based, are at no greater risk for a systemic allergic reaction than patients without egg allergy.[128]

The COVID-19 pandemic has led to the rapid development of 3 new vaccines granted emergency-use authorization by the FDA: Pfizer-BioNTech, Moderna, and Janssen. The Pfizer and Moderna vaccines use mRNA packaged in lipid nanoparticles; the Janssen vaccine uses a modified adenovirus as a vector. Recent data describe an anaphylaxis rate of 5.0 cases per million for the Pfizer-BioNTech, and 2.8 cases per million for the Moderna vaccine.[124] Severe allergic reactions (including anaphylaxis), thrombosis with thrombocytopenia, Guillain–Barré syndrome, and capillary leak syndrome have been reported following administration of the Janssen COVID-19 Vaccine during mass vaccination outside of clinical trials.[129] Etiologies for anaphylaxis to these vaccines are not fully understood. Potential causes include

Table 7 Protocol for graded dose vaccine administration	
(1)	0.05 mL 1:10 Dilution
(2)	0.05 mL full-strength
(3)	0.1 mL full-strength
(4)	0.15 mL full-strength
(5)	0.2 mL full-strength

For a vaccine with a normal dose volume of 0.5 mL, these doses may be administered at 15-min intervals as tolerated under direct medical supervision. Observation should span at least 30 min after the last dose.

Table 8
Polyethylene glycol testing protocol

| | PEG 3350 | | Control | Polysorbate 20 | | Polysorbate 80 | |
	Miralax	Methyl-prednisolone Acetate (Depo-Medrol)	Methyl-prednisolone Sodium Succinate (Solu-medrol)	Hepatitis a Vaccine or Twinrix	Triamcinolone Acetonide	Refresh-Sterile eye drops	Prevnar 13
Step 1 Epicutaneous	1:100 (1.7 mg/ml)	40 mg/mL	40 mg/mL	1:1	40 mg/mL	1:1	1:10
Step 2 Epicutaneous	1:10 (17 mg/mL)						
Step 3 Epicutaneous	1:1 (170 mg/mL)						
Step 4 Intradermal		0.4 mg/mL	0.4 mg/mL	1:100	0.4 mg/mL	1:10	1:100
Step 5 Intradermal		4 mg/mL	4 mg/mL	1:10	4 mg/mL		
Step 6 Intradermal					40 mg/mL		

Adapted from Banerji A, Wickner PG, Saff R, Stone CA Jr, Robinson LB, Long AA, Wolfson AR, Williams P, Khan DA, Phillips E, Blumenthal KG. mRNA Vaccines to Prevent COVID-19 Disease and Reported Allergic Reactions: Current Evidence and Suggested Approach. J Allergy Clin Immunol Pract. 2021 Apr;9(4):1423 to 1437.

an IgE-mediated response to PEG, an ingredient in both mRNA vaccines, complement activation mediated by RNA exposure, contact system activation by nucleic acid, and direct mast cell activation.[124,130] PEG and related macrogols are found as an ingredient in colonoscopy preparations, bowel adjuncts, PEGylated agents and as an excipient in multiple oral and injectable medications. PEG has been previously implicated in anaphylactic reactions.[131] PEG has been reported to cross-react with other macrogols, including polysorbate, which has also been identified as a rare cause of allergic reactions to vaccines.[132] The Janssen vaccine contains polysorbate-80 as an excipient. **Table 8** displays a skin testing protocol for the evaluation of IgE-mediated allergy to PEG and polysorbate. At this time, it is recommended that patients who develop anaphylaxis to a COVID-19 vaccine see a board-certified allergist for further evaluation.

CLINICS CARE POINTS

- Skin testing is well validated for patients with reported penicillin allergy. Individuals with this label should routinely be screened by a board-certified allergist/immunologist for consideration of skin testing and/or oral challenge.

- When deemed favorable from an individualized risk/benefit standpoint, patients with a history of aspirin or NSAID intolerance can in most cases successfully accomplish a challenge or desensitization procedure and be able to take ASA or NSAID as indicated.

- Patients with concern for an IgE mediated reaction to certain biologics or vaccines should seek care with a board-certified allergist, as skin testing and/or desensitization protocols may be available.

DISCLOSURES

R. H. Shah, MD, and M. M. Kuder, MD, have nothing to disclose. D. M. Lang, MD, has received honoraria from, has served as a consultant for, and/or has carried out clinical research with: Astra Zeneca, Sanofi-Regeneron, National Institute of Allergy and Infectious Diseases.

REFERENCES

1. Shaker MS, Wallace DV, Golden DBK, et al. Anaphylaxis—a 2020 practice parameter update, systematic review, and Grading of Recommendations, Assessment, Development and Evaluation (GRADE) analysis. J Allergy Clin Immunol 2020;145(4):1082–123.
2. Wood RA, Camargo CA, Lieberman P, et al. Anaphylaxis in America: the prevalence and characteristics of anaphylaxis in the United States. J Allergy Clin Immunol 2014;133(2):461–7.
3. Wang J, Lieberman JA, Camargo CA, et al. Diverse perspectives on recognition and management of anaphylaxis. Ann Allergy Asthma Immunol 2021;127(1):7–9.
4. Motosue MS, Bellolio MF, Van Houten HK, et al. Risk factors for severe anaphylaxis in the United States. Annals of allergy, asthma and Immunology 2017;119: 356–61.e2.
5. Gonzalez-Estrada A, Silvers SK, Klein A, et al. Epidemiology of anaphylaxis at a tertiary care center. Ann Allergy Asthma Immunol 2017;118(1):80–5.

6. Wong A, Seger DL, Lai KH, et al. Drug hypersensitivity reactions documented in electronic health records within a large health system. J Allergy Clin Immunol Pract 2019;7(4):1253–60.e3.

7. Solé D, Ivancevich JC, Borges MS, et al. Anaphylaxis in Latin America: a report of the online Latin American survey on anaphylaxis (OLASA). Clinics 2011; 66(6):943–7.

8. Turner PJ, Gowland MH, Sharma V, et al. Increase in anaphylaxis-related hospitalizations but no increase in fatalities: An analysis of United Kingdom national anaphylaxis data, 1992-2012. J Allergy Clin Immunol 2015;135(4):956–63.e1.

9. Clark S, Wei W, Rudders SA, et al. Risk factors for severe anaphylaxis in patients receiving anaphylaxis treatment in US emergency departments and hospitals. J Allergy Clin Immunol 2014;134(5):1125–30.

10. Faria E, Rodrigues-Cernadas J, Gaspar Â, et al. Drug-induced anaphylaxis survey in Portuguese allergy departments. J Investig Allergol Clin Immunol 2014; 24(1):40–8.

11. Jerschow E, Lin RY, Scaperotti MM, et al. Fatal anaphylaxis in the United States, 1999-2010: Temporal patterns and demographic associations. J Allergy Clin Immunol 2014;134(6):1318–28.e7.

12. Liew WK, Williamson E, Tang MLK. Anaphylaxis fatalities and admissions in Australia. J Allergy Clin Immunol 2009;123(2):434–42.

13. Dhopeshwarkar N, Sheikh A, Doan R, et al. Drug-induced anaphylaxis documented in electronic health records. J Allergy Clin Immunol Pract 2019;7(1): 103–11.

14. Zhou L, Dhopeshwarkar N, Blumenthal KG, et al. Drug allergies documented in electronic health records of a large healthcare system. Allergy Eur J Allergy Clin Immunol 2016;71(9):1305–13.

15. Lee P, Shanson D. Results of a UK survey of fatal anaphylaxis after oral amoxicillin. J Antimicrob Chemother 2007;60(5):1172–3.

16. Macy E, Contreras R. Health care use and serious infection prevalence associated with penicillin "allergy" in hospitalized patients: A cohort study. J Allergy Clin Immunol 2014;133(3):790–6.

17. Blumenthal KG, Peter JG, Trubiano JA, et al. Antibiotic allergy. Lancet 2019; 393(10167):183–98.

18. Empedrad R. Nonirritating intradermal skin test concentrations for commonly prescribed antibiotics. J Allergy Clin Immunol 2003;112(3):629–30.

19. Solensky R, Jacobs J, Lester M, et al. Penicillin allergy evaluation: a prospective, multicenter, open-label evaluation of a comprehensive penicillin skin test kit. J Allergy Clin Immunol Pract 2019;7(6):1876–85.e3.

20. del Real GA, Rose ME, Ramirez-Atamoros MT, et al. Penicillin skin testing in patients with a history of β-lactam allergy. Ann Allergy Asthma Immunol 2007;98(4): 355–9.

21. Elzagallaai AA, Koren G, Bend JR, et al. In vitro testing for hypersensitivity-mediated adverse drug reactions: Challenges and future directions. Clin Pharmacol Ther 2011;90(3):455–60.

22. Macy E, Ngor EW. Safely diagnosing clinically significant penicillin allergy using only penicilloyl-poly-lysine, penicillin, and oral amoxicillin. J Allergy Clin Immunol Pract 2013;1(3):258–63.

23. Legendre DP, Muzny CA, Marshall GD, et al. Antibiotic hypersensitivity reactions and approaches to desensitization. Clin Infect Dis 2014;58(8):1140–8.

24. White AA, Stevenson DD. Aspirin-exacerbated respiratory disease. In: Longo DL, editor. N Engl J Med 2018;379(11):1060–70.

25. Kowalski ML, Makowska JS, Blanca M, et al. Hypersensitivity to nonsteroidal anti-inflammatory drugs (NSAIDs) - Classification, diagnosis and management: review of the EAACI/ENDA and GA2LEN/HANNA. Allergy Eur J Allergy Clin Immunol 2011;66(7):818–29.

26. Kowalski ML, Woessner K, Sanak M. Approaches to the diagnosis and management of patients with a history of nonsteroidal anti-inflammatory drug-related urticaria and angioedema. J Allergy Clin Immunol 2015;136(2):245–51.

27. Yu RJ, Krantz MS, Phillips EJ, et al. Emerging causes of drug-induced anaphylaxis: a review of anaphylaxis-associated reports in the FDA Adverse Event Reporting System (FAERS). J Allergy Clin Immunol Pract 2021;9(2):819–29.e2.

28. Canto MG, Andreu I, Fernandez J, et al. Selective immediate hypersensitivity reactions to NSAIDs. Curr Opin Allergy Clin Immunol 2009;9(4):293–7.

29. Hirschberg VGSR. Landmark article: Aus der arztlichen praxis, mittleilung uber einen fall von nebenwirkaung des aspirin (a case report on the side effects of aspirin). Allergy Proc 1990;11(5):249–50.

30. Dysart BR. Death following ingestion of five grains of acetylsalicylic acid. J Am Med Assoc 1933;101(6):446.

31. Francis N, Ghent OT, Bullen SS. Death from the grains of aspirin. J Allergy 1935; 6(5):504–6.

32. Samter M, Beers R. Intolerance to aspirin. Ann Intern Med 1968;68(5):975.

33. Stevenson DD, Hougham AJ, Schrank PJ, et al. Salsalate cross-sensitivity in aspirin-sensitive patients with asthma. J Allergy Clin Immunol 1990;86(5): 749–58.

34. Settipane RA, Stevenson DD. Cross sensitivity with acetaminophen in aspirin-sensitive subjects with asthma. J Allergy Clin Immunol 1989;84(1):26–33.

35. Dahlén B, Szczeklik A, Murray JJ. Celecoxib in patients with asthma and aspirin intolerance. N Engl J Med 2001;344(2):142.

36. Rajan JP, Wineinger NE, Stevenson DD, et al. Prevalence of aspirin-exacerbated respiratory disease among asthmatic patients: A meta-analysis of the literature. J Allergy Clin Immunol 2015;135(3):676–81.e1.

37. Kowalski ML, Agache I, Bavbek S, et al. Diagnosis and management of NSAID-Exacerbated Respiratory Disease (N-ERD)—a EAACI position paper. Allergy Eur J Allergy Clin Immunol 2019;74(1):28–39.

38. Bochenek G, Kuschill-Dziurda J, Szafraniec K, et al. Certain subphenotypes of aspirin-exacerbated respiratory disease distinguished by latent class analysis. J Allergy Clin Immunol 2014;133(1):98–103, e6.

39. Lang DM. Antileukotriene agents and aspirin-sensitive asthma: are we removing the second bassoonist or skating to where the puck is gonna be? Ann Allergy Asthma Immunol 2000;85(1):5–8.

40. Lang DM, Aronica MA, Maierson ES, et al. Omalizumab can inhibit respiratory reaction during aspirin desensitization. Ann Allergy Asthma Immunol 2018; 121(1):98–104.

41. Widal F, Abrami P, Lermoyez J. Anaphylaxie et Idiosyncrasie. Allergy Asthma Proc 2006;14(5):373–6.

42. Zeiss CR, Lockey RF. Refractory period to aspirin in a patient with aspirin-induced asthma. J Allergy Clin Immunol 1976;57(5):440–8.

43. Stevenson DD, White AA. Aspirin desensitization in aspirin-exacerbated respiratory disease: consideration of a new oral challenge protocol. J Allergy Clin Immunol Pract 2015;3(6):932–3.

44. Nguyen A, Zuraw BL, Wu C, et al. Intranasal ketorolac, diagnosis, and desensitization for aspirin-exacerbated respiratory disease. Ann Allergy Asthma Immunol 2021;126(6):674–80.

45. Berges-Gimeno MP, Simon RA, Stevenson DD. Long-term treatment with aspirin desensitization in asthmatic patients with aspirin-exacerbated respiratory disease. J Allergy Clin Immunol 2003;111(1):180–6.

46. Gevaert P, Omachi TA, Corren J, et al. Efficacy and safety of omalizumab in nasal polyposis: 2 randomized phase 3 trials. J Allergy Clin Immunol 2020; 146(3):595–605.

47. Bachert C, Han JK, Desrosiers M, et al. Efficacy and safety of dupilumab in patients with severe chronic rhinosinusitis with nasal polyps (LIBERTY NP SINUS-24 and LIBERTY NP SINUS-52): results from two multicentre, randomised, double-blind, placebo-controlled, parallel-group phase 3 trials. Lancet 2019; 394(10209):1638–50.

48. Stevenson DD, Pleskow WW, Simon RA, et al. Aspirin-sensitive rhinosinusitis asthma: A double-blind crossover study of treatment with aspirin. J Allergy Clin Immunol 1984;73(4):500–7.

49. Fruth K, Pogorzelski B, Schmidtmann I, et al. Low-dose aspirin desensitization in individuals with aspirin-exacerbated respiratory disease. Allergy Eur J Allergy Clin Immunol 2013;68(5):659–65.

50. Esmaeilzadeh H, Nabavi M, Aryan Z, et al. Aspirin desensitization for patients with aspirin-exacerbated respiratory disease: a randomized double-blind placebo-controlled trial. Clin Immunol 2015;160(2):349–57.

51. Mortazavi N, Esmaeilzadeh H, Abbasinazari M, et al. Clinical and immunological efficacy of aspirin desensitization in nasal polyp patients with aspirin-exacerbated respiratory disease. Iran J Pharm Res 2017;16(4):1639–47.

52. Swierczyńska-Krępa M, Sanak M, Bochenek G, et al. Aspirin desensitization in patients with aspirin-induced and aspirin-tolerant asthma: A double-blind study. J Allergy Clin Immunol 2014;134(4):883–90.

53. Woessner KM. Aspirin desensitization for cardiovascular disease. Curr Opin Allergy Clin Immunol 2015;15(4):314–22.

54. Mastalerz L, Setkowicz M, Sanak M, et al. Hypersensitivity to aspirin: common eicosanoid alterations in urticaria and asthma. J Allergy Clin Immunol 2004; 113(4):771–5.

55. Kowalski ML, Bienkiewicz B, Woszczek G, et al. Diagnosis of pyrazolone drug sensitivity: clinical history versus skin testing and in vitro testing. Allergy Asthma Proc 1999;20(6):347–52.

56. Bretza JA, Novey HS. Anaphylactoid reactions to tolmetin after interrupted dosage. West J Med 1985;143(1):55–9.

57. Sandler RH. Anaphylactic reactions to zomepirac. Ann Emerg Med 1985;14(2): 171–4.

58. FDA's regulation of Zomax. Intergovernmental Relations and human Resources Subcommittee, Committee on Government Operations, US House of Representatives, 98th Congress, 1st Session, House Report No. 98-584, p.4, 1983.

59. Doña I, Barrionuevo E, Salas M, et al. NSAIDs-hypersensitivity often induces a blended reaction pattern involving multiple organs. Sci Rep 2018;8(1):16710.

60. Sánchez-Borges M, Aberer W, Brockow K, et al. Controversies in drug allergy: radiographic contrast media. J Allergy Clin Immunol Pract 2019;7(1):61–5.

61. Li X, Liu H, Zhao L, et al. Clinical observation of adverse drug reactions to nonionic iodinated contrast media in population with underlying diseases and risk factors. Br J Radiol 2017;90(1070):20160729.

62. Davenport MS, Mervak BM, Ellis JH, et al. Indirect cost and harm attributable to Oral 13-Hour inpatient corticosteroid prophylaxis before contrast-enhanced CT. Radiology 2016;279(2):492–501.

63. Broyles AD, Banerji A, Castells M. Practical guidance for the evaluation and management of drug hypersensitivity: general concepts. J Allergy Clin Immunol Pract 2020;8(9):S3–15.

64. Lerondeau B, Trechot P, Waton J, et al. Analysis of cross-reactivity among radio-contrast media in 97 hypersensitivity reactions. J Allergy Clin Immunol 2016; 137(2):633–5.e4.

65. Fok JS, Smith WB. Hypersensitivity reactions to gadolinium-based contrast agents. Curr Opin Allergy Clin Immunol 2017;17(4):241–6.

66. Rosado Ingelmo A, Doña Diaz I, Cabañas Moreno R, et al. Clinical practice guidelines for diagnosis and management of hypersensitivity reactions to contrast media. J Investig Allergol Clin Immunol 2016;26(3):144–55.

67. Adverse reactions to Gadolinium-Baed contrast media. ACR Man Contrast Media; 2014.

68. Takahashi S, Takada A, Saito K, et al. Fatal anaphylaxis associated with the gadolinium-based contrast agent gadoteridol (ProHance). J Investig Allergol Clin Immunol 2015;25(5):366–7. Available at: http://www.ncbi.nlm.nih.gov/pubmed/26727767.

69. Chiriac A-M, Audurier Y, Bousquet PJ, et al. Clinical value of negative skin tests to gadolinium contrast agents. Allergy 2011;66(11):1504–6.

70. Schiavino D, Murzilli F, Del Ninno M, et al. Demonstration of an IgE-mediated immunological pathogenesis of a severe adverse reaction to gadopentetate di-meglumine. J Investig Allergol Clin Immunol 2003;13(2):140–2. Available at: http://www.ncbi.nlm.nih.gov/pubmed/12968402.

71. Jung J-W, Kang H-R, Kim M-H, et al. Immediate hypersensitivity reaction to gadolinium-based MR contrast media. Radiology 2012;264(2):414–22.

72. Gutta R, Golubski S, Abouhassan S, et al. Anaphylactic reaction to gadopentate dimeglumine (GD-DTPA/Magnevist) confirmed by skin testing. Ann Allergy Asthma Immunol 2011;107(A27).

73. Picard M, Galvão VR. Current knowledge and management of hypersensitivity reactions to monoclonal antibodies. J Allergy Clin Immunol Pract 2017;5(3): 600–9.

74. Rambasek TE, Lang DM, Kavuru MS. Omalizumab: where does it fit into current asthma management? Cleve Clin J Med 2004;71(3):251–61.

75. Cox L, Platts-Mills TAE, Finegold I, et al. American academy of allergy, asthma & immunology/american college of allergy, asthma and immunology joint task force report on omalizumab-associated anaphylaxis. J Allergy Clin Immunol 2007;120(6):1373–7.

76. Lieberman PL, Umetsu DT, Carrigan GJ, et al. Anaphylactic reactions associated with omalizumab administration: Analysis of a case-control study. J Allergy Clin Immunol 2016;138(3):913–5, e2.

77. FDA Approves Xolair (omalizumab) Prefilled Syringe for self-injection across all Indications. Available at: https://www.businesswire.com/news/home/20210412005839/en/FDA-Approves-Xolair-omalizumab-Prefilled-Syringe-for-Self-Injection-Across-All-Indications. Accessed July 25, 2021.

78. Lieberman PL, Jones I, Rajwanshi R, et al. Anaphylaxis associated with omalizumab administration: Risk factors and patient characteristics. J Allergy Clin Immunol 2017;140(6):1734–6.e4.

79. Owens G, Petrov A. Successful desensitization of three patients with hypersensitivity reactions to omalizumab. Curr Drug Saf 2012;6(5):339–42.

80. Gülsen A, Wedi B, Jappe U. Hypersensitivity reactions to biologics (part I): allergy as an important differential diagnosis in complex immune-derived adverse events. Allergo J Int 2020;29(4):97–125.

81. Prescribing information for Nucala. Available at: https://www.accessdata.fda.gov/drugsatfda_docs/label/2015/125526Orig1s000Lbl.pdf. Accessed May 13, 2021.

82. Lugogo N, Domingo C, Chanez P, et al. Long-term efficacy and safety of mepolizumab in patients with severe eosinophilic asthma: a multi-center, open-label, phase IIIb study. Clin Ther 2016;38(9):2058–70.e1.

83. Khatri S, Moore W, Gibson PG, et al. Assessment of the long-term safety of mepolizumab and durability of clinical response in patients with severe eosinophilic asthma. J Allergy Clin Immunol 2019;143(5):1742–51.e7.

84. Pavord ID, Korn S, Howarth P, et al. Mepolizumab for severe eosinophilic asthma (DREAM): A multicentre, double-blind, placebo-controlled trial. Lancet 2012;380(9842):651–9.

85. Castro M, Zangrilli J, Wechsler ME, et al. Reslizumab for inadequately controlled asthma with elevated blood eosinophil counts: Results from two multicentre, parallel, double-blind, randomised, placebo-controlled, phase 3 trials. Lancet Respir Med 2015;3(5):355–66.

86. Murphy K, Jacobs J, Bjermer L, et al. Long-term safety and efficacy of reslizumab in patients with eosinophilic asthma. J Allergy Clin Immunol Pract 2017;5(6):1572–81.e3.

87. Prescribing information for stribild. Available at: https://www.accessdata.fda.gov/drugsatfda_docs/label/2012/125160s189lbl.pdf. Accessed May 13, 2021.

88. Liu W, Ma X, Zhou W. Adverse events of benralizumab in moderate to severe eosinophilic asthma: A meta-analysis. Medicine (Baltimore) 2019;98(22):e15868.

89. Prescribing information for Dupixent. Available at: https://www.accessdata.fda.gov/drugsatfda_docs/label/2017/761055lbl.pdf. [Accessed 13 May 2021]. Accessed.

90. Ou Z, Chen C, Chen A, et al. Adverse events of dupilumab in adults with moderate-to-severe atopic dermatitis: a meta-analysis. Int Immunopharmacol 2018;54:303–10.

91. European Medicines Agency. Assessment report of dupilumab. 2019. Available at: https://www.ema.europa.eu/en/documents/variation-report/dupixent-h-c-4390-ii-0012-epar-assessment-report-variation_en.pdf. Accessed May 20, 2021.

92. Prescribing information for Takhzyro. Available at: https://www.accessdata.fda.gov/drugsatfda_docs/label/2018/761090s000lbl.pdf. Accessed May 13, 2021.

93. Banerji A, Riedl MA, Bernstein JA, et al. Effect of lanadelumab compared with placebo on prevention of hereditary angioedema attacks: a randomized clinical trial. JAMA 2018;320(20):2108–21.

94. Jung JW, Kang HR, Lee SH, et al. The incidence and risk factors of infusion-related reactions to rituximab for treating B cell malignancies in a single tertiary hospital. Oncologist 2014;86(3):127–34.

95. Winkler U, Jensen M, Manzke O, et al. Cytokine-release syndrome in patients with B-cell chronic lymphocytic leukemia and high lymphocyte counts after treatment with an anti-CD20 monoclonal antibody (rituximab, IDEC-C2B8). Blood 1999;94(7):2217–24.

96. Levin AS, Otani IM, Lax T, et al. Reactions to rituximab in an outpatient infusion center: a 5-year review. J Allergy Clin Immunol Pract 2017;5(1):107–13.e1.

97. Vultaggio A, Matucci A, Nencini F, et al. Drug-specific Th2 cells and IgE antibodies in a patient with anaphylaxis to rituximab. Int Arch Allergy Immunol 2012;159(3):321–6.

98. Sloane D, Govindarajulu U, Harrow-Mortelliti J, et al. Safety, costs, and efficacy of rapid drug desensitizations to chemotherapy and monoclonal antibodies. J Allergy Clin Immunol Pract 2016;4(3):497–504.

99. Korycka-Wołowiec A, Wołowiec D, Robak T. Ofatumumab for treating chronic lymphocytic leukemia: a safety profile. Expert Opin Drug Saf 2015;14(12): 1945–59.

100. Goede V, Fischer K, Busch R, et al. Obinutuzumab plus Chlorambucil in Patients with CLL and Coexisting Conditions. N Engl J Med 2014;370(12):1101–10.

101. Prescribing information for Arzerra. Available at: https://www.accessdata.fda. gov/drugsatfda_docs/label/2009/125326lbl.pdf. Accessed May 13, 2021.

102. O'Neil BH, Allen R, Spigel DR, et al. High incidence of cetuximab-related infusion reactions in Tennessee and North Carolina and the association with atopic history. J Clin Oncol 2007;25(24):3644–8.

103. Commins SP, Satinover SM, Hosen J, et al. Delayed anaphylaxis, angioedema, or urticaria after consumption of red meat in patients with IgE antibodies specific for galactose-α-1,3-galactose. J Allergy Clin Immunol 2009;123(2):426–33, e2.

104. Commins SP, James HR, Kelly LA, et al. The relevance of tick bites to the production of IgE antibodies to the mammalian oligosaccharide galactose-α-1,3-galactose. J Allergy Clin Immunol 2011;127(5):1286–93, e6.

105. Maier S, Chung CH, Morse M, et al. A retrospective analysis of cross-reacting cetuximab IgE antibody and its association with severe infusion reactions. Cancer Med 2015;4(1):36–42.

106. García-Menaya J, Cordobés-Durán C, Gómez-Ulla J, et al. Successful desensitization to cetuximab in a patient with a positive skin test to cetuximab and specific IgE to Alpha-gal. J Investig Allergol Clin Immunol 2016;26(2):132–4.

107. Jerath MR, Kwan M, Kannarkat M, et al. A desensitization protocol for the mAb cetuximab. J Allergy Clin Immunol 2009;123(1):260–2.

108. Saif MW, Peccerillo J, Potter V. Successful re-challenge with panitumumab in patients who developed hypersensitivity reactions to cetuximab: Report of three cases and review of literature. Cancer Chemother Pharmacol 2009;63(6): 1017–22.

109. Langerak A, River G, Mitchell E, et al. Panitumumab monotherapy in patients with metastatic colorectal cancer and cetuximab infusion reactions: A series of four case reports. Clin Colorectal Cancer 2009;8(1):49–54.

110. Prescribing information for Enbrel. Available at: https://www.accessdata.fda. gov/drugsatfda_docs/label/2012/103795s5503lbl.pdf. Accessed May 13, 2021.

111. Prescribing information for Simponi. Available at: https://www.accessdata.fda. gov/drugsatfda_docs/label/2011/125289s0064lbl.pdf. Accessed May 13, 2021.

112. Prescribing information for Humira. Available at: https://www.accessdata.fda. gov/drugsatfda_docs/label/2018/125057s406lbl.pdf. Accessed May 13, 2021.

113. Prescribing information for Remicade. Available at: https://www.accessdata.fda. gov/drugsatfda_docs/label/2013/103772s5359lbl.pdf. Accessed May 13, 2021.

114. Ben-Horin S, Yavzori M, Katz L, et al. The immunogenic part of infliximab is the F(ab')2, but measuring antibodies to the intact infliximab molecule is more clinically useful. Gut 2011;60(1):41–8.

115. Fréling E, Peyrin-Biroulet L, Poreaux C, et al. IgE antibodies and skin tests in immediate hypersensitivity reactions to infliximab in inflammatory bowel disease: Impact on infliximab retreatment. Eur J Gastroenterol Hepatol 2015;27(10): 1200–8.

116. Bavbek S, Ataman Ş, Akıncı A, et al. Rapid subcutaneous desensitization for the management of local and systemic hypersensitivity reactions to etanercept and adalimumab in 12 patients. J Allergy Clin Immunol Pract 2015;3(4):629–32.

117. Brennan PJ, Bouza TR, Hsu FI, et al. Hypersensitivity reactions to mAbs: 105 desensitizations in 23 patients, from evaluation to treatment. J Allergy Clin Immunol 2009;124(6):1259–66.

118. González-de-Olano D, Morgado JM, Juárez-Guerrero R, et al. Positive basophil activation test following anaphylaxis to pertuzumab and successful treatment with rapid desensitization. J Allergy Clin Immunol Pract 2016;4(2):338–40.

119. Rocchi V, Puxeddu I, Cataldo G, et al. Hypersensitivity reactions to tocilizumab: Role of skin tests in diagnosis. Rheumatol (United Kingdom) 2014;53(8):1527–9.

120. Justet A, Neukirch C, Poubeau P, et al. Successful rapid tocilizumab desensitization in a patient with still disease. J Allergy Clin Immunol Pract 2014;2(5): 631–2.

121. DeVita MD, Evens AM, Rosen ST, et al. Multiple successful desensitizations to brentuximab vedotin: A case report and literature review. JNCCN J Natl Compr Cancer Netw 2014;12(4):465–71.

122. McNeil MM, Weintraub ES, Duffy J, et al. Risk of anaphylaxis after vaccination in children and adults. J Allergy Clin Immunol 2016;137(3):868–78.

123. McNeil MM, DeStefano F. Vaccine-associated hypersensitivity. J Allergy Clin Immunol 2018;141(2):463–72.

124. Risma KA, Edwards KM, Hummell DS, et al. Potential mechanisms of anaphylaxis to COVID-19 mRNA vaccines. J Allergy Clin Immunol 2021;147(6): 2075–82.e2.

125. Sellaturay P, Nasser S, Islam S, et al. Polyethylene glycol (PEG) is a cause of anaphylaxis to the Pfizer/BioNTech mRNA COVID-19 vaccine. Clin Exp Allergy 2021;51(6):861–3.

126. Stone CA, Rukasin CRF, Beachkofsky TM, et al. Immune-mediated adverse reactions to vaccines. Br J Clin Pharmacol 2019;85(12):2694–706.

127. Kelso JM, Greenhawt MJ, Li JT, et al. Adverse reactions to vaccines practice parameter 2012 update. J Allergy Clin Immunol 2012;130(1):25–43.

128. Greenhawt M, Turner PJ, Kelso JM. Administration of influenza vaccines to egg allergic recipients: A practice parameter update 2017. Ann Allergy Asthma Immunol 2018;120(1):49–52.

129. Janssen COVID-19 vaccine EUA Fact Sheet for Healthcare provider. Available at: https://www.fda.gov/media/146304/download. Accessed August 17, 2021.

130. Kuder MM, Lang DM, Patadia DD. Anaphylaxis to vaccinations: a review of the literature and evaluation of the COVID-19 mRNA vaccinations. Cleve Clin J Med 2021;. 10.3949/ccjm.88a.ccc075.

131. Stone CA, Liu Y, Relling MV, et al. Immediate hypersensitivity to polyethylene glycols and polysorbates: more common than we have recognized. J Allergy Clin Immunol Pract 2019;7(5):1533, 1540.e8.

132. Banerji A, Wickner PG, Saff R, et al. mRNA Vaccines to Prevent COVID-19 disease and reported allergic reactions: current evidence and suggested approach. J Allergy Clin Immunol Pract 2021;9(4):1423–37.

Perioperative Anaphylaxis

Mitchell M. Pitlick, MD*, Gerald W. Volcheck, MD

KEYWORDS

- Anaphylaxis • Perioperative • Intraoperative • Hypersensitivity reaction • Anesthesia

KEY POINTS

- Perioperative anaphylaxis is a potentially life-threatening event caused most commonly by antibiotics, neuromuscular blocking agents (NMBAs), antibiotics, chlorhexidine, latex, and dyes, although any medication or substance used can be a culprit.
- A tryptase level obtained approximately 1 hour after reaction onset can aid in diagnosis, but a normal level does not rule out the diagnosis.
- Comprehensive allergy evaluation and communication with anesthesia and surgical teams are crucial in identifying a culprit agent and outlining a plan for future procedures.

INTRODUCTION

Perioperative anaphylaxis (POA) is a potentially life-threatening event caused by medications and substances used for surgery or anesthesia. Although any substance can cause POA, the most common culprit agents include antibiotics, neuromuscular blocking agents (NMBAs), disinfectants, and latex, although these vary with geographic location.[1–3] Evaluation can be complex and difficult, given that a median of 8 different drugs is used during the average surgical procedure.[4] Despite the fact that a causative agent is not determined in 30% to 50% of cases, comprehensive evaluation and collaboration between allergy/immunology and anesthesia are of paramount importance in formulating a plan to prevent POA during future procedures.[2,5–7]

EPIDEMIOLOGY

The reported incidence of POA varies widely, with estimates ranging from 1 in 300 to 400 to 1 in 20,000 surgical procedures.[8–14] This variability stems from a variety of factors, including nonstandardized diagnostic and reporting criteria, difficulty in determining a denominator of surgical procedures, under-recognition of POA, and regional differences in drug usage. The National Audit Project 6 (NAP6) in the United Kingdom estimated the incidence of severe POA (grade 3–5 on the Ring and Messmer scale) at 1 in 10,000, which is similar to another large study in France.[8,15,16] POA is less

Division of Allergic Diseases, Mayo Clinic, 200 1st St SW, Rochester, MN 55905, USA
* Corresponding author. Division of Allergic Diseases, Mayo Clinic, 200 First Street Southwest, Rochester, MN 55905, USA. ,
E-mail address: pitlick.mitchell@mayo.edu

Immunol Allergy Clin N Am 42 (2022) 145–159
https://doi.org/10.1016/j.iac.2021.09.002
0889-8561/22/© 2021 Elsevier Inc. All rights reserved.

immunology.theclinics.com

common in the pediatric population, as shown by the NAP6 estimate of severe POA in children at 1 in 37,000.[8] There is a female predilection with a female:male ratio of 3:1.[2,17] Possible contributors include the female hormones' influence on the type 1 helper T-cell/type 2 helper T-cell balance or the propensity for female patients to be sensitized to NMBAs through common consumer products.[18] POA carries a higher mortality rate than other causes of anaphylaxis, with estimates ranging from 1.4% to 9%.[1,19]

PATHOPHYSIOLOGY

Approximately 60% of POA episodes are determined to be IgE-mediated, with the remainder due to a nonidentified allergen or non-IgE mechanisms, such as direct mast cell mediator release, kinin system modulation, nonspecific complement activation, and drug-bound IgG interaction with FcγR-expressing neutrophils, macrophages, or platelets.[20–22] Mas-related G protein–coupled receptor X2 (MRGPRX2) is a recently described receptor found on mast cells that can be occupied by a variety of medications, including opioids, NMBAs, vancomycin, amoxicillin–clavulanic acid, and teicoplanin, with resultant activation and degranulation, making it a likely culprit for many non–IgE-mediated POA events.[23,24] Both IgE-mediated and non–IgE-mediated mechanisms can result in similar clinical manifestations and elevation in serum tryptase. They are not reliably distinguished with current clinical methods, thus it is not currently recommended to alter anaphylaxis therapy or future drug avoidance recommendations based on an underlying mechanistic suspicion.[25]

CLINICAL PRESENTATION

All forms of anaphylaxis can present with typical cutaneous, respiratory, and cardiovascular signs and symptoms due to the release of mast cell mediators. The clinical presentation of POA can be unique, however, compared with other causes of anaphylaxis due to the nature of the clinical environment in which it occurs. Early signs and symptoms of anaphylaxis, including cutaneous manifestations, pruritus, dyspnea, and lightheadedness, may be masked due to the patient being draped and intubated. Additionally, the hemodynamic shifts that can occur with anesthesia induction and throughout surgery can hamper early recognition of anaphylaxis.

Isolated cardiovascular symptoms (hypotension or tachycardia) were the presenting feature in nearly 56% of severe cases in NAP6, with isolated respiratory symptoms seen in 18% of cases.[8] Only 56% of cases had documented cutaneous manifestations, and it rarely was a presenting feature.[8] The presence of cutaneous symptoms is highly variable, with regional differences ranging from 50% to 76% in the United States, 84% in Spain, 70% to 95% in France, and 53% to 84% in Belgium.[9,15,26–28] Additionally, cutaneous symptoms tend to be more prevalent in nonsevere or non–IgE-mediated reactions.[15,26] In addition to surgical draping, the lack of cutaneous findings can be the result of decreased effective circulating blood volume or cardiovascular collapse with compensatory sympathetic stimulation and vasoconstriction that prevent flushing and urticaria from manifesting.[29,30] These findings highlight the difficulty in POA recognition. Given the frequency with which POA manifests solely with cardiovascular or respiratory signs and symptoms, it is imperative to consider anaphylaxis if these findings are unexpected or unresponsive to typical therapy.

The severity of POA episodes typically has been graded using a modified Ring and Messmer scale that includes grade I (isolated cutaneous signs), grade II (nonsevere multisystem involvement), grade III (life-threatening multisystem involvement), and grade IV (cardiopulmonary arrest), with grade I and grade II reactions typically attributed to non–IgE-mediated mechanisms and grade III and grade IV reactions ascribed to IgE-mediated mechanisms.[14–16,31] Although other grading systems exist, including a recently published consensus scoring system for diagnosis,[32] it is important to recognize the continuum of anaphylaxis so as to facilitate early recognition and appropriate use of epinephrine.[33,34]

DIFFERENTIAL DIAGNOSIS

The signs and symptoms accompanying POA can be caused by myriad other factors associated with the perioperative period (**Box 1**). Anesthesia induction with inhaled anesthetics or propofol can result in hypotension and compensatory tachycardia that can mimic anaphylaxis with an exaggerated effect in patients taking tricyclic antidepressants or antihypertensive medications.[35,36] Other causes of hemodynamic instability in the perioperative setting can mimic anaphylaxis, including sepsis, hemorrhage or volume depletion, myocardial ischemia, arrythmias, and pulmonary embolism.

Bronchospasm can occur in the absence of POA as a result of airway manipulation in patients with asthma or a recent viral infection or in obese patients.[35,37] Other intubation-associated events, including mucous plugging, aspiration, and mechanical airway obstruction, also can result in bronchospasm.[38] Airway swelling as a result of difficult intubation or angioedema due to angiotensin-converting enzyme (ACE) inhibitors or C1 esterase inhibitor deficiency also can result in respiratory distress.[36]

Approximately 95% of POA episodes occur within 30 minutes of anesthesia induction.[8] Culprit agents in this time frame typically include antibiotics, NMBAs, and hypnotics, whereas POA that manifests more than 30 minutes after anesthesia induction may be more likely due to disinfectants, latex, sugammadex, dyes, colloids, or blood products.[20]

Box 1
Differential diagnosis for signs and symptoms of perioperative anaphylaxis

Hypotension and tachycardia
  Anesthesia induction
  Perioperative antihypertensive or tricyclic antidepressant use
  Sepsis
  Hemorrhage or volume depletion
  Myocardial ischemia
  Arrythmia
  Pulmonary embolism
  Systemic mastocytosis

Bronchospasm
  Asthma
  Recent viral infection
  Obesity
  Mucous plugging
  Aspiration
  Difficult intubation

Urticaria and angioedema
  ACE inhibitor use
  C1 esterase inhibitor deficiency
  Cold-induced urticaria

CULPRIT AGENTS
Neuromuscular Blocking Agents

NMBAs consist of the depolarizing agent succinylcholine and the nondepolarizing agents classified as aminosteroid (rocuronium, vecuronium, and pancuronium) or benzylisoquinolinium (atracurium and cisatracurium) compounds. NMBAs frequently are cited as the most common cause of POA in a large part of the world, including France, Norway, Australia, and New Zealand, where they account for 50% to 70% of POA episodes.[14,39] This is in contrast to reports from the United States, Spain, and Denmark, where antibiotics are the more common culprit and NMBAs account for approximately 30% of POA.[27,28,40,41] The NAP6 report from the United Kingdom recently showed that although antibiotics are the most frequent POA culprit, NMBAs have a higher incidence of POA (1 in 19,070 vs 1 in 26,845 for antibiotics).[8] These regional differences largely are due to differences in style of practice, clinical context, and drug availability at different centers.

NMBAs can cause POA through IgE and non–IgE-mediated mechanisms. NMBAs bind IgE via their substituted tertiary and quaternary ammonium ion structures.[42,43] These ammonium ions are found in a wide array of cosmetics, disinfectants, and over-the-counter medications that can result in sensitization to NMBAs prior to direct clinical exposure. This is hypothesized to account for the increase in POA and NMBA sensitization seen in female patients compared with male patients, which, although incompletely understood, is lent credence by a recent study showing higher rates of sensitization to NMBAs and quaternary ammonium compounds in hairdressers via workplace product exposure.[44] Additional evidence supporting sensitization to NMBAs as a result of exposure to cross-reacting ammonium ion epitopes comes from epidemiologic data regarding pholcodine use. Pholcodine, an opioid antitussive, is an ammonium-containing medication that previously was consumed by as much as 40% of the Norwegian population, is associated with high rates of ammonium ion sensitization, and resulted in high rates of NMBA-induced POA with significant declines in these rates once pholcodine was removed from the market in 2007.[45–47]

NMBAs also can induce anaphylaxis by non–IgE-mediated mechanisms. Atracurium can cause direct histamine release with subsequent hypotension and bronchospasm.[20] NMBAs can bind to MRGPRX2 on mast cells, which results in activation and mediator release. Rocuronium is believed to have the highest affinity for MRGPRX2, which may explain why it is one of the most often implicated NMBAs in POA, although cisatracurium and mivacurium can bind as well.[23,24,48,49] Polymorphisms in the gene encoding MRGPRX2 may have an effect on NMBA binding affinity and mast cell activation.[50] A recent study utilized a MRGPRX2-specific DNA aptamer to prevent anaphylaxis in a rat model, providing foundational evidence that MRGPRX2 could be a therapeutic target in POA prevention.[50]

NMBA-induced POA presents early in the procedure, with a recent report showing 95% of cases occurring within 5 minutes of induction.[8] Succinylcholine and rocuronium are associated with the highest risk of allergic reaction, with atracurium, cisatracurium, vecuronium, and pancuronium having less risk.[8,49,51] It recently has been shown that the incidence of POA with succinylcholine use is twice that of other NMBAs, and it is much more likely to be associated with bronchospasm.[8] Cross-sensitivity between NMBAs is quite variable, with estimates ranging from 36% to 70%, although only 7% are sensitive to all NMBAs.[14,52,53] Cross-sensitivity is seen more commonly in NMBAs within the same molecular class (ie, vecuronium and pancuronium [aminosteroid] and atracurium and cisatracurium [benzylisoquinolinium]), whereas cross-sensitivity between molecular classes potentially is as low as

5%.[14,39,54,55] This highlights the importance of a comprehensive allergy evaluation, because subsequent NMBA use guided by negative skin testing has resulted in low rates of POA recurrence.[5,56,57]

Antibiotics

Antibiotics are the most frequent POA culprit in the United States and Spain, where they account for 40% to 55% of reactions.[20] The frequency of antibiotic-induced POA is increasing, with recent data from France showing an increase from 2% to 20% of all perioperative reactions over the past 30 years.[2] Cefazolin is the antibiotic implicated most frequently in the United States and Spain, whereas NAP6 data from the United Kingdom reported co-amoxiclav (amoxicillin–clavulanic acid) and teicoplanin as the most common culprits, accounting for 46 and 36 of the 92 antibiotic-induced POA cases, respectively.[8,27,28,41] Teicoplanin is not available for use in the United States, but in the European Union it has been implicated in an increasing number of POA cases over the past several years and is estimated to induce POA at an incidence of 1 in 6100 administrations, far higher than any other drug used in the perioperative period.[8,58] In the NAP6 survey, 56% of patients who received teicoplanin had penicillin on their allergy list, which often was a factor in the decision to use teicoplanin.[4,8] This highlights the importance of penicillin allergy evaluation prior to surgery, because up to 98% of penicillin allergy labels are incorrect.[20,59,60]

Antibiotic-induced POA occurs early in surgery, with recent data showing 97% of cases occurring within 15 minutes and 74% of cases occurring within 5 minutes of initiating the procedure.[8] In addition to IgE-mediated mechanisms, many antibiotics, including vancomycin, amoxicillin–clavulanic acid, fluoroquinolones, and teicoplanin, can bind to MRGPRX2 and cause POA in a non–IgE-mediated fashion.[23,24]

Latex

Latex historically has been one of the most common causes of POA, although the frequency is decreasing. This fluctuation is demonstrated in studies from France, where latex was found to be the culprit in 2% of POA cases between 1984 and 1989, 18% of cases from 2005 to 2007, and 5% of cases from 2011 to 2012.[14,61] This decrease has been demonstrated in other studies, and, in the NAP6 survey, there was not a single case of POA attributable to latex.[8,62] This reduction is attributable to several factors, including the adoption of latex-free policies by many health care centers, use of powder-free latex gloves, and Food and Drug Administration mandated labeling of latex-containing products.[63] When it does occur, POA due to latex typically presents later in surgery as a result of a significant and/or cumulative mucocutaneous or serosal exposure.[20] Cutaneous symptoms are common, although aerosolized latex particles can result in bronchospasm.[17]

Sugammadex

Sugammadex is an NMBA reversal agent that recently has emerged as a POA culprit. It was approved for use in the United States in 2015 but has been in use in Europe and Japan since 2008 and 2010, respectively. Sugammadex-induced POA has disproportionately been reported in Japan, where a recent study determined it to be the culprit in 13/46 cases (28.3%) at a single institution between 2012 and 2018.[64] This is in contrast to the UK NAP6 data, where it was the culprit in just 1 case.[8] This is due in part to regional differences in sugammadex use, because Japan uses it in a greater proportion of cases compared with other countries.[20] Sugammadex is a cyclodextrin, and the sensitizing trigger is thought to be due to cyclodextrin exposure via food additives and cosmetics, although this is unproved.[20] Due to its use as an NMBA reversal agent, sugammadex-induced POA occurs late in surgery. The sugammadex-rocuronium complex also is known to cause anaphylaxis in the absence of sensitization to the individual drugs.[65]

Disinfectants

Chlorhexidine is a widely used disinfectant in the procedural and perioperative settings, where it is used as a topical skin disinfectant, as a gel to assist in urinary catheter passage, coated on central venous catheters, and in many other forms. Despite being a common culprit in POA, accounting for 9% to 10% of cases in multiple cohorts, it often is overlooked due to lack of documentation of its use.[8,66] Onset of symptoms typically occurs greater than 30 minutes after anesthesia induction due to its predominant mucocutaneous route of administration, although chlorhexidine impregnated central venous catheters could cause more rapid symptom onset. Chlorhexidine skin testing and specific IgE testing are highly predictive of allergic sensitivity and should be employed in the evaluation of POA.[66] Although less common, bacitracin and povidone-iodine also have been implicated in POA.[20]

Dyes

Blue dyes, commonly used for sentinel lymph node identification, increasingly are implicated in POA and were the third and fourth most common culprits in the French data and NAP6, respectively.[8,14] Patent blue V and isosulfan blue are the dyes used most commonly and are cross-reactive.[67] Methylene blue is a structurally dissimilar dye with less cross-reactivity, although anaphylaxis to methylene blue and cross-reactivity with patent blue V have both been reported.[68] Blue dyes are ubiquitous, and sensitization prior to surgery is thought to be due to exposure to a variety of everyday products, such as toothpaste, topical creams, and food dyes/additives. Onset of POA typically is delayed compared with intravenous medications, likely due to delayed lymphatic or subcutaneous absorption.

Hypnotics

Common hypnotic agents used for induction include propofol, ketamine, etomidate, and midazolam. They rarely are the culprit agent in POA (even less so following removal of polyethyoxylated castor oil (Cremophor EL) as a solvent for propofol) and accounted for only 1 case in NAP6 and 2% of cases in the French data.[8,14,17,20] There were previous concerns regarding propofol use in egg, soy, or peanut allergic patients given the soybean oil, egg lecithin, and glycerol found in propofol. Subsequent studies, however, have shown it safe to use in these populations, with a majority of true allergic reactions being due to the isopropyl groups in propofol.[8,69,70]

Opioids

Opioids are uncommon culprits in POA, with systemic reactions occurring at an estimated rate of 1 in every 100,000 to 200,000 instances of anesthetic administration.[20] Several opioids, morphine, codeine, and meperidine, in particular, can cause histamine release through direct mast cell degranulation, leading to typical cutaneous manifestations of urticaria and pruritus.[3,11,71]

Colloids

Gelatin, dextran, hetastarch, and albumin are the colloids used most commonly in the perioperative period. Of all colloids, gelatin has the highest risk of inducing a systemic reaction followed by dextrans, whereas albumin has the lowest risk.[72] IgE and non–IgE-mediated mechanisms account for colloid-induced POA with previous demonstration of specific IgE antibodies and positive intradermal skin tests against gelatin and detection of IgG and IgM antibodies to hetastarch and dextran in a variety of cases.[3,20] There is no known cross-sensitivity to different colloids, although cross-sensitivity to multiple forms of gelatin has been reported.[20]

Aside from colloid used for intravenous administration, gelatin also is found in topical hemostatic agents, which have been reported as culprit agents in several POA cases.[73–76] Gelatin accounted for 3 of the 192 cases of POA in NAP6.[8] With safer nongelatin colloids available, there has been recent discussion regarding whether the use of intravenous colloids should be reassessed.[77]

Blood Products

Anaphylaxis to blood products is rare, with a rate of 0.6 per 1000 transfusions, although it is higher in patients with IgA deficiency or previously sensitized patients (pregnancy or prior transfusion).[3,78]

Protamine

Protamine is a heparin neutralizing agent used in cardiac and vascular surgery that can cause IgE-mediated and non–IgE-mediated anaphylactic reactions. Sensitization typically is caused by prior intravenous protamine use or use of protamine-containing insulin. Protamine accounted for 1 POA case in NAP6.[8]

EVALUATION
Tryptase

The role of serum tryptase in the acute assessment of POA has been extensively reviewed previously.[17,20] Tryptase peaks 15 minutes to 120 minutes after the onset of reaction, with a half-life of 2 hours. A key point is that a normal tryptase does not rule out an anaphylactic event. Using an international consensus equation to determine acute mast cell degranulation ($[1.2 \times$ serum baseline tryptase$] + 2$ µg/L) showed a 75% sensitivity for POA diagnosis in a French cohort compared with 53% when using a tryptase level greater than 11.4 µg/L without substantial change in specificity or predictive value.[79] This highlights the importance of obtaining a baseline tryptase after recovery from POA. Persistently elevated levels greater than 11.4 µg/mL should prompt evaluation for an underlying mast cell disorder. Other markers of mast cell activation include the urinary metabolites n-methylhistamine, leukotriene E4, prostaglandin D2, and 2,3 dinor β-prostaglandin F2. They are not widely available and have not been evaluated in POA.

Skin Testing

Skin prick testing followed by intradermal skin testing remains the cornerstone of allergen identification in POA. Despite this, the sensitivities, specificities, and predictive values of the various drugs and substances are not well defined, and false-positive results due to irritant reactions can occur. As such, testing typically is done according to published guidelines reporting the maximal nonirritating concentrations **(Table 1)**.[80–82] Skin testing to latex and antibiotics other than penicillins is nonstandardized, but guidelines for nonirritating antibiotic concentrations are available.[83,84]

IgE Testing

Aside from chlorhexidine-specific IgE, which has a sensitivity and specificity nearing 100%, medication-specific IgE testing in POA evaluation is limited due to lack of availability and sensitivity.[66] Latex-specific IgE is commercially available in the United States, with a past report showing a sensitivity of 97% and specificity of 86% in the

Table 1
Nonirritating maximal concentrations for skin prick and intradermal testing

Agent	Undiluted (mg/mL)	Skin Prick Testing (mg/mL)		Intradermal Testing (mg/mL)	
		Dilution	Maximum concentration	Dilution	Maximum concentration
NMBA					
Atracurium	10	1/10	1	1/1000	0.01
Cisatracurium	2	Undiluted	2	1/100	0.02
Mivacurium	2	1/10	0.2	1/100	0.002
Pancuronium	2	Undiluted	2	1/100	0.02
Rocuronium	10	Undiluted	10	1/200	0.05
Vecuronium	4	Undiluted	4	1/100	0.04
Suxamethonium	50	1/5	10	1/500	0.1
Hypnotics					
Etomidate	2	Undiluted	2	1/10	0.2
Midazolam	5	Undiluted	5	1/100	0.05
Propofol	10	Undiluted	10	1/10	1
Thiopental	25	Undiluted	25	1/10	2.5
Ketamine	10	Undiluted	10	1/10	1
Opioids					
Alfentanil	0.5	Undiluted	0.5	1/10	0.05
Fentanyl	0.05	Undiluted	0.05	1/10	0.005
Sufentanil	0.005	Undiluted	0.005	1/10	0.0005
Remifentanil	0.05	Undiluted	0.05	1/10	0.005
Morphine	10	1/10	1	1/2000	0.005
Dyes					
Methylene blue	10	Undiluted	10	1/100	0.1
Patent blue	25	Undiluted	25	1/100	0.25
Antiseptics					
Chlorhexidine	5 (0.5%)	Undiluted	5	1/2500	0.002
NMBA reversal					
Sugammadex	100	Undiluted	100	1/10	10

From Volcheck GW, Hepner DL. Identification and Management of Perioperative Anaphylaxis. J Allergy Clin Immunol Pract. 2019 Sep-Oct;7(7):2134 to 2142; with permission.

diagnosis of latex allergy.[85] A recent review showed that sensitivity and specificity of specific IgE assays for β-lactam antibiotics varied widely, ranging from 0% to 85% and 52% to 100%, respectively.[86] Although the specificity of IgE testing for NMBAs ranges from 85.7% to 100%, its sensitivity is low, ranging from 38.5% to 92%.[86] This lack of consistent sensitivity and specificity makes IgE testing an adjunct to skin testing in the evaluation of POA rather than a primary tool.

Basophil Activation Testing

Basophil activation testing (BAT) is a highly specific in vitro test that measures surface CD63 or CD203c expressed on basophils after stimulation with the culprit agent. It has been used successfully in evaluation of immediate drug hypersensitivity as well as inhalant, food, and venom allergy, but its position in the diagnostic algorithm of these conditions is not established.[87] Although studies have shown 73% to 100% congruency between BAT and skin tests for NMBAs, the widespread adoption of BAT is limited by its lower sensitivity, required specialized equipment, and time-sensitive nature of the assay.[17,52,87,88]

MANAGEMENT
Acute Treatment

The initial management of POA includes withdrawal of the potential culprit agent(s) and early administration of epinephrine. Guidelines exist for dosing based on reaction severity, typically starting at intravenous doses of 10 μg for grade II reactions and titrating based on clinical response (**Table 2**).[36,89] Fluid resuscitation also is of paramount importance.[36,89] Antihistamines and corticosteroids, although commonly used, are not a substitute for epinephrine.[36,89]

Subsequent Procedures

The importance of allergy consultation and communication with the anesthesia and surgical teams cannot be overstated. A thorough review of the perioperative record, including medications used, time and route of administration, and nonmedication substances used (gels, dyes, disinfectants, hemostatic agents, and so forth), is mandatory to identify a culprit agent. There is no validated premedication protocol or evidence supporting premedication with antihistamines or corticosteroids prior to subsequent procedures.[18,31] As discussed previously, a recent study using a DNA aptamer that binds MRGPRX2 was able to prevent anaphylaxis in a rat model and thus potentially

Table 2
Epinephrine dosing recommendations in perioperative anaphylaxis

Ring and Messmer Grade	Epinephrine Dosing[a]
I	Not needed
II	20 μg bolus If suboptimal response, increase to 50 μg Repeat every 2 min as needed
III	50-μg bolus OR 100-μg bolus if previous suboptimal response to other vasopressors If suboptimal response, increase to 200 μg Repeat every 2 min as needed
IV	1 mg Repeat per advanced cardiac life support guidelines
Refractory[b]	Initiate epinephrine infusion at 0.05 μg/kg/min–0.1 μg/kg/min

[a] Intravenous dosing. Preferred intraoperatively when there is access to immediate hemodynamic measurements. Outside of the operating room, standard epinephrine dosing of 0.01 mg/kg intramuscular is recommended.

[b] Refractory POA is defined as inadequate response after 3 epinephrine boluses.

Adapted from Garvey LH, Dewachter P, Hepner DL, Mertes PM, Voltolini S, Clarke R, Cooke P, Garcez T, Guttormsen AB, Ebo DG, Hopkins PM, Khan DA, Kopac P, Krøigaard M, Laguna JJ, Marshall S, Platt P, Rose M, Sabato V, Sadleir P, Savic L, Savic S, Scherer K, Takazawa T, Volcheck GW, Kolawole H. Management of suspected immediate perioperative allergic reactions: an international overview and consensus recommendations. Br J Anaesth. 2019 Jul;123(1):e50-e64.

could serve as a therapeutic target for patients who have had POA in the future.[50] Despite these potential future advances, the key remains identifying the culprit and avoiding it. If no culprit is determined after extensive evaluation and testing, using alternative agents guided by negative skin testing typically is successful in preventing future POA episodes.[5,57]

SUMMARY

POA is a potentially life-threatening and under-recognized event. Although any medication or substance can be causative, antibiotics, NMBAs, chlorhexidine, latex, and dyes are the most common culprits. Early recognition, prompt epinephrine administration, and fluid management are the key components of acute management. Measurement of a serum tryptase at approximately 1 hour after reaction onset is helpful in establishing a diagnosis, although a normal tryptase does not rule out anaphylaxis. A subsequent baseline tryptase should be checked both to establish mast cell degranulation and to assess for persistent elevation suggestive of an underlying mast cell disorder. Comprehensive allergy evaluation, including thorough chart review, communication with anesthesia and surgical teams, and skin testing to possible culprit agents using nonirritating concentrations, is critical in establishing a potential culprit and planning for future procedures. Although this often is successful in preventing future episodes of anaphylaxis, MRGPRX2 offers a potential therapeutic target that could enhance success in the future.

CLINICS CARE POINTS

- POA can present with isolated cardiovascular collapse without cutaneous manifestations.
- When compiling a list of potential culprit agents, do not forget about nonintravenous substances (chlorhexidine, latex, and so forth).
- When determining a management plan for the patient with POA, early collaboration between surgical, anesthesia, and allergy teams is essential.

DISCLOSURE

The authors have no financial or commercial conflicts of interest to disclose.

REFERENCES

1. Mertes PM, Lambert M, Gueant-Rodriguez RM, et al. Perioperative anaphylaxis. Immunol Allergy Clin N Am 2009;29(3):429–51.
2. Mertes PM, Volcheck GW, Garvey LH, et al. Epidemiology of perioperative anaphylaxis. Presse Med 2016;45(9):758–67.
3. Mertes PM, Ebo DG, Garcez T, et al. Comparative epidemiology of suspected perioperative hypersensitivity reactions. Br J Anaesth 2019;123(1):e16–28.
4. Marinho S, Kemp H, Cook TM, et al. Cross-sectional study of perioperative drug and allergen exposure in UK practice in 2016: the 6th National Audit Project (NAP6) Allergen Survey. Br J Anaesth 2018;121(1):146–58.
5. Guyer AC, Saff RR, Conroy M, et al. Comprehensive allergy evaluation is useful in the subsequent care of patients with drug hypersensitivity reactions during anesthesia. J Allergy Clin Immunol Pract 2015;3(1):94–100.

6. Harboe T, Guttormsen AB, Irgens A, et al. Anaphylaxis during anesthesia in Norway: a 6-year single-center follow-up study. Anesthesiology 2005;102(5): 897–903.

7. Laxenaire MC, Mertes PM. Groupe d'Etudes des Reactions Anaphylactoides P. Anaphylaxis during anaesthesia. Results of a two-year survey in France. Br J Anaesth 2001;87(4):549–58.

8. Harper NJN, Cook TM, Garcez T, et al. Anaesthesia, surgery, and life-threatening allergic reactions: epidemiology and clinical features of perioperative anaphylaxis in the 6th National Audit Project (NAP6). Br J Anaesth 2018;121(1):159–71.

9. Berroa F, Lafuente A, Javaloyes G, et al. The incidence of perioperative hypersensitivity reactions: a single-center, prospective, cohort study. Anesth Analg 2015;121(1):117–23.

10. Ebo DG, Fisher MM, Hagendorens MM, et al. Anaphylaxis during anaesthesia: diagnostic approach. Allergy 2007;62(5):471–87.

11. Hepner DL, Castells MC. Anaphylaxis during the perioperative period. Anesth Analg 2003;97(5):1381–95.

12. Mertes PM, Tajima K, Regnier-Kimmoun MA, et al. Perioperative anaphylaxis. Med Clin North Am 2010;94(4):761–789, xi.

13. Savic LC, Kaura V, Yusaf M, et al. Incidence of suspected perioperative anaphylaxis: a multicenter snapshot study. J Allergy Clin Immunol Pract 2015;3(3): 454–455 e451.

14. Tacquard C, Collange O, Gomis P, et al. Anaesthetic hypersensitivity reactions in France between 2011 and 2012: the 10th GERAP epidemiologic survey. Acta Anaesthesiol Scand 2017;61(3):290–9.

15. Mertes PM, Alla F, Trechot P, et al. Groupe d'Etudes des Reactions Anaphylactoides P. Anaphylaxis during anesthesia in France: an 8-year national survey. J Allergy Clin Immunol 2011;128(2):366–73.

16. Ring J, Messmer K. Incidence and severity of anaphylactoid reactions to colloid volume substitutes. Lancet 1977;1(8009):466–9.

17. Kalangara J, Vanijcharoenkarn K, Lynde GC, et al. Approach to perioperative anaphylaxis in 2020: updates in diagnosis and management. Curr Allergy Asthma Rep 2021;21(1):4.

18. Dewachter P, Mouton-Faivre C, Castells MC, et al. Anesthesia in the patient with multiple drug allergies: are all allergies the same? Curr Opin Anaesthesiol 2011; 24(3):320–5.

19. Hsu Blatman KS, Hepner DL. Current knowledge and management of hypersensitivity to perioperative drugs and radiocontrast media. J Allergy Clin Immunol Pract 2017;5(3):587–92.

20. Volcheck GW, Hepner DL. Identification and management of perioperative anaphylaxis. J Allergy Clin Immunol Pract 2019;7(7):2134–42.

21. Bruhns P, Chollet-Martin S. Mechanisms of human drug-induced anaphylaxis. J Allergy Clin Immunol 2021;147(4):1133–42.

22. Cianferoni A. Non-IgE-mediated anaphylaxis. J Allergy Clin Immunol 2021; 147(4):1123–31.

23. McNeil BD, Pundir P, Meeker S, et al. Identification of a mast-cell-specific receptor crucial for pseudo-allergic drug reactions. Nature 2015;519(7542):237–41.

24. Navines-Ferrer A, Serrano-Candelas E, Lafuente A, et al. MRGPRX2-mediated mast cell response to drugs used in perioperative procedures and anaesthesia. Sci Rep 2018;8(1):11628.

25. Ebo DG, Van der Poorten ML, Elst J, et al. Immunoglobulin E cross-linking or MRGPRX2 activation: clinical insights from rocuronium hypersensitivity. Br J Anaesth 2021;126(1):e27–9.

26. Ebo DG, Van Gasse AL, Decuyper II, et al. Acute management, diagnosis, and follow-up of suspected perioperative hypersensitivity reactions in flanders 2001-2018. J Allergy Clin Immunol Pract 2019;7(7):2194–2204 e2197.

27. Gonzalez-Estrada A, Pien LC, Zell K, et al. Antibiotics are an important identifiable cause of perioperative anaphylaxis in the United States. J Allergy Clin Immunol Pract 2015;3(1):101–105 e101.

28. Gurrieri C, Weingarten TN, Martin DP, et al. Allergic reactions during anesthesia at a large United States referral center. Anesth Analg 2011;113(5):1202–12.

29. Dewachter P, Mouton-Faivre C, Hepner DL. Perioperative anaphylaxis: what should be known? Curr Allergy Asthma Rep 2015;15(5):21.

30. Ebo DG, Clarke RC, Mertes PM, et al. Molecular mechanisms and pathophysiology of perioperative hypersensitivity and anaphylaxis: a narrative review. Br J Anaesth 2019;123(1):e38–49.

31. Mertes PM, Malinovsky JM, Jouffroy L, et al. Reducing the risk of anaphylaxis during anesthesia: 2011 updated guidelines for clinical practice. J Investig Allergol Clin Immunol 2011;21(6):442–53.

32. Hopkins PM, Cooke PJ, Clarke RC, et al. Consensus clinical scoring for suspected perioperative immediate hypersensitivity reactions. Br J Anaesth 2019; 123(1):e29–37.

33. Cox LS, Sanchez-Borges M, Lockey RF. World allergy organization systemic allergic reaction grading system: is a modification needed? J Allergy Clin Immunol Pract 2017;5(1):58–62 e55.

34. Rose MA, Green SL, Crilly HM, et al. Perioperative anaphylaxis grading system: 'making the grade'. Br J Anaesth 2016;117(5):551–3.

35. Savic LC, Garvey LH. Perioperative anaphylaxis: diagnostic challenges and management. Curr Opin Anaesthesiol 2020;33(3):448–53.

36. Garvey LH, Dewachter P, Hepner DL, et al. Management of suspected immediate perioperative allergic reactions: an international overview and consensus recommendations. Br J Anaesth 2019;123(1):e50–64.

37. Tassoudis V, Ieropoulos H, Karanikolas M, et al. Bronchospasm in obese patients undergoing elective laparoscopic surgery under general anesthesia. Springerplus 2016;5:435.

38. Hepner DL. Sudden bronchospasm on intubation: latex anaphylaxis? J Clin Anesth 2000;12(2):162–6.

39. Sadleir PH, Clarke RC, Bunning DL, et al. Anaphylaxis to neuromuscular blocking drugs: incidence and cross-reactivity in Western Australia from 2002 to 2011. Br J Anaesth 2013;110(6):981–7.

40. Garvey LH, Roed-Petersen J, Menne T, et al. Danish anaesthesia allergy centre - preliminary results. Acta Anaesthesiol Scand 2001;45(10):1204–9.

41. Lobera T, Audicana MT, Pozo MD, et al. Study of hypersensitivity reactions and anaphylaxis during anesthesia in Spain. J Investig Allergol Clin Immunol 2008; 18(5):350–6.

42. Baldo BA, Fisher MM. Substituted ammonium ions as allergenic determinants in drug allergy. Nature 1983;306(5940):262–4.

43. Gueant JL, Mata E, Namour F, et al. Criteria of evaluation and of interpretation of Sepharose drug IgE-RIA to anaesthetic drugs. Allergy 1999;54(Suppl 58):17–22.

44. Dong S, Acouetey DS, Gueant-Rodriguez RM, et al. Prevalence of IgE against neuromuscular blocking agents in hairdressers and bakers. Clin Exp Allergy 2013;43(11):1256–62.

45. Florvaag E, Johansson SG. The pholcodine story. Immunol Allergy Clin North Am 2009;29(3):419–27.

46. Florvaag E, Johansson SG. The Pholcodine case. cough medicines, IgE-Sensitization, and anaphylaxis: a devious connection. World Allergy Organ J 2012;5(7):73–8.

47. Florvaag E, Johansson SG, Irgens A, et al. IgE-sensitization to the cough suppressant pholcodine and the effects of its withdrawal from the Norwegian market. Allergy 2011;66(7):955–60.

48. Che D, Wang J, Ding Y, et al. Mivacurium induce mast cell activation and pseudoallergic reactions via MAS-related G protein coupled receptor-X2. Cell Immunol 2018;332:121–8.

49. Mertes PM, Volcheck GW. Anaphylaxis to neuromuscular-blocking drugs: all neuromuscular-blocking drugs are not the same. Anesthesiology 2015; 122(1):5–7.

50. Suzuki Y, Liu S, Ogasawara T, et al. A novel MRGPRX2-targeting antagonistic DNA aptamer inhibits histamine release and prevents mast cell-mediated anaphylaxis. Eur J Pharmacol 2020;878:173104.

51. Reddy JI, Cooke PJ, van Schalkwyk JM, et al. Anaphylaxis is more common with rocuronium and succinylcholine than with atracurium. Anesthesiology 2015; 122(1):39–45.

52. Dewachter P, Chollet-Martin S, Mouton-Faivre C, et al. Comparison of basophil activation test and skin testing performances in NMBA Allergy. J Allergy Clin Immunol Pract 2018;6(5):1681–9.

53. Leynadier F, Dry J. Anaphylaxis to muscle-relaxant drugs: study of cross-reactivity by skin tests. Int Arch Allergy Appl Immunol 1991;94(1–4):349–53.

54. Baldo BA, Fisher MM. Anaphylaxis to muscle relaxant drugs: cross-reactivity and molecular basis of binding of IgE antibodies detected by radioimmunoassay. Mol Immunol 1983;20(12):1393 400.

55. Leynadier F, Sansarricq M, Didier JM, et al. Prick tests in the diagnosis of anaphylaxis to general anaesthetics. Br J Anaesth 1987;59(6):683–9.

56. Chiriac AM, Tacquard C, Fadhel NB, et al. Safety of subsequent general anaesthesia in patients allergic to neuromuscular blocking agents: value of allergy skin testing. Br J Anaesth 2018;120(6):1437–40.

57. Miller J, Clough SB, Pollard RC, et al. Outcome of repeat anaesthesia after investigation for perioperative anaphylaxis. Br J Anaesth 2018;120(6):1195–201.

58. Kayode OS, Rutkowski K, Haque R, et al. Teicoplanin hypersensitivity in perioperative anaphylaxis. J Allergy Clin Immunol Pract 2020;8(6):2110–3.

59. Macy E, Ngor EW. Safely diagnosing clinically significant penicillin allergy using only penicilloyl-poly-lysine, penicillin, and oral amoxicillin. J Allergy Clin Immunol Pract 2013;1(3):258–63.

60. Savic LC, Khan DA, Kopac P, et al. Management of a surgical patient with a label of penicillin allergy: narrative review and consensus recommendations. Br J Anaesth 2019;123(1):e82–94.

61. Dong SW, Mertes PM, Petitpain N, et al. Gerap. Hypersensitivity reactions during anesthesia. Results from the ninth French survey (2005-2007). Minerva Anestesiol 2012;78(8):868–78.

62. Habre W, Disma N, Virag K, et al. Incidence of severe critical events in paediatric anaesthesia (APRICOT): a prospective multicentre observational study in 261 hospitals in Europe. Lancet Respir Med 2017;5(5):412–25.

63. Hepner DL, Castells MC. Latex allergy: an update. Anesth Analg 2003;96(4): 1219–29.

64. Horiuchi T, Takazawa T, Orihara M, et al. Drug-induced anaphylaxis during general anesthesia in 14 tertiary hospitals in Japan: a retrospective, multicenter, observational study. J Anesth 2021;35(1):154–60.

65. Ebo DG, Baldo BA, Van Gasse AL, et al. Anaphylaxis to sugammadex-rocuronium inclusion complex: An IgE-mediated reaction due to allergenic changes at the sugammadex primary rim. J Allergy Clin Immunol Pract 2020; 8(4):1410–5, e1413.

66. Opstrup MS, Malling HJ, Kroigaard M, et al. Standardized testing with chlorhexidine in perioperative allergy–a large single-centre evaluation. Allergy 2014; 69(10):1390–6.

67. Scherer K, Studer W, Figueiredo V, et al. Anaphylaxis to isosulfan blue and cross-reactivity to patent blue V: case report and review of the nomenclature of vital blue dyes. Ann Allergy Asthma Immunol 2006;96(3):497–500.

68. Mertes PM, Malinovsky JM, Mouton-Faivre C, et al. Anaphylaxis to dyes during the perioperative period: reports of 14 clinical cases. J Allergy Clin Immunol 2008;122(2):348–52.

69. Dewachter P, Kopac P, Laguna JJ, et al. Anaesthetic management of patients with pre-existing allergic conditions: a narrative review. Br J Anaesth 2019; 123(1):e65–81.

70. Laxenaire MC, Mata-Bermejo E, Moneret-Vautrin DA, et al. Life-threatening anaphylactoid reactions to propofol (Diprivan). Anesthesiology 1992;77(2): 275–80.

71. Kalangara J, Potru S, Kuruvilla M. Clinical manifestations and diagnostic evaluation of opioid allergy labels - a review. J Pain Palliat Care Pharmacother 2019; 33(3–4):131–40.

72. Barron ME, Wilkes MM, Navickis RJ. A systematic review of the comparative safety of colloids. Arch Surg 2004;139(5):552–63.

73. Khoriaty E, McClain CD, Permaul P, et al. Intraoperative anaphylaxis induced by the gelatin component of thrombin-soaked gelfoam in a pediatric patient. Ann Allergy Asthma Immunol 2012;108(3):209–10.

74. Lied GA, Lund KB, Storaas T. Intraoperative anaphylaxis to gelatin-based hemostatic agents: a case report. J Asthma Allergy 2019;12:163–7.

75. Luhmann SJ, Sucato DJ, Bacharier L, et al. Intraoperative anaphylaxis secondary to intraosseous gelatin administration. J Pediatr Orthop 2013;33(5):e58–60.

76. Manrique Espinel AM, Feldman JM, Nelson S, et al. Anaphylaxis to Surgiflo During Posterior Spinal Fusion in an Adolescent Status Post Truncus Arteriosus Repair: A Case Report. A A Pract 2018;10(6):129–32.

77. Charlesworth M, Shelton CL. Should intravenous gelatins have a role in contemporary peri-operative and critical care? Anaesthesia 2020;75(2):266–9.

78. Mertes PM, Bazin A, Alla F, et al. Hypersensitivity reactions to blood components: document issued by the allergy committee of the French medicines and healthcare products regulatory agency. J Investig Allergol Clin Immunol 2011;21(3): 171–8.

79. Vitte J, Amadei L, Gouitaa M, et al. Paired acute-baseline serum tryptase levels in perioperative anaphylaxis: An observational study. Allergy 2019;74(6):1157–65.

80. Brockow K, Garvey LH, Aberer W, et al. Skin test concentrations for systemically administered drugs – an ENDA/EAACI Drug Allergy Interest Group position paper. Allergy 2013;68(6):702–12.
81. Garvey LH, Ebo DG, Mertes PM, et al. An EAACI position paper on the investigation of perioperative immediate hypersensitivity reactions. Allergy 2019;74(10):1872–84.
82. Volcheck GW, Mertes PM. Local and general anesthetics immediate hypersensitivity reactions. Immunol Allergy Clin North Am 2014;34(3):525–546, viii.
83. Khan DA, Banerji A, Bernstein JA, et al. Cephalosporin allergy: current understanding and future challenges. J Allergy Clin Immunol Pract 2019;7(7):2105–14.
84. Broyles AD, Banerji A, Barmettler S, et al. Practical guidance for the evaluation and management of drug hypersensitivity: specific drugs. J Allergy Clin Immunol Pract 2020;8(9S):S16–116.
85. Ebo DG, Stevens WJ, Bridts CH, et al. Latex -specific IgE, skin testing, and lymphocyte transformation to latex in latex allergy. J Allergy Clin Immunol 1997;100(5):618–23.
86. van der Poorten MM, Van Gasse AL, Hagendorens MM, et al. Serum specific IgE antibodies in immediate drug hypersensitivity. Clin Chim Acta 2020;504:119–24.
87. Ebo DG, Bridts CH, Mertens CH, et al. Principles, potential, and limitations of ex vivo basophil activation by flow cytometry in allergology: A narrative review. J Allergy Clin Immunol 2021;147(4):1143–53.
88. Ebo DG, Faber M, Elst J, et al. In vitro diagnosis of immediate drug hypersensitivity during anesthesia: a review of the literature. J Allergy Clin Immunol Pract 2018;6(4):1176–84.
89. Harper NJN, Cook TM, Garcez T, et al. Anaesthesia, surgery, and life-threatening allergic reactions: management and outcomes in the 6th National Audit Project (NAP6). Br J Anaesth 2018;121(1):172–88.

Anaphylaxis to Stinging Insect Venom

Karla E. Adams, MD[a],*, James M. Tracy, DO[b,c], David B.K. Golden, MDCM[d]

KEYWORDS

- Stinging • Insect • Allergy • Anaphylaxis • Hymenoptera • Venom • Immunotherapy

KEY POINTS

- The clinical history of an insect reaction is key to determining the diagnostic evaluation and therapeutic options that are needed.
- Patients with Hymenoptera venom allergy should be assessed for factors that may place them at risk during the diagnostic evaluation and treatment of venom allergy.
- Venom immunotherapy is the treatment of choice to decrease future risk in Hymenoptera venom allergy and should be considered for all patients with insect-triggered anaphylaxis. Patients deemed to be at high risk for relapse should be candidates for lifelong immunotherapy.

INTRODUCTION

Stings from insects are a common nuisance throughout the world. For some, insect stings carry significant morbidity due to the development of severe allergic reactions. Stinging insects from the order Hymenoptera are common triggers for allergic reactions. **Fig. 1** shows the important taxonomic relationships within the Hymenoptera order, with 3 distinct families of importance: Apidae (bees), Vespidae (yellow jackets [YJ], hornets, wasps), and Formicidae (stinging ants of several genera).

PREVALENCE

The prevalence of Hymenoptera venom allergy (HVA) in adults is 0.3% to 3.3% in the United States and 0.3% to 7.5% in Europe.[1,2] In children, prevalence of insect sting allergy is estimated to be 0.8%.[3] Based on survey data, anaphylaxis to the imported fire ant (IFA) is seen in 2% of the population in endemic areas of the United States.[4]

[a] Allergy & Immunology Division, Department of Medicine, Wilford Hall Ambulatory Surgical Center, 1100 Wilford Hall Loop, Building 4554, Lackland AFB, San Antonio, TX 78236, USA; [b] University of Nebraska College of Medicine; [c] Allergy, Asthma and Immunology Associates, P. C., 2808 South 80th Avenue, Suite 210, Omaha, NE 68133, USA; [d] Johns Hopkins University, 25 Crossroads Drive #410, Owings Mills, MD 21117, USA
* Corresponding author.
E-mail address: karla.e.adams2.mil@mail.mil

Immunol Allergy Clin N Am 42 (2022) 161–173
https://doi.org/10.1016/j.iac.2021.09.003
0889-8561/22/Published by Elsevier Inc.

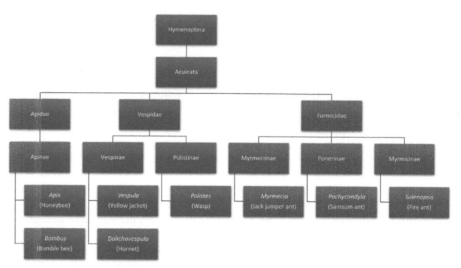

Fig. 1. Hymenoptera taxonomy.

Fatal reactions occur at an annual rate of 0.1 cases per million.[5] Although the incidence of all-cause anaphylaxis and HVA has increased over decades, the fatality case rate has remained stable. In the United States, male sex, older age, and white race were noted as risk factors for fatal insect reactions.[6]

CLINICAL PRESENTATION

Important historical information needs to be gathered from patients to determine the culprit stinging insect and the clinical pattern of reaction. Some Hymenoptera species will only sting if feeling threatened (eg, *Polistes* spp), so occupations that are more likely to disturb nests in trees or in the ground may experience increased stings from these insects. Other species (eg, *Vespula* spp) are commonly found in areas where humans are eating and can sting with little provocation.

Reactions to stinging insects range from painful, localized cutaneous symptoms to anaphylaxis. For IFA stings, normal local reactions also include the development of a sterile pseudopustule at the site of the sting. Large local reactions (LLRs) are typically defined as erythema and induration of 10 cm or larger starting 12 to 24 hours after a sting and lasting 3 to 10 days. Generalized reactions range from single organ system involvement (eg, systemic cutaneous reactions characterized by generalized urticaria with or without angioedema) to anaphylaxis, which has multiorgan involvement. Biphasic reactions are uncommon with insect stings, although the reason for this may be that they are underreported. In a prospective study, Hymenoptera stings were the cause of 25% of biphasic reactions.[7]

NATURAL HISTORY OF STINGING INSECT REACTIONS

The natural history of stinging insect reactions will determine what, if any, additional evaluation or treatment is needed. For example, asymptomatic venom sensitization or evidence of specific IgE (sIgE) without a correlating reaction history has been noted in up to 15% of adults.[2] The risk of future sting anaphylaxis in individuals with asymptomatic sensitization is relatively small, and thus no testing or venom immunotherapy

(VIT) is required. The natural history in other (symptomatic) sensitized individuals is reviewed later in the article.

Large Local Reactions

LLRs are late-phase IgE-mediated reactions that are typically self-limited but can cause significant morbidity. Historical data have shown that patients with LLRs are likely to have recurrent LLRs with repeat stings and only a 1.4% to 7% risk for systemic symptoms.[8,9] However, in a recent European study of patients with LLRs to Hymenoptera, repeat stings led to systemic reactions (SRs) in 24% of patients.[10] Additional testing or VIT is generally not recommended in patients with LLRs; however, it may be considered in cases in which unavoidable stings cause recurrent LLRs that affect quality of life (QOL).

Systemic Cutaneous Reactions and Anaphylaxis

The single best predictor for recurrent reactions is the severity of a previous insect-related reaction. For example, most individuals with a history of a cutaneous SR to a stinging insect go on to have the same or less severe symptoms on a subsequent sting. The risk of a more severe reaction is best estimated up to 3%, although some studies with limited data suggest risk up to 15%.[9,11–13] Although adults with previous cutaneous SRs to stings have been historically advised to receive VIT, in the most recent stinging insect allergy practice parameter, both children and adults with cutaneous SRs are advised that routine testing or VIT are not needed because the risk with future stings is relatively low.[14] As with LLR, VIT may be considered for those with cutaneous SRs due to other risk factors or impaired QOL. By comparison, patients with anaphylaxis to Hymenoptera have a 30% to 67% risk for recurrent anaphylaxis on a subsequent sting and thus require evaluation and VIT.[9,11,12]

EVALUATION

The decision to test for HVA is based on the detailed history of a stinging insect reaction, an assessment of current and future risks, and a consideration for medical and lifestyle factors that may place someone at increased risk with future stings. As patients may not be proficient at correctly identifying flying insects, it is recommended that testing for all available flying Hymenoptera (FH) species is done.

Skin Testing and Serologic Testing

Standard testing options include an assessment for venom sIgE through skin test (SKT) or serologic testing. Given the significant morbidity associated with HVA, the variability of venom SKT responses and limited concordance between testing modalities, patients with negative results on one type of test should have repeat testing via the other modality because they may still be at risk for subsequent Hymenoptera reactions.[15] Similarly, if all initial testing results are negative, then repeat testing after 1 to 2 months should be done. Neither the SKT sensitivity nor the absolute serum sIgE level is predictive of the severity of a Hymenoptera sting reaction.

Although SKT is generally considered safe, testing protocols can be time consuming and may be limited in certain populations due to discomfort. A single-step intradermal (ID) test at a concentration of 1 μg/mL was noted to be safe in a retrospective study.[16] Simultaneous ID testing (ie, placement of multiple ID concentrations) has also been deemed safe.[17] Concurrent or single-step testing protocols seem to be safe, faster, and more cost-effective methods in assessing for HVA compared with the standard sequential approach of testing.

Imported Fire Ant Hypersensitivity Testing

IFA testing follows the same protocol as for FH. Testing for IFA alone is reasonable in patients who live in an endemic area and can clearly identify IFA as the culprit insect. IFA whole-body extracts (WBE) that include *Solenopsis invicta, Solenopsis richteri,* or a mixture are commercially available for SKT. Similar to FH, in vitro testing for IFA sIgE is also available and should be considered for patients who are not SKT candidates or in patients who have a negative SKT despite a convincing history of IFA-triggered systemic symptoms.

Serum Basal Tryptase

Obtaining a serum basal tryptase (sBT) level should be considered in all patients with HVA because an elevated sBT level is a marker for mast cell burden and mast cell disease (MCD). Elevated sBT levels are associated with increased risk for HVA, sting reaction severity, side effects during VIT in both children and adults, and relapse after VIT.[18-20] Moreover, although the accepted upper limit for a normal sBT level is 11.4 ng/mL, this cutoff may be inadequate because levels greater than 5 ng/mL may be predictive of sting reaction severity.[18] In fact, sBT levels can be used to risk stratify patients with HVA.[21]

A recent study noted that elevated sBT levels may be due to hereditary α-tryptasemia (HαT). HαT, a genetic condition with multiple copies of the α-tryptase gene, is seen in 5.6% of healthy individuals. HαT is more frequent in patients with Hymenoptera reaction (with increased severity of reaction), in those with mastocytosis, and in idiopathic anaphylaxis.[22] For patients with HVA, even those with normal sBT levels, an additional biomarker identified is the detection of the *KIT* p.D816V mutation in peripheral blood, which correlated with a higher frequency of severe symptoms.[23] Additional data regarding the limitations and advantages of these tests is needed before recommending their routine use in HVA evaluations.

Component Resolved Diagnostics

Evidence of sIgE to multiple venoms may be due to clinically relevant cosensitization, cross-reactive carbohydrate determinants (CCDs), or homologous venom protein epitopes leading to cross-reactivity. The use of CCD-free, species-specific recombinant allergens has been described as a way to increase the accuracy and sensitivity of venom testing. In vitro testing with YJ venom spiked with recombinant Ves v 5 (rVes v 5) increases the sensitivity of the test from 83.4% to 96.8%.[24] However, testing with single recombinant allergens may not suffice. In a cohort of honeybee (HB) allergic patients, evidence of sIgE to single recombinant allergens (rApi 1–3, rApi m 5, and rApi m 10) ranged from 47.9% to 72.2%. However, when taken together, positive tests to at least 1 recombinant HB allergen was noted in 94.4% of patients.[25] Recently, component resolved diagnostics (CRD) for Hymenoptera venoms has been approved by the US Food and Drug Administration and has become more available, although limitations still exist, which prevent its use routinely. For example, the clinical availability of full panels of recombinant allergens is needed to ensure that diagnostic sensitivity is improved with the use of CRD. In addition, component testing needs to take into account the geographic distribution of Hymenoptera whereby component panels for all relevant species in a location need to be commercially available to be clinically useful. If available, the main clinical application of venom CRD is in elucidating dual sensitization patterns in patients with HB and YJ sensitivity.[26,27] CRD can distinguish those who need both HB and YJ for VIT and those who need only the one that is their primary allergen. This approach will be more useful in the United

States when it can be applied to *Polistes*/YJ dual sensitivity. **Table 1** has a listing of recombinant allergens and their corresponding native allergens. Finally, as there remains a single commercial supplier of venom for testing and treating there may be a cost savings opportunity by treating with a single venom versus multiple venoms.

Basophil Activation Test

The basophil activation test (BAT) is a functional test of basophil reactivity that measures upregulation of CD63 or CD203c on basophils after allergen exposure. The BAT is a sensitive test that can detect sensitization in patients with HVA with inconclusive serologic and SKT results and in those with double sensitization.[28] Decreased BAT sensitivity (ie, percent CD63 basophil response) is associated with successful VIT induction of tolerance and thus serves as an in vitro marker for VIT effectiveness and for treatment failure.[29,30] Finally, high BAT sensitivity as measured by concentration-dependent activation ratios was noted to be predictive for reactions during VIT in children and adults.[31,32] Although the characteristics of the BAT make it a potentially useful test, current limitations include a lack of commercial availability and inconsistent methodology, analysis, and reporting of results. However, at this time BAT has begun to evolve as a more available diagnostic tool.

RISK FACTORS

In addition to the clinical history of a stinging insect reaction, there are several factors that may predispose individuals to increased risks for HVA. Some risk factors may be modifiable (eg, underlying asthma control), whereas other nonmodifiable risk factors (eg, age) still need to be accounted for and used to determine an individual's risk profile.

Medications

Medications such as β-blockers (BB) or angiotensin-converting enzyme (ACE) inhibitors (ACE-I) may be associated with an increased risk for severe anaphylaxis due to interference of the endogenous compensatory mechanisms or exogenous therapeutic interventions (eg, epinephrine) use to treat anaphylaxis. Data from Europe showed that both ACE-I and BB were associated with increased severity of anaphylaxis in patients with HVA and non-HVA patients, although the medication effect may have been related to underlying cardiovascular disease.[33] On the other hand, there was no

Table 1 Hymenoptera venom allergens and recombinant component allergens			
Genus and Species	**Allergen**	**Name/Function**	**Recombinant Allergen**
Apis mellifera	Api m 1	Phospholipase 2	rApi m 1
	Api m 2	Hyaluronidase	rApi m 2
	Api m 3	Acid phosphatase	rApi m 3
	Api m 5	Dipeptidyl peptidase	rApi m 5
	Api m 10	Carbohydrate-rich protein	rApi m 10
Vespula vulgaris	Ves v 1	Phospholipase 1	rVes v 1
	Ves v 3	Dipeptidyl peptidase	rVes v 3
	Ves v 5	Antigen 5	rVes v 5
Polistes dominulus	Pol d 1	Phospholipase 1	rPol d 1
	Pol d 5	Antigen 5	rPol d 5

correlation between HVA reaction severity and the use of BB, ACE-I, or both in a retrospective review of 657 patients with HVA.[20] There is now increasing evidence that points to the safety of these medications in patients on VIT.[34,35] In the largest prospective study to date, neither BB nor ACE-I use were associated with increased risk for SRs or severity of SRs on VIT.[36] Furthermore, efficacy of VIT was not affected for patients on these medications, which adds supporting data to the notion that BB and ACE-I can be safely continued during VIT.

Mast Cell Disease

The close relationship between MCD and HVA has been elucidated over the last 3 decades. Insect stings are a leading cause for anaphylaxis in patients with underlying MCD. The prevalence of clonal MCD in patients with SRs to Hymenoptera is 1% to 7.9%.[37] Conversely, 88.2% of patients with HVA with an elevated sBT level were subsequently diagnosed with MCD.[38] Although an elevated sBT level may indicate the possibility of MCD, cases of MCD in patients with HVA with normal sBT levels have also been described.[39] In patients with normal sBT levels, insect-triggered hypotension without cutaneous symptoms may be the most critical historical factor to identify concurrent MCD.[39] Because SKT and serologic testing may be negative in patients with MCD, use of CRD or a decrease in the threshold sIgE cutoff may help to establish a diagnosis of HVA.[40,41]

MCD also predisposes patients to increased severity of sting-related reactions with rare fatal stings described.[41] VIT is the treatment of choice for HVA in patients with MCD. Systemic side effects with VIT are seen in up to 13.9% of patients with MCD.[37] Successful conventional and rush immunotherapy using IFA WBE in patients with MCD has also been described.[42] Finally, MCD is also a risk factor for relapse in patients who have completed a course of VIT.[43] For this reason, patients with MCD and HVA should be considered candidates for prolonged VIT courses.

Trigger Insect

The particular insect that triggered the allergic reaction may also impact risk. For example, vespid stings were associated with increased risk for field sting reaction severity before VIT, whereas HB allergy was an independent predictor of side effects during VIT.[18,19] HB allergy has historically been considered higher risk, although the exact reasons are unclear. One reason may be related to the increased venom content released by HBs compared with vespids (50–140 µg vs 2–17 µg, respectively). It is also theorized that venom composition in extracts used to diagnose HB allergy (eg, lack of Api m 10) as well as differences in individual sensitization profiles may play a role.[25,44] Predominant Api m 10 sensitization was the best predictor for treatment failure in patients on HB VIT confirmed via a sting challenge.[45]

THERAPEUTICS

Acute treatment of anaphylaxis follows the same algorithm as other triggers of anaphylaxis. Once acute symptoms are resolved, patients require a referral to an allergy specialist for further evaluation of HVA. Patients also need to be educated on avoidance measures, wearing of medical alert jewelry, and carrying self-injectable epinephrine in case of future stings. **Fig. 2** is a flow diagram for the evaluation and management of insect-triggered reactions that takes into account clinical history and risk factors.

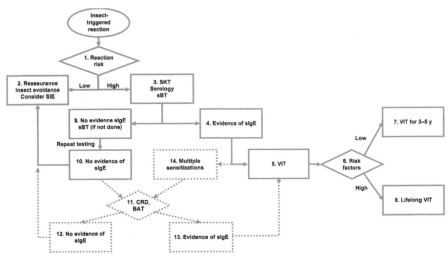

Fig. 2. Flow diagram for the evaluation and management of insect-triggered reactions. BAT, basophil activation test; CRD, component resolved diagnostics; SIE, self-injectable epineph-rine. Solid lines describe current clinical practice; dashed lines indicate the potential work-flow with the availability of adjunct tests. (1) The first decision point is an assessment of a patient's future risk with a subsequent insect sting. (2) Low-risk reactions (eg, large local re-actions) require reassurance and education on insect avoidance. In select cases, SIE may be prescribed. (3) For high-risk reactions (eg, anaphylaxis), SKT and/or serology is recommen-ded. An sBT is recommended because it will help with risk stratification. (4 and 5) Evidence of sIgE that is consistent with the clinical history requires VIT. (6–8) Risk stratification that takes into account the reaction history and the patient's medical history is needed to deter-mine duration of treatment. (9) If no evidence of sIgE is discovered, the tests should be repeated in 1 to 2 months. An sBT can be considered at this stage if not already done. (10) If repeat testing still fails to show evidence of sIgE, then it is recommended that patients be counseled on insect avoidance and have SIE prescribed. (11) If available, CRD or BAT testing should be considered. (12) If additional tests fail to show evidence of sIgE, then it is recommended that patients be counseled on insect avoidance and have SIE prescribed. (13) Evidence of sIgE after CRD or BAT testing that is consistent with the clinical history re-quires VIT. (14) If multiple sensitizations are noted without a correlating history, then CRD and BAT testing should be considered to further delineate true sensitization versus cross-reacting carbohydrate determinants.

Venom Immunotherapy

VIT is the single best therapy to decrease the risk of anaphylaxis with future stings in HVA. VIT reduces the risk of subsequent sting-related reactions to 3% to 5%, although the efficacy may be lower for high-risk groups (eg, 75% to 85% efficacy for VIT for HB allergy or in MCD).[9,37,46,47]

Dosing and Schedules

For FH, the maintenance dose (MD) is 100 µg, although a higher MD of 200 µg may be considered in refractory cases (eg, field sting triggered symptoms while on MD VIT). Once MD is reached, the schedule can be spaced to every 4 weeks. Extended main-tenance intervals (EMI) of 6 to 8 weeks can be considered after 12 to 18 months of monthly MDs. EMI of up to 12 weeks have been shown to be safe and effective after 3 to 4 years on MD treatment.[48]

Duration

Current recommendations for length of VIT treatment is 3 to 5 years in both children and adults, although longer treatment courses may be superior. Higher risk for recurrence was noted in patients experiencing more severe initial sting reactions, those with SRs to VIT injection, in HB allergic individuals, and in those with MCD.[49] Longer VIT treatment duration should be considered for patients deemed to be at high risk for relapse. Lifetime treatment is recommended to patients with mastocytosis because of the reported risk of fatal reaction. There are no long-term data to determine how long to extend VIT in high-risk patients. The risk of sting reaction remains even when the SKT becomes negative.[50]

Safety

Adverse reactions to VIT include minor local reactions, LLRs, and SRs that occur mostly during the build-up phase. Compared with accelerated schedules for aeroallergen immunotherapy, accelerated VIT protocols have not been associated with a similarly increased risk of side effects.[51] Risk factors for reactions include treatment with HB venom, an elevated sBT level, and use of an ultrarush build-up protocol.[19] The use of H1 and H2 antagonists for premedication can decrease the risk of local and systemic side effects during VIT.[52] Finally, omalizumab has been used as a pretreatment and concurrent treatment strategy for patients with and without MCD who experience recurrent reactions to VIT.[53]

Whole-Body Extract Immunotherapy

Immunotherapy using crushed FH was not shown to be better than placebo, whereas IFA WBE has been shown to reduce the risk of subsequent sting reactions to 2.1%.[46,54] The MD for IFA WBE is 0.5 mL of a 1:100 weight/volume extract concentration.[54,55] The build-up schedule for IFA WBE is less well defined compared with that for FH VIT. In general, build-up occurs with once to twice per week doses until MD is reached at which point the interval can be extended to monthly doses.[14] The suggested duration of IFA WBE treatment is 3 to 5 years. In one small retrospective study, patients receiving less than 3 years of IFA WBE noted a similar level of protection as patients who received 3 or more years.[56] Larger controlled studies are needed to delineate the optimal duration of IFA WBE treatment. Because frequency of exposure is considered a risk factor, and the attack rate for IFA is much higher than for FH, extended treatment may be considered.

Venom Extracts and Availability

Venom extracts are the cornerstone for the evaluation and treatment of HVA. Knowledge of location and relevant species is key because this will determine whether commercial extracts will be diagnostically and therapeutically useful (eg, because *Polistes dominulus* has incomplete cross-reactivity with other *Polistes* spp; availability of a *P dominulus* extract is desirable in locations where this species is present).[57]

Concern about the availability of venom extracts was highlighted by the shortage of extracts in 2016 after the loss of an extract supplier in North America.[58] Mitigation strategies such as the use of EMI or the switch to a different manufacturer's extracts are both feasible plans. Safety and efficacy of lowered MDs (eg, 50 μg) has been studied and shown to provide good efficacy in children, although the data in adults are conflicting.[59–61] Other long-term strategies include improvement in diagnostics such as CRD to ensure that patients are only treated with extracts that are clinically relevant. Other venom extract preparations such as depot and dialyzed venoms are currently not available in North America. Access to VIT is also an issue. For instance, insurance reimbursement has not kept pace with the cost of venom extracts, contributing to a decrease in the number of allergy clinics that offer venom testing and treatment. Finally, delays in provision of VIT can also arise from a lack of demand as seen during the coronavirus 2019 pandemic, which necessitated the need to space out or even stop VIT in some locations to slow the spread of the virus.

SUMMARY

Allergic reactions to members of the Hymenoptera order of insects are associated with significant morbidity for the world's population. Knowledge of taxonomic relationships is key to understanding and interpreting diagnostic tests and management of HVA. The clinical history of an insect-triggered reaction is the most important aspect to the diagnosis of HVA because it impacts what evaluation and treatments are required. A risk assessment for all patients needs to occur because it will guide recommendations for evaluation and treatment duration. Finally, although much is known about HVA, questions still remain that need further research to move the field to one of precise and individualized medical care.

CLINICS CARE POINTS

- The details of the clinical history of an insect-triggered reaction are the most important factors that will determine if evaluation and treatment of HVA is indicated.
- Patients with insect reactions should be referred to an allergist/immunologist for education and to conduct an assessment of risk factors to determine the risk of anaphylaxis, the need for evaluation and VIT, and the duration of VIT treatment.
- For patients with a convincing history of HVA, an sBT level should be ordered to rule out MCD. When initial skin or serologic test results are negative, testing should be repeated. Additional testing modalities (eg, CRD, BAT, peripheral *KIT* p.D816V mutation) should be considered if available.
- VIT is the treatment of choice to decrease future risk for cases of HVA. Although it is important to identify risk factors, in general the risk of untreated HVA outweighs the risks associated with chronic medical conditions, antihypertensive medication use, or MCD.

DISCLOSURE

K.E. Adams has nothing to disclose. J.M. Tracy serves on the advisory boards for Pharming, Biocrist, and Thermo-Fischer; Honoraria: UptoDate. D.B.K. Golden serves on the speaker bureau for Genentech; as a consultant to ALK, Stallergenes, Allergy Therapeutics, Kaleo, and Aquestive; as a section editor for UpToDate and receives clinical trials support from Genentech, Novartis, and Allergy Therapeutics.

REFERENCES

1. Bilo BM, Rueff F, Mosbech H, et al. Diagnosis of hymenoptera venom allergy. Allergy 2005;60(11):1339–49.
2. Golden DB, Marsh DG, Kagey-Sobotka A, et al. Epidemiology of insect venom sensitivity. JAMA 1989;262(2):240–4.
3. Settipane GA, Newstead GJ, Boyd GK. Frequency of hymenoptera allergy in an atopic and normal population. J Allergy Clin Immunol 1972;50(3):146–50.

4. Stafford CT, Hutto LS, Rhoades RB, et al. Imported fire ant as a health hazard. South Med J 1989;82(12):1515–9.

5. Turner PJ, Jerschow E, Umasunthar T, et al. Fatal anaphylaxis: mortality rate and risk factors. J Allergy Clin Immunol Pract 2017;5(5):1169–78.

6. Jerschow E, Lin RY, Scaperotti MM, et al. Fatal anaphylaxis in the United States, 1999-2010: temporal patterns and demographic associations. J Allergy Clin Immunol 2014;134(6):1318–1328 e7.

7. Ellis AK, Day JH. Incidence and characteristics of biphasic anaphylaxis: a prospective evaluation of 103 patients. Ann Allergy Asthma Immunol 2007; 98(1):64–9.

8. Mauriello PM, Barde SH, Georgitis JW, et al. Natural history of large local reactions from stinging insects. J Allergy Clin Immuno 1984;74(4 Pt 1):494–8.

9. Golden DB, Kagey-Sobotka A, Norman PS, et al. Outcomes of allergy to insect stings in children, with and without venom immunotherapy. N Engl J Med 2004; 351(7):668–74.

10. Bilo MB, Martini M, Pravettoni V, et al. Large local reactions to Hymenoptera stings: outcome of re-stings in real life. Allergy 2019;74(10):1969–76.

11. Reisman RE. Natural history of insect sting allergy: relationship of severity of symptoms of initial sting anaphylaxis to re-sting reactions. J Allergy Clin Immunol 1992;90(3 Pt 1):335–9.

12. Lange J, Cichocka-Jarosz E, Marczak H, et al. Natural history of hymenoptera venom allergy in children not treated with immunotherapy. Ann Allergy Asthma Immunol 2016;116(3):225–9.

13. Valentine MD, Schuberth KC, Kagey-Sobotka A, et al. The value of immunotherapy with venom in children with allergy to insect stings. N Engl J Med 1990;323(23):1601–3.

14. Golden DB, Demain J, Freeman T, et al. Stinging insect hypersensitivity: a practice parameter update 2016. Ann Allergy Asthma Immunol 2017;118(1):28–54.

15. Golden DB, Kagey-Sobotka A, Norman PS, et al. Insect sting allergy with negative venom skin test responses. J Allergy Clin Immunol 2001;107(5):897–901.

16. Quirt JA, Wen X, Kim J, et al. Venom allergy testing: is a graded approach necessary? Ann Allergy Asthma Immunol 2016;116(1):49–51.

17. Strohmeier B, Aberer W, Bokanovic D, et al. Simultaneous intradermal testing with hymenoptera venoms is safe and more efficient than sequential testing. Allergy 2013;68(4):542–4.

18. Rueff F, Przybilla B, Bilo MB, et al. Predictors of severe systemic anaphylactic reactions in patients with hymenoptera venom allergy: importance of baseline serum tryptase-a study of the European Academy of Allergology and Clinical Immunology Interest Group on Insect Venom Hypersensitivity. J Allergy Clin Immunol 2009;124(5):1047–54.

19. Rueff F, Przybilla B, Bilo MB, et al. Predictors of side effects during the buildup phase of venom immunotherapy for Hymenoptera venom allergy: the importance of baseline serum tryptase. J Allergy Clin Immunol 2010;126(1):105–11.e5.

20. Stoevesandt J, Hain J, Kerstan A, et al. Over- and underestimated parameters in severe Hymenoptera venom-induced anaphylaxis: cardiovascular medication and absence of urticaria/angioedema. J Allergy Clin Immunol 2012;130(3): 698–704 e1.

21. Farioli L, Losappio LM, Schroeder JW, et al. Basal tryptase levels can predict clinical severity in hymenoptera venom anaphylaxis and ischemic cardiovascular disorders. J Investig Allergol Clin Immunol 2019;29(2):162–4.

22. Lyons JJ, Chovanec J, O'Connell MP, et al. Heritable risk for severe anaphylaxis associated with increased alpha-tryptase-encoding germline copy number at TPSAB1. J Allergy Clin Immunol 2021;147(2):622–32.
23. Selb J, Rijavec M, Erzen R, et al. Routine KIT p.D816V screening identifies clonal mast cell disease in Hymenoptera allergic patients regularly missed using baseline tryptase levels alone. J Allergy Clin Immunol 2021. https://doi.org/10.1016/j.jaci.2021.02.043.
24. Vos B, Kohler J, Muller S, et al. Spiking venom with rVes v 5 improves sensitivity of IgE detection in patients with allergy to Vespula venom. J Allergy Clin Immunol 2013;131(4):1225–7.e1.
25. Kohler J, Blank S, Muller S, et al. Component resolution reveals additional major allergens in patients with honeybee venom allergy. J Allergy Clin Immunol 2014; 133(5):1383–9, 1389.e1–6.
26. Eberlein B, Krischan L, Darsow U, et al. Double positivity to bee and wasp venom: improved diagnostic procedure by recombinant allergen-based IgE testing and basophil activation test including data about cross-reactive carbohydrate determinants. J Allergy Clin Immunol 2012;130(1):155–61.
27. Selb J, Bidovec Stojkovic U, Bajrovic N, et al. Limited ability of recombinant Hymenoptera venom allergens to resolve IgE double sensitization. J Allergy Clin Immunol Pract 2018;6(6):2118–20.
28. Korosec P, Silar M, Erzen R, et al. Clinical routine utility of basophil activation testing for diagnosis of hymenoptera-allergic patients with emphasis on individuals with negative venom-specific IgE antibodies. Int Arch Allergy Immunol 2013;161(4):363–8.
29. Erzen R, Kosnik M, Silar M, et al. Basophil response and the induction of a tolerance in venom immunotherapy: a long-term sting challenge study. Allergy 2012; 67(6):822–30.
30. Peternelj A, Silar M, Erzen R, et al. Basophil sensitivity in patients not responding to venom immunotherapy. Int Arch Allergy Immunol 2008;146(3):248–54.
31. Kosnik M, Silar M, Bajrovic N, et al. High sensitivity of basophils predicts side effects in venom immunotherapy. Allergy 2005;60(11):1401–6.
32. Zitnik SE, Vesel T, Avcin T, et al. Monitoring honeybee venom immunotherapy in children with the basophil activation test. Pediatr Allergy Immunol 2012;23(2): 166–72.
33. Francuzik W, Rueff F, Bauer A, et al. Phenotype and risk factors of venom-induced anaphylaxis: a case-control study of the European Anaphylaxis Registry. J Allergy Clin Immunol 2021;147(2):653–662 e9.
34. Muller UR, Haeberli G. Use of beta-blockers during immunotherapy for hymenoptera venom allergy. J Allergy Clin Immunol 2005;115(3):606–10.
35. Stoevesandt J, Hain J, Stolze I, et al. Angiotensin-converting enzyme inhibitors do not impair the safety of hymenoptera venom immunotherapy build-up phase. Clin Exp Allergy 2014;44(5):747–55.
36. Sturm GJ, Herzog SA, Aberer W, et al. beta-blockers and ACE inhibitors are not a risk factor for severe systemic sting reactions and adverse events during venom immunotherapy. Allergy 2021. https://doi.org/10.1111/all.14785.
37. Niedoszytko M, Bonadonna P, Oude Elberink JN, et al. Epidemiology, diagnosis, and treatment of hymenoptera venom allergy in mastocytosis patients. Immunol Allergy Clin North Am 2014;34(2):365–81.
38. Bonadonna P, Perbellini O, Passalacqua G, et al. Clonal mast cell disorders in patients with systemic reactions to hymenoptera stings and increased serum tryptase levels. J Allergy Clin Immunol 2009;123(3):680–6.

39. Zanotti R, Lombardo C, Passalacqua G, et al. Clonal mast cell disorders in patients with severe hymenoptera venom allergy and normal serum tryptase levels. J Allergy Clin Immunol 2015;136(1):135–9.

40. Michel J, Brockow K, Darsow U, et al. Added sensitivity of component-resolved diagnosis in hymenoptera venom-allergic patients with elevated serum tryptase and/or mastocytosis. Allergy 2016;71(5):651–60.

41. Vos B, van Anrooij B, van Doormaal JJ, et al. Fatal anaphylaxis to yellow jacket stings in mastocytosis: options for identification and treatment of at-risk patients. J Allergy Clin Immunol Pract 2017;5(5):1264–71.

42. Nath P, Adams K, Schapira R, et al. Imported fire ant hypersensitivity and mastocytosis: a case series of successful venom immunotherapy. Ann Allergy Asthma Immunol 2019;122(5):541–2.

43. Bonadonna P, Zanotti R, Pagani M, et al. Anaphylactic reactions after discontinuation of hymenoptera venom immunotherapy: a clonal mast cell disorder should be suspected. J Allergy Clin Immunol Pract 2018;6(4):1368–72.

44. Blank S, Seismann H, Michel Y, et al. Api m 10, a genuine A. Mellifera venom allergen, is clinically relevant but underrepresented in therapeutic extracts. Allergy 2011;66(10):1322–9.

45. Frick M, Fischer J, Helbling A, et al. Predominant Api m 10 sensitization as risk factor for treatment failure in honey bee venom immunotherapy. J Allergy Clin Immunol 2016;138(6):1663–71.e9.

46. Hunt KJ, Valentine MD, Sobotka AK, et al. A controlled trial of immunotherapy in insect hypersensitivity. N Engl J Med 1978;299(4):157–61.

47. Muller U, Helbling A, Berchtold E. Immunotherapy with honeybee venom and yellow jacket venom is different regarding efficacy and safety. J Allergy Clin Immunol 1992;89(2):529–35.

48. Goldberg A, Confino-Cohen R. Maintenance venom immunotherapy administered at 3-month intervals is both safe and efficacious. J Allergy Clin Immunol 2001;107(5):902–6.

49. Keating MU, Kagey-Sobotka A, Hamilton RG, et al. Clinical and immunologic follow-up of patients who stop venom immunotherapy. J Allergy Clin Immunol 1991;88(3 Pt 1):339–48.

50. Golden DB, Kagey-Sobotka A, Lichtenstein LM. Survey of patients after discontinuing venom immunotherapy. J Allergy Clin Immunol 2000;105(2 Pt 1):385–90.

51. Cox L, Nelson H, Lockey R, et al. Allergen immunotherapy: a practice parameter third update. J Allergy Clin Immunol 2011;127(1 Suppl):S1–55.

52. Brockow K, Kiehn M, Riethmuller C, et al. Efficacy of antihistamine pretreatment in the prevention of adverse reactions to hymenoptera immunotherapy: a prospective, randomized, placebo-controlled trial. J Allergy Clin Immunol 1997;100(4):458–63.

53. Galera C, Soohun N, Zankar N, et al. Severe anaphylaxis to bee venom immunotherapy: efficacy of pretreatment and concurrent treatment with omalizumab. J Investig Allergol Clin Immunol 2009;19(3):225–9.

54. Freeman TM, Hylander R, Ortiz A, et al. Imported fire ant immunotherapy: effectiveness of whole body extracts. J Allergy Clin Immunol 1992;90(2):210–5.

55. Tankersley MS, Walker RL, Butler WK, et al. Safety and efficacy of an imported fire ant rush immunotherapy protocol with and without prophylactic treatment. J Allergy Clin Immunol 2002;109(3):556–62.

56. Forester JP, Johnson TL, Arora R, et al. Systemic reaction rates to field stings among imported fire ant-sensitive patients receiving >3 years of immunotherapy versus <3 years of immunotherapy. Allergy Asthma Proc 2007;28(4):485–8.

57. Severino M, Bonadonna P, Bilo MB, et al. Safety and efficacy of immunotherapy with Polistes dominulus venom: results from a large Italian database. Allergy 2009;64(8):1229–30.
58. Golden DB, Bernstein DI, Freeman TM, et al. AAAAI/ACAAI joint venom extract shortage task force report. Ann Allergy Asthma Immunol 2017;118(3):283–5.
59. Houliston L, Nolan R, Noble V, et al. Honeybee venom immunotherapy in children using a 50-mug maintenance dose. J Allergy Clin Immunol 2011;127(1):98–9.
60. Golden DB, Kagey-Sobotka A, Valentine MD, et al. Dose dependence of Hymenoptera venom immunotherapy. J Allergy Clin Immunol 1981;67(5):370–4.
61. Reisman RE, Livingston A. Venom immunotherapy: 10 years of experience with administration of single venoms and 50 micrograms maintenance doses. J Allergy Clin Immunol 1992;89(6):1189–95.

Anaphylaxis

Access to Epinephrine in Outpatient Setting

Emma Westermann-Clark, MD, MA[a],*, Amber N. Pepper, MD[a,1],
Richard F. Lockey, MD[a,b,1]

KEYWORDS

- Epinephrine • Anaphylaxis • Costs • Price • Economics • EpiPen • Shortage

KEY POINTS

- Epinephrine autoinjectors (EAIs) are expensive.
- Access to EAIs is limited worldwide.
- Lower cost alternatives to EAIs exist.

INTRODUCTION

Epinephrine is a lifesaving treatment of systemic allergic reactions (SARs) and anaphylaxis to foods, insect stings or bites, medications, and other allergens. Cox and colleagues[1] updated the World Allergy Organization (WAO) grading system for SARs as summarized in **Table 1** to clarify the early signs and symptoms of a SAR and to encourage the early administration of epinephrine. The term systemic allergic reaction applies to all grades of reactions with the term "anaphylaxis" appropriate for grades 4 or 5. The early use of epinephrine in SARs is important to maximize the likelihood of successful treatment, whereas delayed use is associated with increased incidence of death.[2–4]

Epinephrine autoinjectors (EAIs) were developed in the 1970s and first approved by the Food and Drug Administration (FDA) in the United States in 1987 (EpiPen, Mylan, Canonsburg, PA, USA). EAIs available in the United States include EpiPen and its authorized generic (Mylan, Canonsburg, PA, USA); Auvi-Q (Kaléo, Richmond, VA, USA); as well as epinephrine injection USP autoinjector (Teva, Tel Aviv, Israel, and

[a] Division of Allergy and Immunology, Department of Internal Medicine, University of South Florida Morsani College of Medicine, Tampa, FL, USA; [b] James A. Haley Veterans Affairs Hospital, Tampa, FL, USA
[1] Present address: Division of Allergy and Immunology, Department of Internal Medicine, University of South Florida Morsani College of Medicine, Joy McCann Culverhouse Airway Disease Research Center, James A. Haley V.A. Medical Center, 13000 Bruce B. Downs Blvd (111D), Tampa, FL 33612.
* Corresponding author. 601 5th Street South, Suite 301, St. Petersburg, FL 33701.
E-mail address: ewester1@usf.edu

Immunol Allergy Clin N Am 42 (2022) 175–186
https://doi.org/10.1016/j.iac.2021.09.004
0889-8561/22/© 2021 Elsevier Inc. All rights reserved.
immunology.theclinics.com

Table 1
Proposed modification of the 2010 World Allergy Organization grading system

Grade 1: Any of the Following Symptoms	Grade 2	Grade 3	Grade 4	Grade 5
Upper respiratory: Nasal symptoms: sneezing, rhinorrhea, nasal pruritus/congestion	Symptoms/signs from ≥ 2 organ systems listed in grade 1	Lower airway: Mild bronchospasm, eg, cough, wheezing, shortness of breath, which responds to treatment and/or	Lower airway: Severe bronchospasm, eg, not responding or worsening in spite of treatment	Lower or upper airway: respiratory failure
Cutaneous: Urticaria and/or erythema/warmth/ pruritus other than localized at injection site, tingling of lips, angioedema (not laryngeal)		Abdominal: Abdominal cramps and/or vomiting/ diarrhea and/or uterine cramps	Upper airway: laryngeal edema with stridor	Cardiovascular: collapse, hypotension, or loss of consciousness
Throat clearing/itchy throat				
Cough				
Tingling, itching of lips				
Angioedema (not laryngeal)				
Conjunctival erythema, pruritus, tearing				
Nausea				
Metallic taste				

Adapted from Cox LS, Sanchez-Borges M, Lockey RF. World Allergy Organization Systemic Allergic Reaction Grading System: Is a modification needed? J Allergy Clin Immunol Pract. 2017;5(1):58–62.e5.

Parsippany, NJ, USA), Adrenaclick (Amneal Specialty), and the authorized generic of Adrenaclick, epinephrine injection, USP autoinjector (Impax Generics, Hayward, CA, USA/Amneal Pharmaceuticals, Bridgewater, NJ, USA). An epinephrine syringe developed as a lower-cost alternative is Symjepi epinephrine injection (Adamis Pharmaceuticals, San Diego, CA, USA). Other EAIs available in Europe include Jext (ALK-Abelló Ltd, Berkshire, UK) and Emerade, developed by Medeca Pharma AB (Uppsala, Sweden) and produced/sold by Bausch & Lomb (Kingston upon Thames, UK). Emerade is available in Sweden, Norway, Denmark, Finland, France, Spain, the Netherlands, the United Kingdom, Ireland, and Germany. As of 2021, Emerade is seeking a partner to market this device in the United States.

Mylan's EpiPen intermittently has been in short supply since November 2017[5]; the FDA officially posted notice of this shortage on May 9, 2018.[6] An editorial in *The Lancet*, October 2018, entitled "The EpiPen Shortage: How Has It Come to This?" reports on national shortages of the EpiPen in Australia, Canada, United States, and the United Kingdom. Some countries reported being completely out of stock of the "junior" version of the EpiPen indicated for younger children. Responses to the shortages include prescription of alternative EAIs as listed earlier, permitting use of devices past their expiration date, prescribing only 1 rather than 2 EAIs per subject, and reducing the minimum weight for use of the adult dose from 30 to 25 kg.[5] The *Lancet* editorial challenges Mylan's explanation that its manufacturer, Meridian Medical Technologies, was fully responsible for the shortage and states that the reason for the shortage "remains a mystery."[5] Furthermore, the editors point out that Mylan's dominance of the EAI market (90%) has public health consequences and ethical implications, when cost and availability become insurmountable barriers to access a lifesaving medication.[5]

Manufacturing issues have at times plagued most, if not all, companies that make EAIs and these issues have contributed to EAI shortages. A voluntary recall of EpiPens occurred in 2018 due to 2 reports of "failure to activate the device due to a potential defect in a supplier component."[7] In March 2020, the FDA issued a notice making consumers aware of potential malfunction of the EpiPen related to "device failure from spontaneous activation caused by using sideways force to remove the blue safety release, device failure from inadvertent or spontaneous activation due to a raised blue safety release, difficulty removing the device from the carrier tube, or user errors."[8] A notice from the FDA dated June 1, 2020, warns consumers who "received" EAIs manufactured by Impax/Amneal (Adrenaclick and its generic) after December 20, 2018, of a manufacturing issue.[9] Consumers were instructed to inspect the product for lack of a yellow "stop collar," which is intended to prevent the devices from delivering a double dose of epinephrine. It is not clear if this manufacturing issue affected availability of Adrenaclick and its generic. Auvi-Q had a voluntary recall in 2015 due to potential dosing issues.[10]

Several factors limit the ability of newer products to garner and maintain market share versus Mylan's EpiPen. First, the EpiPen has name recognition. Second, training for the use of each device is different. To illustrate, the epinephrine injection, USP autoinjector from Amneal Pharmaceuticals/Impax Generics requires the removal of 2 caps rather than just 1. Although learning to use a new device can be challenging, novel design elements can improve safety and usability. An example is Auvi-Q, which has unique features including its rectangular shape intended to fit in a pocket, a retractable needle, and voice instructions. Untrained adults were more likely to use Auvi-Q correctly versus the EpiPen Jr, when given only written instructions and the voice instructions inherent in the Auvi-Q device.[11] Symjepi also has a compact design, compared with the EpiPen, and fits more easily into a pocket or purse. Third, insurance coverage differs for each EAI. According to the Managed Markets Insight and

Technology Database, the EpiPen had unrestricted access for 61% of commercial lives as of 2018.[12] In contrast, Auvi-Q had unrestricted access for "19% of commercial lives in all locations" among these same commercial health plans. Even though Auvi-Q was not covered by as many commercial insurance plans, the manufacturer offers it with $0 to $25 copayment to all commercially insured subjects and has a patient assistance program for uninsured and Medicaid subjects. Fourth, EAIs are rated "BX" by the FDA indicating that "data that have been reviewed by the Agency are insufficient to determine therapeutic equivalence" and when ordered may not be substituted by a pharmacist one for another.[13] Therefore, if a health care professional prescribes an "EpiPen," the pharmacist is obligated to prescribe the Mylan brand. One issue that has not yet been addressed in the literature is the ease of ordering different EAIs in the electronic medical record (EMR). When health care professionals order EAIs, they may use the term EpiPen due to brand familiarity, and other brands of EAIs may or may not be easily searchable or even included in the EMR ordering system.

The annual direct costs in the year 2010 in the United States for EAIs were estimated to be $294 million, accounting for about 25% of the $1.2 billion annual cost to treat SARs including anaphylaxis.[14,15] The average wholesale price (AWP) and wholesale acquisition cost (WAC) of each EAI is included in **Table 2**, except for the Auvi-Q. Accurate wholesale pricing for the Auvi-Q is not available because it is distributed through a single specialty pharmacy network and one commercial pharmacy to minimize costs. Many of the products' AWP and WAC have not been updated since 2015 to 2016; the most recent AWP and WAC available data are presented. Costs for the EpiPen were relatively stable until Mylan acquired this product from Merck (Kenilworth, NJ, USA) in 2007. The AWP since that time for 2 EpiPens increased 545% from $113.27 to $730.33 as of 2016, based on the most recent AWP available.[16] This price increase persists even after accounting for inflation (**Fig. 1**).[16,17] Although the out-of-pocket expenses for individual subjects may have decreased since the public outcry about EpiPen costs in 2016, the effective date of the most recent AWP available is May 16, 2016, and does not reflect the impact of price cuts or patient assistance programs.[16] Another source of costing data called ProspectoRx, published by Elsevier, promises "real-time" drug pricing, but academic institutions typically do not have access to this resource. Marketing information for Symjepi provides WACs for several devices as of December 2020 and cites ProspectoRx as the source[18]; however, the WACs derived from ProspectoRx in this document are identical to those listed in the Redbook, with dates ranging from October 1, 2015, to January 16, 2019. Therefore, it is unlikely that new WAC or AWP have been posted for the EAIs in the United States since the Redbook values available at the time of this writing.

Use of the AWP is controversial, but it is often used as a proxy for societal cost in cost-effectiveness analyses.[19] An economic analysis published in 2011 used the 2006 to 2007 AWP of the EpiPen to estimate the annual cost of EAIs for food-induced SARs. According to the International Society for Pharmacoeconomics and Outcomes Research good research practices guidelines from 2010, "Pharmaceutical prices used in the vast majority of cost-effectiveness analyses are either based on average wholesale prices (AWPs) in the United States or government-negotiated prices in Europe. The former are not only imperfect measures of actual prices paid (eg, ignoring discounts and rebates), but may also greatly overestimate societal opportunity costs because of the implicit inclusion of producer surplus created through patent-protected monopoly pricing."[20] In summary, AWP is used as an approximation for societal drug costs, despite its limitations. The United States Department of Veterans Affairs Health Economics Resource Center (HERC) discusses the challenge of

Table 2
Average wholesale prices and wholesale acquisition costs for epinephrine autoinjectors, epinephrine prefilled syringes, and epinephrine kits in the United States

Manufacturer	Drug Name	NDC Number	Pkg Size	Dose	AWP Pkg price(US$)	WAC	Effective Date
Mylan	EpiPen	49502-0500-02	2s ea	0.3 mg/0.3 mL	730.33	608.61	May 16, 2016
Mylan	EpiPen Jr.	49502-0501-02	2s ea	0.15 mg/0.3 mL	730.33	608.61	May 16, 2016
Mylan	Epinephrine injection, USP autoinjector	49502-0102-02	2s ea	0.3 mg/0.3 mL	375	300	December 15, 2016
Mylan	Epinephrine injection, USP autoinjector	49502-0101-02	2s ea	0.15 mg/3 mL	375	300	December 15, 2016
Kaleo	Auvi-Q	60842-0022-01	2s ea	0.15 mg/0.15 mL	n/a*	n/a*	n/a
Kaleo	Auvi-Q	60842-0023-02	2s ea	0.3 mg/0.3 mL	n/a*	n/a*	n/a
Adamis[a]	Symjepi epinephrine injection	00781-3442-20	2s ea	0.3 mg/0.3 mL	312.5	250	January 16, 2019
Teva	Epinephrine injection, autoinjector	00093-5986-27	2s ea	0.3 mg/0.3 mL	693.81	300	November 27, 2018
Teva	Epinephrine injection, autoinjector	00093-5985-27	2s ea	0.15 mg/0.3 mL	693.81	300	August 20, 2019
Amneal Specialty	Adrenaclick	52054-0804-02	2s ea	0.3 mg/0.3 mL	553.12	460.93	October 1, 2015
Amneal Specialty	Adrenaclick	52054-0803-02	2s ea	0.15 mg/0.15 mL	553.12	460.93	October 1, 2015
Amneal/Impax	Epinephrine injection, autoinjector	54505-0102-02	2s ea	0.3 mg/0.3 mL	494.01	395.21	October 1, 2015
Amneal/Impax	Epinephrine injection, autoinjector	54505-0101-02	2s ea	0.15 mg/0.15 mL	494.01	395.21	October 1, 2015
Certa Dose, Inc[b]	Epinephrine convenience kit	71754-0001-01	1 mL	1mg/mL	89.99	89.99	November 26, 2018
Focus Health Group[b]	Epinephrine Snap-V	24357-0911-01	1 ea	1mg/1 mL	156	130	June 16, 2016

Abbreviations: n/a, not available; NDC, National Drug Code; Pkg, package.

* Accurate AWP and WAC for Auvi-Q were not available.
[a] At the time of this Redbook listing, Symjepi was distributed by Sandoz. Adamis reacquired rights of manufacturing, commercialization, and distribution on May 11, 2020.
[b] These products are available only for licensed health care professionals to administer in a health care setting.

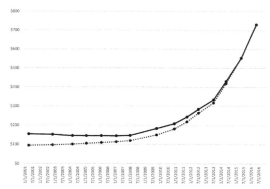

Fig. 1. AWP for the EpiPen 2001 to 2016. AWP of an EpiPen 2-pack or AWP of 2 EpiPens when sold individually, 2001 to 2016. The dotted line represents AWP in actual US dollars. The solid line represents AWP in constant year 2016 US dollars to adjust for inflation. Data were obtained from the Red Book Online System[16] and converted into constant US dollars using the Consumer Price Index for medical care from the US Bureau of Labor Statistics.[45] The most recent AWP available was effective date May 16, 2016 (verified August 12, 2021).

determining medication costs for research purposes. The HERC states, "We recommend using 121% of the drug costs reported in the Federal Supply Schedule, 152% of the VA cost, or 64% of AWP. To find the cost of a generic label prescription drug, we recommend using 27% of AWP."[19] Federal Supply Schedule prices are publicly available.[21] WACs, which have other methodologic advantages and disadvantages, may also be used to compare prices among different medications.[22]

Decision analysis software (TreeAge Pro, Williamstown, MA, USA) has been used to evaluate the cost of generic EAIs versus the EpiPen using a model that tracked spending for individual subjects over 20 years, with the assumption that each subject needs two 2-packs yearly, one each for home and school or work.[23] The cost for the EpiPen over a 20-year model duration totals $58,667 (95% confidence interval [CI], $57,745–$59,588) versus $45,588 for the generic EAI (95% CI, $44,873–$46,304). The model also incorporates other food allergy-related costs, such as specialist visits, grocery costs, and loss of work time for parents of food-allergic children. These costs are assumed to be the same for all subjects regardless of the type of EAI prescribed.

Cost-effectiveness analyses (CEAs) are computer simulations that incorporate the cost of, for example, a medication or a procedure, and the benefits of said intervention, often measured in quality-adjusted life years (QALYs) gained. A CEA published in 2021 found that prescribing 2 EAIs to all subjects with a history of peanut *allergy* was not cost effective; however, among patients with a history of *anaphylaxis* to peanut, prescribing 2 EAIs was more cost-effective.[24] The investigators therefore suggest limiting the second EAI to patients with a history of *anaphylaxis* to peanut. The incremental cost of prescribing a second EAI to all patients with peanut allergy was US $10 million per QALY. Allergists/immunologists in clinical practice, however, know that SARs to food can be unpredictable, that the severity of prior SARs does not necessarily predict the severity of future SARs, and that subjects without a history of anaphylaxis may need 2 doses of epinephrine to manage a SAR. A 2020 review of epinephrine use in anaphylaxis states that all patients at risk for anaphylaxis should carry 2 EAIs.[25] A European Academy of Allergy and Clinical Immunology task force on the clinical epidemiology of anaphylaxis surveyed experts and found that 68% of experts prescribe only 1 device, whereas 32% prescribe 2 devices.[26] The investigators point out a lack of consensus that needs to be resolved and note that prescribing habits were affected by the patient's past medical history. Shortages of EAIs have also contributed to prescribing habits, with some health care professionals prescribing only one EAI instead of 2 in times of shortage.[5]

Research demonstrates that subjects do not always fill their prescriptions when medical professionals prescribe EAIs, and that cost is a factor in subject decision making. Only 50% of subjects prescribed epinephrine on discharge from pediatric emergency rooms filled the prescription in one study.[27] The impact of copayments, coupons, and assistance programs on prices at the pharmacy counter requires further research. Pourang and colleagues[28] (2017) found that copayments did not affect the likelihood of an EAI being dispensed once it was prescribed in the Kaiser Permanente Health Maintenance Organization. However, although the investigators indicate that nearly 30% of copayments exceeded $30, they did not consider higher copayments. Data are not available on prescription:dispense ratios for subjects with exceedingly high copayments or for uninsured and underinsured subjects who can pay retail prices. More than 50% of EpiPen prescriptions are abandoned or not filled when the cost exceeds $300 for a 2-pack.[14] Two generic EAIs manufactured by Mylan have an AWP of $375. Two generic EAIs manufactured by Impax Generics have an AWP of $494.01. Subjects with any commercial insurance plan receive Auvi-Q for $0–$25 copayment through Walgreens pharmacy or the specialty pharmacy network, ASPN Pharmacies LLC (200 Park Avenue, Suite 300, Florham Park, NJ 07932, USA. (973) 295-3289) that distributes Auvi-Q. Kaléo, which manufactures Auvi-Q, works with this organization to reduce costs associated with traditional distribution routes. All uninsured subjects who make less than $100,000 annually and Medicaid-eligible subjects can apply to a patient assistance program through Kaléo. Symjepi is the most affordable epinephrine device on the US market, perhaps owing to its simpler design.

Socioeconomic factors impact access to EAIs. Children from high-income versus lower-income homes are 8.35 times more likely to be prescribed EAIs.[29] Medicaid-enrolled children are less likely to receive EAIs before arrival at an emergency department.[30] In another study, white versus non-white children were more likely to receive epinephrine early during a SAR.[31] Early use of epinephrine is defined as epinephrine administered before arrival to the emergency department. Owning an EAI greatly increased the odds of early epinephrine treatment (odds ratio, 12.67; 95% CI, 4.46–35.96). The investigators did not assess insurance status but indicate that this finding suggests that there might be an economic influence on access to EAIs.[31] Fleming and colleagues[31] examined the out-of-pocket costs for medications associated with food allergy and found higher costs for Caucasian and higher-income subjects. The investigators hypothesize that Medicaid-enrolled children may have lower out-of-pocket costs, that is, lower copayments. To reduce or eliminate insurance copayments, Fromer[14] suggest that epinephrine be classified as a preventive medicine by the US Preventive Services Task Force (USPSTF).

The price of EAIs also affects school districts and communities. The Michigan legislature mandated that all public schools stock EAIs in 2014. The legislature estimated the cost for 2 EAI 2-packs, one adult and one pediatric, at $140, whereas the "recently reported costs for commercial sources" was $1200, according to the investigators. The annual calculated cost to Michigan public schools based on these 2 cost estimates ranges from $565,460 to $4,846,800.[32]

A 2007 WAO survey of its House of Delegates indicates that EAIs are available in 59% of 44 countries surveyed.[33] A 2020 study by Tanno and colleagues[34] found that only 32% of the 195 countries in the world have access to EAIs, which suggests that access may be decreasing over time. Those without EAIs may use other, albeit less convenient, methods for the self-administration of epinephrine.[35] These methods include the use of ampules of epinephrine 1:1000 (1 mg/mL) with an empty 1-mL syringe to be drawn up as needed or epinephrine prefilled syringes (EPSs) containing various amounts of epinephrine. Both options are much less expensive than EAIs; for example, an ampule of epinephrine 1:1000 (1 mg/mL) (Hospira, Lake Forest, IL, USA) has an AWP of $2.52 and retail price of approximately $12.[16] Both options also allow for tailored dosing of epinephrine, greater than or less than the standard 0.15 mg or 0.3 mg doses contained in most FDA-approved EAIs.

The ability to tailor dosing can theoretically be beneficial for children weighing less than 15 kg (33 pounds) or for large or obese subjects. Of note, in November 2017, the FDA approved an infant version of the Auvi-Q, Auvi-Q 0.1 mg, for children weighing 7.5 to 15 kg (16.5–33 pounds). This version has a shorter needle and a smaller dose of epinephrine (0.1 mg, vs 0.15 mg contained in other "junior" products). This is the only EAI available for infants and toddlers weighing less than 15 kg.

Low-cost alternatives to EAIs are needed, and a few are discussed here. Symjepi (Adamis, San Diego, CA, USA) is an EPS that contains 0.3 mg epinephrine (or 0.15 mg, for patients weighing 15–30 kg) with a user-friendly design; it was approved by the FDA in June 2017 for subjects 30 kg (66 pounds) or more, and the 0.15 mg dose followed. The Ana-Kit (Hollister-Stier Laboratories, Spokane, WA, USA), which is no longer available, consisted of a syringe filled with 1 mL epinephrine 1:1000 (1 mg/mL) housed in a protective case for subcutaneous injection before it was removed from the US market.[36,37] The Ana-Kit syringe had 0.1-mL graduations so that smaller doses could be administered depending on the subject's age. The instructions recommended the following doses: "Adults and children over 12 years: 0.3 mL; 6-12 years: 0.2 mL; 2-6 years: 0.15 mL; Infants to 2 years: 0.05 to 0.1 mL."[38] An appropriate dose could be administered by pushing the syringe plunger until it stopped. A second dose could be administered as appropriate, after rotating the rectangular plunger one-fourth turn to the right, to line up with a rectangular slot in the syringe.[38] An advantage of the prefilled Symjepi syringe is that it is housed in a dark blue plastic encasement to protect the epinephrine from ultraviolet light degradation. Epinephrine degrades with exposure to ultraviolet light, oxygen in ambient air, and excessive heat.[39–41] EPSs stored at room temperature in a pencil box maintain acceptable US Pharmacopeia concentrations (90%–115% of label claim), pH, and sterility for 3 months.[35] The stability is limited to 2 months in high-temperature and low-humidity climates.[35,42] In addition, some physicians and other health care professionals provide subjects with EPSs wrapped in aluminum foil,[41,43] and these can be transported in a crush-resistant eyeglass case.

More affordable epinephrine convenience kits have been developed for use by emergency medical technicians and other health care professionals. Snap Medical Industries (Dublin, OH, USA) has developed EpinephrineSnap-V (a kit containing a vial of epinephrine 1:1000 [1 mg/mL] and empty syringes) and the EpinephrineSnap convenience kit (a kit containing an ampule of epinephrine 1:1000 [1 mg/mL] and empty syringes). The Focus Health Group, located in Knoxville, TN, USA, was contracted to commercialize these products. The AWP of this product is $156,[16] although information from company officials states that the average prices of EpinephrineSnap EpinephrineSnap-V are $80 and $130, respectively, with discounted group purchasing organization pricing available (personal communication, EWC, November 1, 2017). Another epinephrine convenience kit is manufactured by Certa Dose, Inc, with an

AWP of $89.99 (see **Table 2**). Use of these options may not be as practical as is an EAI. The reason is that an epinephrine ampule or vial with an empty syringe requires more skill to properly draw up the epinephrine and administer it under emergency circumstances. Parents of individuals with a history of a SAR take longer to draw up epinephrine from an ampule (average 142 ± 13 seconds) compared with emergency department nurses (29 ± 0.09 seconds; $P < .05$).[44] The epinephrine dose drawn up by parents also ranged 40-fold when compared with 2-fold for emergency department nurses.[44] This is not an exhaustive list of epinephrine syringes and convenience kits available to health care professionals. These kits do not alleviate the cost or availability burden for the average consumer.

The rising cost of EAIs has made self-administered epinephrine potentially unavailable to some subjects. Lower-cost alternatives such as EPSs are entering the US market. EAIs have advantages, such as ease of use, but they are expensive, and shortages of EAIs exacerbate the problem of access. Some EAI manufacturers strive to improve patient access via innovative distribution mechanisms that bypass complex incentives, which can drive up prices. Classifying EAIs as USPSTF preventive medicines, or adding them to the World Health Organization Model List of Essential Medicines, could improve access by reducing or eliminating copayments.[34]

CLINICS CARE POINTS

- Epinephrine is a lifesaving medication when used early to manage systemic allergic reactions
- EAIs and EPSs facilitate epinephrine administration
- EAIs are expensive, and costs have increased exponentially since 2007
- EAIs are not available in every country, and shortages of EAIs have exacerbated the problem of access
- EPSs such as Symjepi are a lower-cost alternative to EAIs
- The only product available for infants weighing 7 to 15 kg is the Auvi-Q 0.1 mg EAI
- Prescribing 1 rather than 2 EAIs is common and is at least partly a response to cost and access limitations
- Global access to EAIs and EPSs is an equity issue that needs to be addressed by policymakers

DISCLOSURE

The authors report no conflicts of interest in this work.

REFERENCES

1. Cox LS, Sanchez-Borges M, Lockey RF. World allergy organization systemic allergic reaction grading system: is a modification needed? J Allergy Clin Immunol Pract 2017;5(1):58–62.e55.
2. Bock SA, Munoz-Furlong A, Sampson HA. Fatalities due to anaphylactic reactions to foods. J Allergy Clin Immunol 2001;107(1):191–3.
3. Sampson HA, Mendelson L, Rosen JP. Fatal and near-fatal anaphylactic reactions to food in children and adolescents. N Engl J Med 1992;327(6):380–4.
4. Pumphrey R. When should self-injectible epinephrine be prescribed for food allergy and when should it be used? Curr Opin Allergy Clin Immunol 2008;8(3): 254–60.

5. The Lancet Child Adolescent H. The EpiPen shortage: how has it come to this? Lancet Child Adolesc Health 2018;2(12):839.

6. Food and Drug Administration Database of Drug Shortages. Available at: https://www.accessdata.fda.gov/scripts/drugshortages/dsp_ActiveIngredientDetails.cfm?AI=Epinephrine%20Injection,%20Auto-Injector&st=c. Accessed August 26, 2021.

7. Mylan provides update on Meridian medical Technologies', a Pfizer Company, Expanded Voluntary Worldwide Recall of EpiPen® Auto-Injector. Available at: https://www.fda.gov/safety/recalls-market-withdrawals-safety-alerts/mylan-provides-update-meridian-medical-technologies-pfizer-company-expanded-voluntary-worldwide. Accessed August 27, 2021.

8. FDA alerts patients and health care professionals of EpiPen auto-injector errors related to device malfunctions and user administration. Available at: https://www.fda.gov/drugs/drug-safety-and-availability/fda-alerts-patients-and-health-care-professionals-epipen-auto-injector-errors-related-device. Accessed August 27, 2021.

9. Epinephrine auto-injector devices by amneal and Impax: CDER alert - FDA alerts patients and health care professionals about device malfunction. United States Food and Drug Administration; 2020. Available at: https://www.fda.gov/safety/medical-product-safety-information/epinephrine-auto-injector-devices-amneal-and-impax-cder-alert-fda-alerts-patients-and-health-care. Accessed August 26, 2021 2021.

10. Auvi Q. (epinephrine injection, USP): recall - potential inaccurate dosage delivery. 2015. Available at: https://www.pbm.va.gov/PBM/vacenterformedicationsafety/nationalpbmcommunication/Auvi_Q_epinephrine_injection_USP_Recall_Potential_Inaccurate_Dosage_Delivery_National_PBM_Patient_Level_Recall_Communication_FINAL_103015.pdf. Accessed August 27, 2021.

11. Kessler C, Edwards E, Dissinger E, et al. Usability and preference of epinephrine auto-injectors: Auvi-Q and EpiPen Jr. Ann Allergy Asthma Immunol 2019;123(3): 256–62.

12. Managed Markets Insight and Technology database. Available at: https://formularylookup.com. Accessed November 1, 2017.

13. U.S. Food and Drug Administration orange book preface. Available at: http://www.fda.gov/Drugs/DevelopmentApprovalProcess/ucm079068.htm. Accessed August 26, 2016.

14. Fromer L. Prevention of anaphylaxis: the role of the epinephrine auto-injector. Am J Med 2016;129(12):1244–50.

15. Dunn JD, Sclar DA. Anaphylaxis: a payor's perspective on epinephrine autoinjectors. Am J Med 2014;127(1 Suppl):S45–50.

16. Red Book online system (electronic version). Colorado, USA: Truven Health Analytics. Available at: http://micromedexsolutions.com/.

17. Pepper AN, Westermann-Clark E, Lockey RF. The high cost of epinephrine auto-injectors and possible alternatives. J Allergy Clin Immunol Pract 2017;5(3): 665–8.e1.

18. The Low-Price Leader Among Available Epinephrine Devices. Symjepi (epinephrine) injection vol USWMSYMJ-0021 2021.

19. Determining the cost of pharmaceuticals for a cost-effectiveness analysis. Available at: https://www.herc.research.va.gov/include/page.asp?id=pharmaceutical-costs. Accessed November 1, 2017.

20. Garrison LP Jr, Mansley EC, Abbott TA 3rd, et al. Good research practices for measuring drug costs in cost-effectiveness analyses: a societal perspective: the ISPOR Drug Cost Task Force report–Part II. Value Health 2010;13(1):8–13.
21. Pharmaceutical Pricing for Federal Supply Schedule and National Contracts. United States Department of Veterans Affairs Office of Acquisition and Logistics. Available via United States Department of Veterans Affairs Office of Acquisition and Logistics. https://www.va.gov/oal/business/fss/pharmPrices.asp. Accessed November 3, 2017.
22. Levy J, Rosenberg M, Vanness D. A transparent and consistent approach to assess US outpatient drug costs for use in cost-effectiveness analyses. Value Health 2018;21(6):677–84.
23. Shaker M, Bean K, Verdi M. Economic evaluation of epinephrine auto-injectors for peanut allergy. Ann Allergy Asthma Immunol 2017;119(2):160–3.
24. Shaker M, Turner PJ, Greenhawt M. A cost-effectiveness analysis of epinephrine autoinjector risk stratification for patients with food allergy-one epinephrine auto-injector or two? J Allergy Clin Immunol Pract 2021;9(6):2440–2451 e3.
25. Brown JC, Simons E, Rudders SA. Epinephrine in the management of anaphylaxis. J Allergy Clin Immunol Pract 2020;8(4):1186–95.
26. Kraft M, Dolle-Bierke S, Turner PJ, et al. EAACI task force clinical epidemiology of anaphylaxis: experts' perspective on the use of adrenaline autoinjectors in Europe. Clin Transl Allergy 2020;10:12.
27. Cohen JS, Agbim C, Hrdy M, et al. Epinephrine autoinjector prescription filling after pediatric emergency department discharge. Allergy Asthma Proc 2021;42(2):142–6.
28. Pourang D, Batech M, Sheikh J, et al. Anaphylaxis in a health maintenance organization: International Classification of Diseases coding and epinephrine auto-injector prescribing. Ann Allergy Asthma Immunol 2017;118(2):186–90.e1.
29. Coombs R, Simons E, Foty RG, et al. Socioeconomic factors and epinephrine prescription in children with peanut allergy. Paediatr Child Health 2011;16(6):341–4.
30. Huang F, Chawla K, Jarvinen KM, et al. Anaphylaxis in a New York City pediatric emergency department: triggers, treatments, and outcomes. J Allergy Clin Immunol 2012;129(1):162–8, e161–3.
31. Fleming JT, Clark S, Camargo CA Jr, et al. Early treatment of food-induced anaphylaxis with epinephrine is associated with a lower risk of hospitalization. J Allergy Clin Immunol Pract 2015;3(1):57–62.
32. Steffens C, Clement B, Fales W, et al. Evaluating the cost and utility of mandating schools to stock epinephrine auto-injectors. Prehosp Emerg Care 2017;21(5):563–6.
33. Simons FE. Lack of worldwide availability of epinephrine autoinjectors for outpatients at risk of anaphylaxis. Ann Allergy Asthma Immunol 2005;94(5):534–8.
34. Tanno LK, Demoly P, Joint Allergy A. Action plan to ensure global availability of adrenaline autoinjectors. J Investig Allergol Clin Immunol 2020;30(2):77–85.
35. Kerddonfak S, Manuyakorn W, Kamchaisatian W, et al. The stability and sterility of epinephrine prefilled syringe. Asian Pac J Allergy Immunol 2010;28(1):53–7.
36. Browner BD, Gupton CL, editors. (2002) Allergic reactions and envenomations. In: Browner BD, Pollak AN, Gupton CI, editors. Emergency care and transportation of the sick and injured, 8th edition.
37. Auerbach P (2009) Medicine for the outdoors: the essential guide to first aid and medical emergencies, 5th edition Allergic reaction. Philadelphia, PA: Mosby Elsevier.

38. Ana-kit drug information. Available at: http://www.kiessig.com/drugs/druginfo. aspx?id=1207. Accessed November 27, 2017.

39. EPIPEN (epinephrine injection, USP), auto-injector 0.3 mg, EPIPEN Jr (epinephrine injection, USP) auto-injector 0.15 mg. Morgantown, WV: Mylan Inc; 2016.

40. Rachid O, Simons FE, Rawas-Qalaji M, et al. Epinephrine doses delivered from auto-injectors stored at excessively high temperatures. Drug Dev Ind Pharm 2016;42(1):131–5.

41. Parish HG, Bowser CS, Morton JR, et al. A systematic review of epinephrine degradation with exposure to excessive heat or cold. Ann Allergy Asthma Immunol 2016;117(1):79–87.

42. Rawas-Qalaji M, Simons FE, Collins D, et al. Long-term stability of epinephrine dispensed in unsealed syringes for the first-aid treatment of anaphylaxis. Ann Allergy Asthma Immunol 2009;102(6):500–3.

43. Waserman S, Avilla E, Ben-Shoshan M, et al. Epinephrine autoinjectors: new data, new problems. J Allergy Clin Immunol Pract 2017;5(5):1180–91.

44. Simons F, Chan ES, Gu X, et al. Epinephrine for the out-of-hospital (first-aid) treatment of anaphylaxis in infants: is the ampule/syringe/needle method practical? J Allergy Clin Immunol 2001;108(6):1040–4.

45. United States Department of Labor Bureau of Labor Statistics Consumer Price Index. Available at: https://www.bls.gov/cpi/. Accessed December 4, 2017.

Anaphylaxis
Data Gaps and Research Needs

Timothy E. Dribin, MD[a,b,*], Mariana Castells, MD, PhD[c]

KEYWORDS

- Anaphylaxis • Basic science • Biomarkers • Emergency department
- Long-term management • Population science • Research • Translational science

KEY POINTS

- There are significant anaphylaxis data and knowledge gaps across key clinical care and research domains—Population Science, Basic and Translational Sciences, Acute Management, and Long-Term Management—that contribute to suboptimal patient outcomes.
- Population science: refine anaphylaxis diagnostic criteria and develop reliable ways to record and measure it using multinational datasets.
- Basic and translational sciences: identify reliable diagnostic, predictive, and prognostic anaphylaxis biomarkers to standardize and optimize short and long-term management strategies.
- Acute management: develop clinical prediction models to standardize post-anaphylaxis observation periods and hospitalization criteria.
- Long-term management: determine immunotherapy best practices including oral immunotherapy for patients with food allergy.

Funding: The project described was supported by the National Center for Advancing Translational Sciences of the National Institutes of Health, under Award Number 2UL1TR001425 - 05A1. The content is solely the responsibility of the authors and does not necessarily represent the official views of the NIH. The project described was supported by the National Center for Advancing Translational Sciences of the National Institutes of Health, under Award Number 2KL2TR001426 -05A1. The content is solely the responsibility of the authors and does not necessarily represent the official views of the NIH.
[a] Division of Emergency Medicine, Cincinnati Children's Hospital Medical Center, 3244 Burnet Avenue, Cincinnati, OH 45229, USA; [b] Department of Pediatrics, University of Cincinnati College of Medicine, Cincinnati, OH, USA; [c] Division of Allergy and Clinical Immunology, Department of Medicine, Brigham and Women's Hospital, Harvard Medical School, Hale BTM Building Room 5002N, 60 Fenwood Road, Boston, MA 02115, USA
* Corresponding author. Cincinnati Children's Hospital, 3244 Burnet Avenue, Cincinnati, OH 45229.
E-mail address: Timothy.Dribin@cchmc.org

Immunol Allergy Clin N Am 42 (2022) 187–200
https://doi.org/10.1016/j.iac.2021.10.002
0889-8561/22/© 2021 Elsevier Inc. All rights reserved.

BACKGROUND

Anaphylaxis is an acute, potentially life-threatening systemic allergic reaction with an increasing burden in the United States and abroad.[1] During the past decade there have been significant advances in the understanding of the epidemiology, pathogenesis, acute management, and long-term prevention of anaphylaxis among high-risk patients.[2] These advances have resulted in improved care for patients with and at risk of anaphylaxis; however, pressing data gaps and research needs remain that should be addressed to optimize patient care and clinical outcomes and to reduce the societal burden of this disease.[2]

To this end, a 25-member multidisciplinary panel of anaphylaxis experts was convened in 2020 to systematically describe and appraise anaphylaxis knowledge gaps and research priorities.[2] This study group previously used Delphi methodology to develop consensus anaphylaxis outcome definitions, including persistent, refractory, and biphasic anaphylaxis (**Box 1**) as well as persistent and biphasic non-anaphylactic reactions (**Box 2**).[3] The panel used similar methodology to develop a consensus severity grading system for acute allergic reactions to standardize their severity and

---

Box 1
Clinical criteria for diagnosing persistent, refractory, and biphasic anaphylaxis

Persistent anaphylaxis is highly likely when the following criterion is fulfilled: [a]

Presence of symptoms/examination findings that fulfill the 2006 NIAID/FAAN anaphylaxis criteria that persist for at least 4 hours.

Refractory anaphylaxis is highly likely when both of the following 2 criteria are fulfilled: [b]
1. Presence of anaphylaxis following appropriate epinephrine dosing <u>and</u> symptom-directed medical management (eg, intravenous [IV] fluid bolus for hypotension).
2. The initial reaction must be treated with 3 or more appropriate doses of epinephrine (or initiation of an IV epinephrine infusion).[c]

Biphasic anaphylaxis is highly likely when all of the following 4 criteria are fulfilled:[d]
1. New/recurrent symptoms/examination findings must fulfill the 2006 NIAID/FAAN anaphylaxis criteria.
2. Initial symptoms/examination findings must completely resolve before the onset of new/recurrent symptoms/examination findings.
3. There cannot be allergen reexposure before the onset of new/recurrent symptoms/examination findings.
4. New/recurrent symptoms/examination findings must occur within 1 to 48 hours from complete resolution of initial symptoms/examination findings.

[a]The diagnosis of persistent anaphylaxis is independent of the management of the initial reaction. For reactions that do not fulfill persistent anaphylaxis criteria, please refer to **Box 2** (clinical criteria for diagnosing persistent nonanaphylactic reactions).

[b]Refractory anaphylaxis is <u>not</u> dependent on the duration of symptoms/examination findings.

[c]Appropriate epinephrine dosing: 0.01 mg/kg intramuscular epinephrine, maximum single dose 0.5 mg. Also includes manufacturer recommended dosing for epinephrine auto-injectors.

[d]The diagnosis of biphasic anaphylaxis is independent of the management of the initial reaction. For reactions that do not fulfill biphasic anaphylaxis criteria, please refer to **Box 2** (clinical criteria for diagnosing biphasic nonanaphylactic reactions).

From Dribin TE, Sampson HA, fCamargo CA Jr, Brousseau DC, Spergel JM, Neuman MI, Shaker M, Campbell RL, Michelson KA, Rudders SA, Assa'ad AH, Risma KA, Castells M, Schneider LC, Wang J, Lee J, Mistry RD, Vyles D, Vaughn LM, Schumacher DJ, Witry JK, Viswanathan S, Page EM, Schnadower D. Persistent, refractory, and biphasic anaphylaxis: A multidisciplinary Delphi study. J Allergy Clin Immunol. 2020 Nov;146(5):1089-1096; with permission.

Box 2
Clinical criteria for diagnosing persistent and biphasic nonanaphylactic reactions

Persistent allergic reactions are highly likely when the following criterion is fulfilled:[a]

Presence of symptoms/examination findings that do not fulfill the 2006 NIAID/FAAN anaphylaxis criteria that persist for at least 4 hours.

Biphasic allergic reactions are highly likely when all of the following 4 criteria are fulfilled:[b]
1. New/recurrent symptoms/examination findings do not fulfill the 2006 NIAID/FAAN anaphylaxis criteria.
2. Initial symptoms/examination findings must completely resolve before the onset of new/recurrent symptoms/examination findings.
3. There cannot be allergen reexposure before the onset of new/recurrent symptoms/examination findings.
4. New/recurrent symptoms/examination findings must occur within 1 to 48 hours from complete resolution of initial symptoms/examination findings.

[a]The diagnosis of persistent allergic reaction is independent of the management of the initial reaction.

[b]The diagnosis of biphasic allergic reaction is independent of the management of the initial reaction.

From Dribin TE, Sampson HA, Camargo CA Jr, Brousseau DC, Spergel JM, Neuman MI, Shaker M, Campbell RL, Michelson KA, Rudders SA, Assa'ad AH, Risma KA, Castells M, Schneider LC, Wang J, Lee J, Mistry RD, Vyles D, Vaughn LM, Schumacher DJ, Witry JK, Viswanathan S, Page EM, Schnadower D. Persistent, refractory, and biphasic anaphylaxis: A multidisciplinary Delphi study. J Allergy Clin Immunol. 2020 Nov;146(5):1089-1096; with permission.

---

harmonize language used in clinical care and research (**Fig. 1**).[4] The severity grading system for acute allergic reactions (SGS-AR) is novel in that it can be used to assess the severity of allergic reactions on a continuum from mild local reactions to anaphylactic shock. It can also be used to evaluate reaction severity of initial and biphasic reactions. These studies, including the perspectives from the multidisciplinary panel, underscore that significant anaphylaxis research and knowledge gaps exist that may hinder clinical care and can result in suboptimal patient outcomes. As such, these same experts sought to systematically outline and appraise anaphylaxis knowledge gaps and research priorities by asking panelists to generate knowledge gaps/research priority statements. Panelists were then asked to review and revise all statements after which they rated the potential impact and feasibility of addressing statements on a 0 to 100 scale. The panel generated 98 statements across 4 anaphylaxis themes: Population Science, Basic and Translational Sciences, Emergency Department Care/Acute Management, and Long-term Management Strategies and Prevention. This study provides the framework for collaborative scientific pursuits to address these and other anaphylaxis knowledge and research gaps to improve the care and outcomes of patients with anaphylaxis.[2]

The objective of this review is to summarize anaphylaxis data gaps and research needs consistent with the aforementioned study by Dribin and colleagues, given it is the most comprehensive, systematic appraisal of anaphylaxis research and knowledge gaps to date.[2] Addressing these gaps will result in improved care of patients with or at risk of anaphylaxis with the ultimate goal of optimizing patient outcomes and lessening the burden of anaphylaxis on patients, families, communities, and the health care system. Of note, some anaphylaxis data gaps and research needs do not directly reference *anaphylaxis* but instead conditions that predispose to anaphylaxis, such as food, venom, and medication allergy; this is intentional, given that reducing the risk

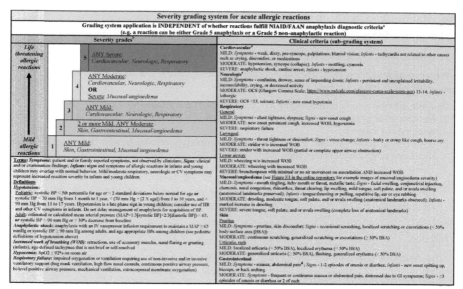

Fig. 1. Severity grading system for acute allergic reactions. [a] The severity grading system is designed for use across the spectrum of acute allergic reactions as depicted by the vertical arrow (mild to life-threatening reactions), whether they fulfill NIAID/FAAN criteria for anaphylaxis or not. [b] For patients with multiple symptoms, reaction severity is based on the most severe symptom; symptoms that constitute more severe grades always supersede symptoms from less severe grades. The grading system can be used to assign reaction severity at any time during the course of reactions; reactions may progress rapidly (within minutes) from one severity grade to another. The grading system does not dictate management decisions; reactions of any severity grade may require treatment with epinephrine. [c] Patients with severe cardiovascular and/or neurologic involvement may have urinary or stool incontinence. However, the significance of incontinence as an isolated symptom is unclear, and it is therefore not included as a symptom in the subgrading system. [d] Abdominal pain may also result from uterine cramping. (*From* Dribin TE, Schnadower D, Spergel JM, Campbell RL, Shaker M, Neuman MI, Michelson KA, Capucilli PS, Camargo CA Jr, Brousseau DC, Rudders SA, Assa'ad AH, Risma KA, Castells M, Schneider LC, Wang J, Lee J, Mistry RD, Vyles D, Pistiner M, Witry JK, Zhang Y, Sampson HA. Severity grading system for acute allergic reactions: A multidisciplinary Delphi study. J Allergy Clin Immunol. 2021 Jul;148(1):173-181; with permission.)

and burden of anaphylaxis is predicated on preventing and treating allergic conditions.[2,5,6]

DISCUSSION

The aforementioned themes align with principal anaphylaxis research and clinical domains. It will only be possible to address these gaps and improve patient care and clinical outcomes through integrated research strategies that align expertise in basic science, translational, and clinical research as well as epidemiology, public health, implementation science,[7] drug development, and bioengineering.

Population Science

Background

The incidence of anaphylaxis is increasing globally, although there does not seem to be an increase in deaths. It is difficult to assess the true rate of anaphylaxis-induced deaths for a variety of reasons, including difference in diagnostic codes globally.[8] Increasing cases of anaphylaxis are attributed to nonsteroidal antiinflammatory drugs, monoclonal antibodies, and chemotherapeutic agents.[9-11] Food-induced anaphylaxis has also increased, particularly in children and adolescents. Between 1.6% and 5.1% of the US population have had anaphylaxis, and 1% of hospitalizations and 0.1% of emergency department (ED) encounters result in fatalities.[12] ED visits for anaphylaxis doubled among all ages and tripled in children during the past decade in the United States.[13] There is need for an accurate population database to support disease surveillance, to assess trends in anaphylaxis across diverse, broad populations and geographies, and to develop targeted interventions to mitigate disease burden and evaluate the effectiveness of these interventions longitudinally.

Data gaps and research needs
A review of central data gaps and research needs for Population Science is described in (**Box 3**). The 2006 National Institute of Allergy and Infectious Disease and Food Allergy and Anaphylaxis Network (NIAID/FAAN) anaphylaxis diagnostic criteria are widely used in clinical practice and research and are retrospectively and prospectively validated. However, there is a lack of universal consensus whether or not the NIAID/FAAN criteria should be modified based on new data and proposed recommendations from the World Allergy Organization.[1,14-19] This includes how to account for isolated respiratory involvement after a known/suspected allergen exposure in sensitive patients, mild symptoms (eg, "throat tightness and nausea") reported in food allergic patients, and how to define persistent gastrointestinal symptoms associated with the route of exposure (eg, food ingestion). Refining and achieving an international consensus as to the definition of anaphylaxis will promote improved disease surveillance globally.[2]

There also is a need to evaluate global anaphylactic practice variations, including Emergency Medical Services protocols, access to and use of epinephrine auto-injectors (EAIs), and EAI prescription patterns. There is a need to evaluate barriers to patient access to allergy/immunology care, particularly in research-deficient settings/geographies, and the long-term management of anaphylaxis and predisposing conditions such as that occurs with food, medication, and venom allergy. Investigations pursuing this line of research should account for differences in resource allocation/availability, particularly in resource-limited communities and countries. This work should support novel, efficacious, cost-effective, and sustainable community and public health interventions to mitigate the burden of anaphylaxis by accounting for socioeconomic, infrastructure, and environmental differences.[2]

Basic and Translational Sciences

Background
There have been exciting advances in the understanding of anaphylaxis and its pathogenesis during the past decade[20]; however, these have not been translated into reliable or improved bedside care of patients. Promising breakthroughs include identifying the role of anaphylaxis effector cells (mast cells, basophils, neutrophils, monocytes/macrophages) and their mediators (histamine, tryptase, platelet-activating factor, prostaglandins, interleukins, complement) as well as immunoglobulin E (IgE) and non-IgE pathways.[21-24] In addition, there is now an improved understanding of risk factors, including hereditary alpha tryptasemia (the only presently known genetic risk factor) caused by the duplication of alpha tryptase genes at the TPSAB1 gene locus on chromosome 16. The prevalence in Western populations is believed to be between 4% and 6%.[25,26] Mast cell activation disorders, including mastocytosis, are

---

Box 3
Population Science data gaps and research needs

Population Science
There is a need to
1. Establish international consensus about what constitutes anaphylaxis to support population research, including disease surveillance.
2. Evaluate the barriers (eg, geographic, socioeconomic) of patient access to allergists/immunologists for the long-term management (eg, venom immunotherapy, oral immunotherapy) of anaphylaxis and related conditions (eg, food, medication, venom allergies).
3. Better evaluate for socioeconomic disparities in the risk of, care, and outcomes of patients with anaphylaxis. There is a need to develop novel personal and community interventions to target these sectors of the population and to address these disparities to improve health outcomes for all patients with anaphylaxis.
4. Clarify geographic practice variation in anaphylaxis management (eg, emergency medical service, protocols, access to epinephrine auto-injectors, prescription patterns for epinephrine auto-injectors).
5. Evaluate the epidemiology of anaphylaxis severity, fatal anaphylaxis, as well as persistent, refractory, and biphasic anaphylaxis; this includes evaluating the association between specific allergens and these outcomes, as well as individual patient characteristics.
6. Understand the influence of prior anaphylaxis on quality of life and allergen avoidance behavior.
7. Better understand primary care physician's understanding of anaphylaxis and specific allergy management.
8. Identify risk factors for future anaphylaxis severity, including tools that can identify patients/individuals who are at low risk of future anaphylaxis.
9. Evaluate the role of epinephrine auto-injectors in public spaces. Assuming there is a role for epinephrine auto-injectors in public spaces, what is the best way to implement such programs accounting for location (restaurants, schools, planes, stadiums) and specific costs (eg, pricing models, cost-effectiveness)?
10. Evaluate the long-term follow-up care of patients with anaphylaxis (eg, proportion of patients who follow-up with allergists/immunologists, have up-to-date epinephrine auto-injectors, and undergo testing to identify eliciting allergens), including barriers, facilitators, and strategies for improvement. Such evaluation would need to be sensitive to the differing resources available in different contexts (eg, developed vs developing countries, urban vs rural areas)

Modified from Dribin TE, Schnadower D, Wang J, Camargo CA Jr, Michelson KA, Shaker M, Rudders SA, Vyles D, Golden DBK, Spergel JM, Campbell RL, Neuman MI, Capucilli PS, Pistiner M, Castells M, Lee J, Brousseau DC, Schneider LC, Assa'ad AH, Risma KA, Mistry RD, Campbell DE, Worm M, Turner PJ, Witry JK, Zhang Y, Sobolewski B, Sampson HA. Anaphylaxis knowledge gaps and future research priorities: A consensus report. J Allergy Clin Immunol. 2021 Aug 12:S0091-6749(21)01209-4; with permission.

---

associated with an increased frequency of anaphylaxis. Anaphylaxis can be the presenting manifestation that leads to the diagnosis of clonal and nonclonal mast cell activation disorders.[27–29] Research as to the role of the intestinal microbiome in protecting infants from developing food allergies, the most common cause of anaphylaxis in children, has also evolved during the past decade.[30,31]

Data gaps and research needs
A review of central data gaps and research needs for *Basic and Translational Sciences* is described in **Box 4**.[2] Despite the identification of promising anaphylaxis biomarkers, there is a need to determine how biomarkers, for example, histamine and tryptase, can be incorporated into routine clinical care and to identify novel biomarkers to improve

---

Box 4
Basic and Translational Sciences data gaps and research needs

Basic and Translational Sciences
There is a need to
  1. Develop strategies (eg, therapies, early food exposures) to prevent the development of food allergies in infancy.
  2. Determine whether the basophil activation test can be configured (with standardized technique, reporting of results, and clinical threshold) to predict risk for anaphylaxis occurrence, severity, and course.
  3. Evaluate the clinical usefulness of current biomarkers (tryptase, basophil activation test, urinary histamine, or leukotrienes) in confirming the diagnosis of anaphylaxis and in predicting future reaction severity, clinical courses, and informing optimal management strategies (eg, when to administer epinephrine, observation periods).
  4. Clarify the compensatory mechanisms responsible for anaphylaxis recovery, the impact of anaphylaxis risk factors and triggers on these mechanisms, and how timing of epinephrine administration, intravenous fluid, and oxygen affect these mechanisms before and after the onset of multiorgan involvement.
  5. Determine what other mediators are important in anaphylaxis that may serve as more reliable biomarkers for identification of anaphylaxis (during the episode) and risk of anaphylaxis (before the episode).
  6. Develop biomarkers to indicate who is at risk for severe anaphylactic reactions.
  7. There is a need to explore the role of cytokines, histamine, leukotrienes, metabolomics, and other factors in the severity and response to allergic triggers and therapies used to treat allergic reactions.
  8. Determine why some foods are more likely to induce severe/fatal anaphylaxis (eg, peanut, cashew, seafood) than others (eg, egg, soybean).
  9. Define clinically meaningful and reliable thresholds to screen/detect specific allergens in food for patients with life-threatening allergies.
  10. Evaluate how the use of tryptase as a biomarker can be improved (eg, optimal timing).

Modified from Dribin TE, Schnadower D, Wang J, Camargo CA Jr, Michelson KA, Shaker M, Rudders SA, Vyles D, Golden DBK, Spergel JM, Campbell RL, Neuman MI, Capucilli PS, Pistiner M, Castells M, Lee J, Brousseau DC, Schneider LC, Assa'ad AH, Risma KA, Mistry RD, Campbell DE, Worm M, Turner PJ, Witry JK, Zhang Y, Sobolewski B, Sampson HA. Anaphylaxis knowledge gaps and future research priorities: A consensus report. J Allergy Clin Immunol. 2021 Aug 12:S0091-6749(21)01209-4; with permission.

---

the diagnosis and treatment of anaphylaxis. Although anaphylaxis is a clinical diagnosis, identifying accurate, easy to obtain biomarkers would improve and help standardize care, particularly when there is diagnostic uncertainty, for example, "Is this allergen induced asthma or anaphylaxis?" Biomarkers would also help to standardize observation periods to monitor for persistent and biphasic reactions by allowing clinicians to trend biomarker levels and optimize treatment strategies as to if and when persistent and biphasic symptoms warrant additional treatment with epinephrine. Developing and translating the use of biomarkers into routine care would be the first step in transitioning the current model of care to a precision medicine care model that also incorporates host characteristics, for example, phenotypes, comorbidities, causative agents, and endotypes to predict and prognosticate management strategies both for short- and long-term care.[32] In addition, identifying novel biological markers/mediators is an important first step to develop targeted, mechanistic-based therapies to treat refractory anaphylaxis, prevent anaphylaxis among high-risk individuals, and possibly cure common predisposing allergic conditions such as food, medication, and venom allergy.[2]

However, conducting basic and clinical research during human anaphylaxis is difficult because of the challenge of timely enrolling patients in EDs, collecting serial biospecimens, and the need to simultaneously collect short- and long-term phenotypic and outcome data.[2] An additional challenge is that mature mast cells, the key effector cells of anaphylaxis, are tissue based and not in the circulation and therefore difficult to obtain during reactions. Therefore, it is important that scientists with expertise in animal-based research collaborate with clinical/translational researchers to study human anaphylaxis. Likewise, there is a need for large prospective studies to facilitate the collection and banking of clinical and biological data to accelerate scientific discoveries and support grant applications.[2]

Acute Management

Background
Anaphylaxis continues to be underrecognized, misdiagnosed, and mismanaged,[6] and this includes the underuse of epinephrine, the first line of therapy to treat primary and biphasic reactions, and the overuse of "second-line therapies" (antihistamines and glucocorticosteroids) for which there are insufficient data to support their use.[6,33] Likewise, there are no validated data for the use of epinephrine, specifically for persistent and biphasic reactions. In addition, practice variations exist regarding the lengths of observation following initial reaction onset and/or treatment with epinephrine to monitor for a biphasic reaction, nor are there validated clinical criteria to standardize hospitalization criteria and care. These gaps may contribute to unnecessary hospitalizations, increasing health care costs, and undo personal and financial strain on patients and families.[2,13,34,35]

A limitation of conducting rigorous research specific to acute anaphylaxis management, including the prevalence of and risk factors for biphasic reactions, is the lack of consensus definitions for adverse anaphylaxis outcomes. To address this gap, a 19-member panel developed consensus definitions of persistent, refractory, and biphasic anaphylaxis (see **Box 1**) as well as persistent and biphasic nonanaphylactic reactions (see **Box 2**).[3] Dissemination and application of these definitions in research and clinical care will serve as a foundation to optimize and standardize clinical management and patient outcomes for future investigations. This project also highlighted the need to develop a consensus severity grading system for acute allergic reactions, including anaphylaxis and nonanaphylactic reactions. The same researchers, using Delphi methodology, developed the SGS-AR (see **Fig. 1**).[4] Validation, dissemination, and application of the grading system will help standardize the language and outcomes used in clinical care and research and will serve as a tool to standardize adverse reaction reporting for clinical trials.[2,4]

Data gaps and research needs
A review of central data gaps and research needs for *Acute Management* are described in **Box 5**.[2] An important first step is to validate the SGS-AR in different clinical settings, for example, EDs and allergy/immunology centers, to ensure it can be used universally and is reliable. Successful validation of the SGS-AR will help harmonize clinical care language and standardize outcomes in observational and interventional trials. It may also lead to the development of SGS-AR–embedded patient technologies and result in standardized reporting of acute allergic reactions in non–health care settings. Validation of the SGS-AR may also have the positive impact of improving real-time management decisions in non–health care settings for patients and their families, including when to administer epinephrine or seek emergent medical care.[4]

There is also a need to improve anaphylaxis diagnostic criteria as discussed in the *Population Science* section of this review, which includes modifying diagnostic criteria

---

Box 5
Acute Management **data gaps and research needs**

Acute Management
There is a need to
1. Validate the severity grading system for acute allergic reactions.
2. Improve the evidence-based practice of the emergency treatment of anaphylaxis.
3. Conduct a randomized controlled trial to evaluate the efficacy of adjunctive systemic glucocorticoids in treating anaphylaxis, including reducing initial reaction severity, and preventing biphasic reactions.
4. Develop tools and strategies to improve anaphylaxis recognition by caregivers and health care professionals.
5. Develop clinical prediction models to determine if hospitalization is indicated after initial reaction management and to inform patient-centric periods of observation.
6. Identify shortcomings of current anaphylaxis action plans used in the ED, inpatient and outpatient settings, and develop optimal, patient-centered anaphylaxis action plans for these settings; this includes determining the minimum number of elements to be included in the action plan to achieve efficacy.
7. Identify signs and symptoms of anaphylaxis in infants/young children accounting for:
   a. The challenge of recognizing signs and symptoms of anaphylaxis in nonverbal children (challenges: lack of subjective symptoms; assessing mental status, eg, inconsolability, lethargy).
   b. Differences in cardiovascular involvement in infants/young children compared with adults (eg, hypotension in children is a late finding of decompensated shock, and tachycardia may be the only sign of compensated shock in children).
   c. Signs and symptoms of anaphylaxis in infants/young children can overlap with normal behavior.
8. Develop an anaphylaxis management guideline specific to treatment with epinephrine that takes into account all patient ages and care settings to address the following questions:
   a. After treatment of anaphylaxis with epinephrine, which recurrent/new signs and/or symptoms should be treated with epinephrine versus those that can be monitored without treatment with epinephrine?
   b. Can mild anaphylactic reactions be safely managed without epinephrine?
   c. What constitutes delayed epinephrine administration and the degree to which this increases the risk for adverse outcomes including refractory and/or biphasic reactions?
   d. What is the optimal timing for repeat epinephrine administration?
9. Develop a model (including information such as past medical history, reaction severity, response to treatment with epinephrine) to identify patients with anaphylaxis who can be safely managed at home instead necessitating emergency care evaluation.
10. Evaluate the role of alternative epinephrine delivery mechanisms (beyond currently available epinephrine auto-injectors) to treat anaphylaxis.

Modified from Dribin TE, Schnadower D, Wang J, Camargo CA Jr, Michelson KA, Shaker M, Rudders SA, Vyles D, Golden DBK, Spergel JM, Campbell RL, Neuman MI, Capucilli PS, Pistiner M, Castells M, Lee J, Brousseau DC, Schneider LC, Assa'ad AH, Risma KA, Mistry RD, Campbell DE, Worm M, Turner PJ, Witry JK, Zhang Y, Sobolewski B, Sampson HA. Anaphylaxis knowledge gaps and future research priorities: A consensus report. J Allergy Clin Immunol. 2021 Aug 12:S0091-6749(21)01209-4; with permission.

---

to account for signs/symptoms of infant anaphylaxis, which may overlap with normal infant behavior, for example, crying, irritability, spitting up, and back arching.[36] Likewise, cardiovascular or neurologic signs/symptoms in infants and young children may represent a more severe/advanced disease state than in adults.[4,36,37]

There is also a need to derive and validate clinical prediction models to standardize ED observation periods and hospitalization criteria.[2] Such models would positively affect the length of observation periods and potentially prevent unnecessary, costly hospitalizations. Furthermore, given the importance of timely epinephrine administration, there is a need to better understand the pharmacodynamics, pharmacokinetics, and the clinical outcomes of epinephrine administered by different devices and routes. This includes evaluating the efficacy of noninjectable epinephrine delivery systems, which would may preferable to patients and families compared with EAIs. Furthermore, although delayed epinephrine use is a potential risk factor for biphasic anaphylaxis, there is a need to determine what constitutes "delay" and the degree to which it increases the risk of adverse anaphylaxis outcomes, including fatal, refractory, persistent, and biphasic reactions.[2,38,39]

Although epinephrine is the first-line anaphylaxis therapy it is often underused and replaced by second-line therapies, such as H_1 and H_2 antagonists and systemic glucocorticosteroids, for which there are insufficient data to support their use.[6] Therefore, there is a need for randomized controlled trials to evaluate the efficacy of these therapies at reducing reaction severity and preventing biphasic reactions. Such a line of investigation is difficult to conduct, given the obstacles associated with ED enrollment, randomization, and because of the perceived lack of equipoise, given the routine use of these medications in clinical care.[2,33] There is also a need to evaluate how to best standardize and implement anaphylaxis action plans for patients and families and to identify best practices for EAI prescription programs to ensure access to EAIs.[2]

In summary, there is a need for large, prospective observational and interventional trials to address research gaps specific for the management of acute anaphylaxis. Such research will allow investigators to collect accurate longitudinal data using novel techniques and patient-friendly technologies. In addition, it would be ideal to consent patients to biobank specimens at the time of study enrollment to accelerate basic and translational research discoveries. Finally, it is essential to incorporate the perspectives of patients and families when designing prospective ED-based research to ensure study findings translate into equitable and patient-centric outcomes.[2]

Long-Term Management

Background
The long-term management and prevention of anaphylaxis is contingent on allergen avoidance, drug desensitization, allergen immunotherapy, and appropriate observation periods for patients at high risk of acute allergic reactions or anaphylaxis.[5,6] Providing a diagnosis of mast cell activation disorders is critical. Despite the benefit of allergen immunotherapy in mitigating the risk of anaphylaxis, particularly for food allergy, patients are at risk of immunotherapy-induced anaphylaxis. A central tenet of the long-term management and prevention is the need for clinicians to appropriately discuss the potential benefits and risks of different therapies and treatment strategies with patients and families.[2]

Data gaps and research needs
A review of central data gaps and research needs for Long-Term Management is described in **Box 6**.[2] There is a need to determine immunotherapy best practices, including oral immunotherapy for food allergies. Immunotherapy protocols must be patient-centered and modified to meet the needs of patients and families from diverse communities and backgrounds. For example, there is a potential for maintenance immunotherapy to be available in nonmedical facilities. There is also a need to evaluate practice differences that contribute to patients being labeled or delabeled with drug allergy and the underutilization of drug desensitization protocols.[2]

Box 6
Long-Term Management data gaps and research needs

Long-Term Management
There is a need to

1. Delabel individuals who are unnecessarily labeled as medication allergic/at risk of anaphylaxis, particularly to antibiotics, due to vague reactions or reactions that occurred a long time ago. Use of expensive, broader spectrum antibiotics, due to incorrect or outdated diagnosis, is very costly and may promote more antimicrobial resistance.
2. Determine how risk perceptions influence quality of life for patients at risk for anaphylaxis and determine what anaphylaxis outcomes matter most to patients. These patient-oriented outcomes are key to evaluating the effectiveness of current and novel anaphylaxis therapies and management strategies.
3. Evaluate the impact of device cost and pragmatic device limitations as a barrier to effective anaphylaxis treatment in the community.
4. There is a need to understand barriers to self-injectable epinephrine carriage and use and how these barriers can be addressed.
5. Determine best practices for oral immunotherapy in patients with food allergy.
6. Understand how the health literacy of patients from diverse racial, cultural, and socioeconomic backgrounds affects their understanding of and application of written anaphylaxis action plans to provide anaphylaxis self-management.
7. Develop validated decision aids (eg, use of therapies/strategies to prevent anaphylaxis) to address the needs of patients/families from diverse racial, cultural, and socioeconomic backgrounds.
8. Identify and address barriers to early allergen introduction to prevent food allergies that lead to risk of recurrent anaphylaxis.
9. Understand the psychological impact of anaphylaxis and anaphylaxis therapies on patients and caregivers and develop novel interventions and/or strategies to address them.
10. Understand the unwarranted geographic practice variation in the underutilization of drug desensitization, particularly in high-risk populations (eg, patients with cystic fibrosis treated with β-lactam antibiotics, patients treated with carboplatin).

Modified from Dribin TE, Schnadower D, Wang J, Camargo CA Jr, Michelson KA, Shaker M, Rudders SA, Vyles D, Golden DBK, Spergel JM, Campbell RL, Neuman MI, Capucilli PS, Pistiner M, Castells M, Lee J, Brousseau DC, Schneider LC, Assa'ad AH, Risma KA, Mistry RD, Campbell DE, Worm M, Turner PJ, Witry JK, Zhang Y, Sobolewski B, Sampson HA. Anaphylaxis knowledge gaps and future research priorities: A consensus report. J Allergy Clin Immunol. 2021 Aug 12:S0091-6749(21)01209-4; with permission.

Identifying and addressing barriers to early allergen introduction to prevent food allergies, the most common cause of anaphylaxis in children, is also necessary.[40] There are practice guideline variations for such recommendations, which are confusing to families and clinicians and lead to suboptimal care and patient outcomes. When designing investigations specific to the long-term management of patients at risk for anaphylaxis, it is imperative to include patients and families from diverse backgrounds to ensure that study procedures, outcomes, and interventions result in optimal health outcomes.[2]

SUMMARY

This article outlines central anaphylaxis data gaps and research needs related to the following anaphylaxis themes: Population Science, Basic and Translational Sciences, Acute Management, and Long-Term Management. There is need for multidisciplinary collaboration among basic, translational, clinical, and population scientists with input from patients/families, policymakers, and other stakeholders to address these gaps with the ultimate goal of reducing the societal burden of anaphylaxis.[2]

CLINICS CARE POINTS

There have been promising advances in the care of patients with or at risk of anaphylaxis, including the long-term management and prevention of common predisposing allergic conditions. Despite these advances, significant data gaps and research needs remain. These needs include the need to refine anaphylaxis diagnostic criteria; identify accurate and reliable diagnostic, predictive, and prognostic biomarkers; standardize postanaphylaxis care, for example, observation periods, hospitalization criteria; and determine allergen/immunotherapy best practices. Addressing these and other gaps through multidisciplinary research collaborations will result in improved clinical care and optimal outcomes for patients with or at risk of anaphylaxis.

DISCLOSURE

T.E. Dribin receives funding from the NIH. M. Castells is the BWH PI for the PIONEER BluePrint Clinical trial for Indolent Systemic Mastocytosis.

REFERENCES

1. Sampson HA, Muñoz-Furlong A, Campbell RL, et al. Second symposium on the definition and management of anaphylaxis: Summary report–Second National Institute of Allergy and Infectious Disease/Food Allergy and Anaphylaxis Network symposium. J Allergy Clin Immunol 2006;117(2):391–7.
2. Dribin TE, Schnadower D, Wang J, et al. Anaphylaxis knowledge gaps and future research priorities: a consensus report. J Allergy Clin Immunol 2021. https://doi.org/10.1016/j.jaci.2021.07.035.
3. Dribin TE, Sampson HA, Camargo CA Jr, et al. Persistent, refractory, and biphasic anaphylaxis: a multidisciplinary Delphi study. J Allergy Clin Immunol 2020. https://doi.org/10.1016/j.jaci.2020.08.015.
4. Dribin TE, Schnadower D, Spergel JM, et al. Severity grading system for acute allergic reactions: a multidisciplinary Delphi study. J Allergy Clin Immunol 2021;148.
5. Cardona V, Ansotegui IJ, Ebisawa M, et al. World Allergy Organization Anaphylaxis Guidance 2020. World Allergy Organ J 2020;13(10):100472. Available at: https://www.sciencedirect.com/science/article/pii/S1939455120303756.
6. Shaker MS, Wallace DV, Golden DBK, et al. Anaphylaxis–a 2020 practice parameter update, systematic review, and Grading of Recommendations, Assessment, Development and Evaluation (GRADE) analysis. J Allergy Clin Immunol 2020;145(4):1082–123.
7. Bauer MS, Damschroder L, Hagedorn H, et al. An introduction to implementation science for the non-specialist. BMC Psychol 2015;3(1):32.
8. Turner PJ, Campbell DE, Motosue MS, et al. Global Trends in Anaphylaxis Epidemiology and Clinical Implications. J Allergy Clin Immunol Pract 2020;8(4):1169–76. Available at: http://www.sciencedirect.com/science/article/pii/S2213219819309675.
9. Sloane D, Govindarajulu U, Harrow-Mortelliti J, et al. Safety, Costs, and Efficacy of Rapid Drug Desensitizations to Chemotherapy and Monoclonal Antibodies. J Allergy Clin Immunol Pract 2016;4(3):497–504. Available at: https://www.sciencedirect.com/science/article/pii/S2213219816000118.

10. Isabwe GAC, Garcia Neuer M, de las Vecillas Sanchez L, et al. Hypersensitivity reactions to therapeutic monoclonal antibodies: phenotypes and endotypes. J Allergy Clin Immunol 2018;142(1):159–70.e2. Available at: https://www.sciencedirect.com/science/article/pii/S0091674918303063.

11. Aun MV, Blanca M, Garro LS, et al. Nonsteroidal Anti-Inflammatory Drugs are Major Causes of Drug-Induced Anaphylaxis. J Allergy Clin Immunol Pract 2014;2(4): 414–20. Available at: https://www.sciencedirect.com/science/article/pii/S2213219814001354.

12. Turner PJ, Gowland MH, Sharma V, et al. Increase in anaphylaxis-related hospitalizations but no increase in fatalities: An analysis of United Kingdom national anaphylaxis data, 1992-2012. J Allergy Clin Immunol 2015;135(4):956–63.e1. Available at: http://www.sciencedirect.com/science/article/pii/S0091674914015164.

13. Michelson KA, Dribin TE, Vyles D, et al. Trends in emergency care for anaphylaxis. J Allergy Clin Immunol Pract 2020;8(2):767–8.e2.

14. Turner PJ, Worm M, Ansotegui IJ, et al. Time to revisit the definition and clinical criteria for anaphylaxis? World Allergy Organ J 2019;12(10):100066. Available at: https://pubmed.ncbi.nlm.nih.gov/31719946.

15. Motosue MS, Bellolio MF, Van Houten HK, et al. Outcomes of Emergency Department Anaphylaxis Visits from 2005 to 2014. J Allergy Clin Immunol Pract 2017; 6(3):1002–9.e2.

16. Brauer CEL, Motosue MS, Li JT, et al. Prospective Validation of the NIAID/FAAN Criteria for Emergency Department Diagnosis of Anaphylaxis. J Allergy Clin Immunol Pract 2016;4:1220–6.

17. Campbell RL, Hagan JB, Manivannan V, et al. Evaluation of National Institute of Allergy and Infectious Diseases/Food Allergy and Anaphylaxis Network criteria for the diagnosis of anaphylaxis in emergency department patients. J Allergy Clin Immunol 2012;129:748–52.

18. Cox L, Larenas-Linnemann D, Lockey RF, et al. Speaking the same language: The World Allergy Organization Subcutaneous Immunotherapy Systemic Reaction Grading System. J Allergy Clin Immunol 2010;125(3):569–74.e7.

19. Cox LS, Sanchez-Borges M, Lockey RF. World Allergy Organization Systemic Allergic Reaction Grading System: Is a Modification Needed? J Allergy Clin Immunol Pract [Internet] 2017;5(1):58–62.e5. Available at: http://www.sciencedirect.com/science/article/pii/S2213219816305669.

20. Muraro A, Lemanske RF, Castells M, et al. Precision medicine in allergic disease — food allergy , drug allergy , and anaphylaxis — PRACTALL document of the European Academy of Allergy and Clinical Immunology and the American Academy of Allergy , Asthma and Immunology. Allergy 2017;72:1006–21.

21. Reber LL, Hernandez JD, Galli SJ. The pathophysiology of anaphylaxis. J Allergy Clin Immunol 2017;140(2):335–48. Available at: https://www.sciencedirect.com/science/article/pii/S0091674917310205.

22. Brown SGA, Stone SF, Fatovich DM, et al. Anaphylaxis: Clinical patterns, mediator release, and severity. J Allergy Clin Immunol 2013;132(5):1141–9.e5. Available at: http://www.sciencedirect.com/science/article/pii/S0091674913009834.

23. Cianferoni A. Non–IgE-mediated anaphylaxis. J Allergy Clin Immunol 2021; 147(4):1123–31.

24. Finkelman FD, Khodoun MV, Strait R. Human IgE-independent systemic anaphylaxis. J Allergy Clin Immunol 2016;137(6):1674–80. Available at: https://www.sciencedirect.com/science/article/pii/S0091674916003821.

25. Lyons JJ, Chovanec J, O'Connell MP, et al. Heritable risk for severe anaphylaxis associated with increased α-tryptase–encoding germline copy number at TPSAB1. J Allergy Clin Immunol 2020;147(2):622–32. Available at: http://www.sciencedirect.com/science/article/pii/S0091674920310290.

26. Luskin KT, White AA, Lyons JJ. The Genetic Basis and Clinical Impact of Hereditary Alpha-Tryptasemia. J Allergy Clin Immunol Pract 2021;9(6):2235–42. Available at: https://www.sciencedirect.com/science/article/pii/S2213219821003068.

27. Giannetti MP, Weller E, Bormans C, et al. Hereditary alpha-tryptasemia in 101 patients with mast cell activation-related symptomatology including anaphylaxis. Ann Allergy Asthma Immunol 2021;126(6):655–60.

28. Fuchs D, Kilbertus A, Kofler K, et al. Scoring the Risk of Having Systemic Mastocytosis in Adult Patients with Mastocytosis in the Skin. J Allergy Clin Immunol Pract 2021;9(4):1705–12.e4. Available at: https://www.sciencedirect.com/science/article/pii/S2213219820313544.

29. Valent P, Akin C, Bonadonna P, et al. Proposed Diagnostic Algorithm for Patients with Suspected Mast Cell Activation Syndrome. J Allergy Clin Immunol Pract 2019;7(4):1125–33.e1. Available at: https://www.sciencedirect.com/science/article/pii/S221321981930056X.

30. Feehley T, Plunkett CH, Bao R, et al. Healthy infants harbor intestinal bacteria that protect against food allergy. Nat Med 2019;25(3):448–53.

31. Huang YJ, Marsland BJ, Bunyavanich S, et al. The microbiome in allergic disease: Current understanding and future opportunities–2017 PRACTALL document of the American Academy of Allergy, Asthma & Immunology and the European Academy of Allergy and Clinical Immunology. J Allergy Clin Immunol 2017;139(4):1099–110.

32. Castells M. Diagnosis and management of anaphylaxis in precision medicine. J Allergy Clin Immunol 2017;140:321–33.

33. Michelson KA, Monuteaux MC, Neuman MI. Variation and Trends in Anaphylaxis Care in United States Children's Hospitals. Acad Emerg Med 2016;23(5):623–7.

34. Rudders SA, Banerji A, Vassallo MF, et al. Trends in pediatric emergency department visits for food-induced anaphylaxis. J Allergy Clin Immunol 2010;126(2):385–8.

35. Robinson LB, Arroyo AC, Faridi MK, et al. Trends in US hospitalizations for anaphylaxis among infants and toddlers: 2006 to 2015. Ann Allergy Asthma Immunol 2021;126(2):168–74.e3. Available at: https://www.sciencedirect.com/science/article/pii/S1081120620310024.

36. Greenhawt M, Gupta RS, Meadows JA, et al. Guiding Principles for the Recognition , Diagnosis , and Management of Infants with Anaphylaxis : An Expert Panel Consensus. J Allergy Clin Immunol Pract 2019;7(4):1148–56.e5.

37. Pistiner M, Mendez-Reyes JE, Eftekhari S, et al. Caregiver Reported Presentation of Severe Food-induced Allergic Reactions in Infants and Toddlers. J Allergy Clin Immunol Pract 2020. https://doi.org/10.1016/j.jaip.2020.11.005.

38. Lee JM, Greenes DS. Biphasic Anaphylactic Reactions in Pediatrics. Pediatrics 2000;106(4):762–6.

39. Lee S, Peterson A, Lohse CM, et al. Further Evaluation of Factors That May Predict Biphasic Reactions in Emergency Department Anaphylaxis Patients. J Allergy Clin Immunol Pract 2017;5(5):1295–301.

40. Schroer B, Groetch M, Mack DP, et al. Practical Challenges and Considerations for Early Introduction of Potential Food Allergens for Prevention of Food Allergy. J Allergy Clin Immunol Pract 2021;9(1):44–56.e1.

Patient Communications

Why Is It Important to Quickly Use Epinephrine at the Onset of Symptoms and Signs of Anaphylaxis?

James C. Collie, MD[a],[1],*, Richard F. Lockey, MD[b]

KEYWORDS

- Anaphylaxis • Systemic allergic reaction • Epinephrine • Adrenaline
- Adverse effects

KEY POINTS

- Intramuscular epinephrine is extremely safe for management of anaphylaxis.
- Epinephrine should be administered at the first symptoms and signs of anaphylaxis, including any systemic allergic reaction (SAR).
- Affected individuals or caregivers should be educated on the safety profile of epinephrine and the importance of epinephrine use early in SAR and anaphylaxis.

INTRODUCTION

The authors define a systemic allergic reaction (SAR) and anaphylaxis as an acute, potentially fatal systemic allergic or nonallergic reaction expressed as a continuum encompassing grades 1 to 5 in the proposed modified World Allergy Organization (WAO) grading system.[1] Grades 4 and 5 meet the definition of anaphylaxis per the National Institute of Allergy and Infectious Diseases/Food Allergy and Anaphylaxis Network Expert Panel criteria.[1,2] Although most cases of SAR and anaphylaxis resolve without treatment, it is impossible to accurately predict which subjects will develop SAR versus those who may progress to anaphylaxis and possibly death.[3] The early administration of epinephrine in the potential course of SAR and anaphylaxis not only reduces mortality, but results in a reduction of its progression and can negate the onset of anaphylaxis.[4]

Although there is a trend toward an increasing lifetime prevalence of SAR and anaphylaxis, succumbing from this disease is rare with mortality rates between 0.63

[a] Department of Internal Medicine, University of South Florida, Tampa, FL, USA; [b] Division of Allergy and Immunology, Department of Internal Medicine, University of South Florida Morsani College of Medicine, 13000 Bruce B. Downs Blvd (111D), Tampa, FL 33612, USA
[1] Present address: 17 Davis Blvd, Suite 308, Tampa, Fl 33606.
* Corresponding author.
E-mail address: Collie@usf.edu

Immunol Allergy Clin N Am 42 (2022) 201–217
https://doi.org/10.1016/j.iac.2021.09.009 immunology.theclinics.com
0889-8561/22/© 2021 Elsevier Inc. All rights reserved.

and 0.76 per million population in the United States.[5] Mortality occurs from respiratory or cardiovascular compromise and often occurs in the absence of or delayed administration of epinephrine.[2,6,7] The latter is also associated with increased biphasic reactions, that is, reactions that occur initially and reoccur 1 to 72 hours later, rarely longer, some of which are severe and even fatal.[8]

DISCUSSION

It is the responsibility of the affected subject, parent, or caregiver to recognize the symptoms and signs of SAR and anaphylaxis and to appropriately administer epinephrine intramuscularly into the anterolateral thigh.[3] The symptoms and signs of SAR or anaphylaxis are illustrated in **Table 1**, including reactions grades 1 to 5. Symptoms and signs generally appear in escalating order, but not necessarily. Some individuals can present with a feeling of impending doom, respiratory problems, or a drop in blood pressure, without any other symptoms or signs of SAR or anaphylaxis.[3]

Educating affected subjects or their parents and caregivers about SAR and anaphylaxis as a continuum, as illustrated in the cited modified WAO classification, allows physicians and other health care professionals to clearly indicate when to administer this drug. This is not only to stop the reaction, but to prevent its progression to potential death.[4] Likewise, understanding the risk factors for SAR and anaphylaxis and death is necessary. Risk factors for severe or fatal anaphylaxis include asthma, cardiovascular disease, mast cell disorders, older age, route of administration of the allergen (parenteral greater than oral), dose of allergen administered, and time of onset.[3,10] In addition, in 2020 Cardona and colleagues[3] summarized possible cofactors that may contribute to "anaphylaxis" including exercise, medication use (β-blockers, angiotensin-converting enzyme inhibitors), active infection, sleep deprivation, alcohol use, and psychological factors. Risk factors for SAR or anaphylaxis following subcutaneous immunotherapy (SCIT) used to treat allergic rhinoconjunctivitis, atopic eczema, and allergic asthma include: prior anaphylactic reaction to SCIT, uncontrolled asthma, rush immunotherapy, high degree of sensitivity, and seasonal exacerbations.[11,12] Intramuscular (IM) epinephrine, administered at the first symptom or sign of SAR associated with SCIT in a retrospective study of SARs following approximately 28,000 SCIT injections, resulted in the quick resolution of these reactions.[13] With early IM epinephrine, none progressed beyond WAO grade 2 of 5 reactions. Timing of the onset of the reaction also is of utmost importance. Although SAR or anaphylaxis rarely can begin up to several hours, even longer, following allergen exposure, the earlier the onset of the reaction, the more potential for it to be serious.[6] Major barriers to subjects appropriately using epinephrine include a lack of universal symptoms and signs as to when it should be administered, trypanophobia, administration via injection, and perceived or potential side effects.[14]

IM epinephrine is safe when administered in the appropriate dose, body site, and time interval. The recommended dose is 0.01 mg/kg with a maximum dose of 0.5 mg/kg body weight.[2,3,10] The appropriate site is the anterolateral region of the middle third of the thigh.[2] The dose is repeated at increments of 5 to 15 minutes, as necessary, depending on the continuing or worsening symptoms and signs of SAR or anaphylaxis.[2,3,10]

Approximately one in five individuals experience side effects from epinephrine.[15] Side effects include transient tremors, restlessness, increased anxiety, headache, and palpitations.[15,16] Other more uncommon adverse events (AEs) include needle lacerations; inappropriate injections sites; and, rarely, a secondary infection at the

Table 1
Proposed modification of the 2010 WAO grading system

	Grading System for SAR			
			Grade 4	Grade 5
			Anaphylaxis	
Grade 1	Grade 2	Grade 3		Grade 5
Administer epinephrine at the first symptom or sign of any of the following[c]				
Symptoms/signs from 1 organ system present	Symptoms/signs from ≥2 organ systems listed in grade 1	Lower airway	Lower airway	Lower or upper airway
Cutaneous		Mild bronchospasm (eg, cough, wheezing, shortness of breath) that responds to treatment	Severe bronchospasm (eg, not responding or worsening despite treatment)	Respiratory failure
Urticaria and/or erythema-warmth and/or pruritus, other than localized at the injection site				and/or
		And/or	And/or	Cardiovascular
And/or		Gastrointestinal	Upper airway	Collapse/hypotension[b]
Tingling, or itching of the lips[a] or		Abdominal cramps[a] and/or or vomiting/diarrhea	Laryngeal edema with stridor	And/or
Angioedema (not laryngeal)[a]		Other	Any symptoms/signs from grades 1 or 3 would be included	Loss of consciousness (vasovagal excluded)
		Uterine cramps		Any symptoms/signs from grades 1, 3, or 4 would be included
Or		Any symptoms/signs from grade 1 would be included		
Upper respiratory				
Nasal symptoms (eg, sneezing, rhinorrhea, nasal pruritus, and/or nasal congestion)				
And/or				
Throat-clearing (itchy throat)[a]				
And/or				
Cough not related to bronchospasm				

(continued on next page)

Table 1
(continued)

	Grading System for SAR			
Grade 1	Grade 2	Grade 3	Grade 4	Grade 5
				Anaphylaxis
Or				
Conjunctival				
Erythema, pruritus, or tearing				
Or				
Other				
Nausea				
Metallic taste				

The final grade of the reaction is not determined until the event is over, regardless of the medication administered to treat the reaction. The final report should include the first symptoms/signs and the time of onset after the causative agent exposure and a suffix reflecting if and when epinephrine was or was not administered: a, ≤5 minutes; b, >5 minutes to ≤10 minutes; c, >10 to ≤20 minutes; d, >20 minutes; z, epinephrine not administered.

Final report: grade 1 to 5; a-d, or z; first symptoms/signs; time of onset of first symptoms/signs.

Case example. Within 10 minutes of receiving an allergen-specific immunotherapy injection, a patient develops generalized urticaria followed by a tickling sensation in the posterior pharynx. Intramuscular epinephrine is administered within 5 minutes of symptoms/signs resulting in complete resolution of the reaction. The final report would be: grade 2; a; urticaria; 10 minutes.

A) Infants and children: low systolic blood pressure (age-specific) or >30% decrease in systolic blood pressure. Low systolic blood pressure for children is defined as follows.

- 1 month–1 year: <70 mm Hg
- 1–10 years: <70 mm Hg + [2 × age]
- 11–17 years: <90 mm Hg

B) Adults: systolic blood pressure of <90 mm Hg or >30% decrease from that person's baseline.

a Application-site reactions would be considered local reactions. Oral mucosa symptoms, such as pruritus, after sublingual immunotherapy (SLIT) administration, or warmth and/or pruritus at a subcutaneous immunotherapy injection site would be considered a local reaction. However, tingling or itching of the lips or mouth could be interpreted as SAR if the known allergen (eg, peanut) is inadvertently placed into the mouth or ingested in a subject with a history of a peanut-induced SAR. Gastrointestinal tract reactions after SLIT or oral immunotherapy would also be considered local reactions, unless they occur with other systemic manifestations. SLIT or oral immunotherapy reactions associated with gastrointestinal tract and other systemic manifestations would be classified as SARs. SLIT local reactions would be classified according to the WAO grading system for SLIT local reactions.[9] A fatal reaction would not be classified in this grading system but rather reported as a serious adverse event.

b Hypotension is defined per the National Institute of Allergy and Infectious Disease/Food Allergy and Anaphylaxis Network Expert Panel criteria[2]: reduced blood pressure after exposure to known allergen for that subject (minutes to several hours).

c Recommendations as to when to use epinephrine were added by the authors and were not included in the original table cited.

From Cox LS, Sanchez-Borges M, Lockey RF. World Allergy Organization Systemic Allergic Reaction Grading System: Is a Modification Needed? J Allergy Clin Immunol Pract. 2017 Jan-Feb;5(1):58-62.e5.

injection site.[17,18] These latter are not side effects from the epinephrine but sequalae from its parenteral administration. Severe AEs, usually associated with excessive intravenous administration, include arrythmias; chest pain; QT prolongation; cardiac ischemia; and, rarely, death.[15,16] Severe AEs occur more commonly in older subjects and subjects with cardiovascular disease.[16] When given appropriately, the medical literature does not support the commonality of significant adverse effects. Therefore, there is no absolute contraindication to its use, even in subjects with older age or cardiovascular disease.

To reiterate, those at highest risk for epinephrine side effects are those subjects with cardiovascular disease.[16] However, the drug of choice for an individual with cardiovascular disease who is having SAR or anaphylaxis is epinephrine. With that and possibly other rare exceptions, the dose of epinephrine administered is safe.[16]

Affected individuals who self-administer or parents or caregivers who administer epinephrine should be counseled on how and when to use it and on its safety profile. Receiving such counseling yearly or even more frequent may help negate the inappropriate fear of using it and may reassure the subject, parent, or caregiver of their ability to administer it. Where available, epinephrine autoinjectors (EAIs) should be prescribed.[3] These autoinjectors are designed to be easy to use and to ensure standardized dosing.[16] They are available in 0.1-mg, 0.15-mg, and 0.3-mg doses in the United States and other parts of the world, whereas the 0.5-mg EAIs are only available in limited countries. Even when appropriately used, underdosing of epinephrine remains of great concern.[3] This is compounded by obesity. More than 70% of adults older than the age of 20 years in the United States meet the criteria for being overweight, and an estimated 42.5% meet criteria for obesity, defined as a body mass index of more than 30 kg/m^2, in a 2018 report.[19] For subjects weighing greater than 36 kg, a 0.3-mg dose from an EAI is an inadequate dose of epinephrine, based on the expert consensus dose of 0.01 mg/kg up to a maximum of 0.5 mg.[3]

Although EAIs are convenient and easy to use, they are not readily available throughout the world, particularly in developing countries.[20] Less than 35% of the worldwide population has access to EAIs.[20] Even when they are available, cost is prohibitive. Cost-efficient alternatives include ampules of epinephrine with an empty syringe or an epinephrine prefilled syringe (EPS).[21] The EPS is the preferred alternative because an affected individual or caregiver does not have to accurately draw up the epinephrine into a syringe.[21] The shelf life of an EPS is approximately 3 months when stored at room temperature.[21] However, EAIs retain nearly 90% of their epinephrine potency 30 months past the labeled expiration date, a tremendous advantage over an EPS.[22]

Alternative methods to administer epinephrine are under investigation, and two promising routes include intranasal and sublingual delivery. Early studies indicate that such administration results in plasma concentrations equivalent to IM epinephrine.[23] Five milligrams of intranasal epinephrine in healthy human subjects and 40 mg of sublingual in animals achieves comparable concentrations when compared with 0.3 mg of IM epinephrine.[24,25] Further human studies are needed to ensure their clinical efficacy and respective safety profiles. In theory, these delivery systems may be more user friendly and safer than the current use of EAIs, mainly through the avoidance of needles.

It is up to the affected individual, parent, or caregiver to know when and how to administer epinephrine because most SARs and anaphylaxis begin in the community from foods, medications, or insect stings to which an individual is allergic.[3] However, affected individuals often have difficulty determining when to administer it.[26] In a survey of SAR and anaphylaxis survivors, 73% did not self-administer epinephrine, and of those who did, almost a third questioned the appropriate time as to when it should be administered.[26]

This problem is secondary to an unclear consensus among physicians and other health care professionals as to the time it should be used with the initial symptoms and signs of a SAR and anaphylaxis. Treatment of rare events may limit general applicability of the resulting rare observations. Proving that a given treatment or timing of treatment is essential is nearly impossible with anaphylaxis because of rapid onset, variability, and high rate of spontaneous resolution. IM epinephrine is safe, and use before development of definitive anaphylaxis is potentially life-saving.[27] However, recommendations to administer epinephrine before symptoms in a community setting is controversial. The art of anaphylaxis treatment requires risk assessment and individualization, and some physicians do not agree that IM epinephrine should be used for expected or anticipated symptoms in a community setting.

A discussion of risk should occur, incorporating such factors as route of allergen exposure (eg, insect sting or allergen immunotherapy injection vs food ingestion), comorbidities that increase risk (eg, asthma or underlying heart disease), anaphylaxis history including severity and pace of development, likelihood of allergen exposure (eg, known ingestion vs eating a food that "may contain" allergen), access to emergency health care, patient and family anxiety level, and baseline tryptase. The recommended timing of epinephrine administration varies based on these variables and not on a universal, one-size-fits-all approach. For example, most physicians would agree that a subject who receives an IM injection of penicillin and develops generalized urticaria and erythema within 5 minutes should receive epinephrine. Likewise, so too with peanut ingestion in an individual with peanut allergy. However, not everyone agrees when to give epinephrine to an individual with peanut allergy who presents with nausea and vomiting. Another example is a Boy Scout on the Appalachian Trail who receives an *Hymenoptera* insect sting and 1 hour later has the onset of generalized urticaria. A fourth example is an individual who has a past history of anaphylaxis secondary to peanut ingestion. He or she is at a summer camp and inadvertently ingests a cookie that contains peanuts. The prophylactic administration of epinephrine in this case in the authors' opinion, is warranted. Each case is different, and this often leads to confusion as to whether epinephrine should or should not be given at the onset of the first symptoms and signs of SAR and anaphylaxis.

Therefore, the authors believe that epinephrine should be given at the first symptoms or signs of any SAR and anaphylaxis, in particular, those reactions that begin within an hour of an alleged administration of an allergen or suspected allergen. The quicker the onset of the reaction, the more potential it has to be serious.[6] In such cases, it is absolutely necessary to administer epinephrine. The senior author tells his patients, when in doubt, administer epinephrine. He also informs them that epinephrine is safe and stops the reaction before it progresses beyond a WAO grade 1, 2, or 3 reaction, that is, anaphylaxis. He has each patient repeat three times, "Epinephrine is safe." He also indicates that if the subject is not improving within several minutes, to administer the second dose of epinephrine.

The concept of when to administer epinephrine is further complicated by online resources from many different organizations with a wide variety of definitions of anaphylaxis and recommendations as to when to administer epinephrine. **Table 2** illustrates recommendations from 13 different organizations about the symptoms and signs of anaphylaxis and when to administer epinephrine. This information was derived from the patient-directed educational material on respective Web sites. Most of the organizations recommend epinephrine as soon as anaphylaxis is recognized, but the threshold and definition of anaphylaxis between them differ. For example, the Allergy

Table 2
Organization recommendations for the symptoms and signs of anaphylaxis and epinephrine administration

Organization	Symptoms and Signs of Anaphylaxis after an Exposure to an Allergen	When to Administer Epinephrine
Allergy & Asthma Network[28]	Symptoms typically involve more than 1 organ system of the body and can include: Skin: itching, redness, swelling, hives Mouth: itching, swelling of lips, tongue Stomach: vomiting, diarrhea, cramps Respiratory: shortness of breath, wheezing, coughing, chest pain, and/or tightness Heart: weak pulse, dizziness, faintness, cardiac arrest Headache, nasal congestion, watery eyes, sweating Confusion, feeling of impending doom Loss of consciousness	At the first symptom or sign of a reaction
Food Allergy Research & Education[29]	Severe symptoms: Lung: shortness of breath, wheezing, repetitive cough Heart: pale or bluish skin, faintness, weak pulse, dizziness Throat: tight or hoarse throat, trouble breathing or swallowing Mouth: significant swelling of the tongue or lips Skin: many hives over the body, widespread redness Gut: repetitive vomiting, severe diarrhea Other: feeling something bad is about to happen, anxiety, confusion Mild symptoms from more than 1 system area Nose: itchy or runny nose, sneezing Mouth: itchy mouth Skin: a few hives, mild itch Gut: mild nausea or discomfort	For any of the severe symptoms For mild symptoms from more than 1 system area

(continued on next page)

Table 2
(continued)

Organization	Symptoms and Signs of Anaphylaxis after an Exposure to an Allergen	When to Administer Epinephrine

Allergy UK[30]	1 or more of the following:
	Airway:
	  Swollen tongue
	  Difficulty swallowing/ speaking
	  Throat tightness
	  Change in voice (hoarse or croaky sounds)
	Breathing:
	  Difficult or noisy breathing
	  Chest tightness
	  Persistent cough
	  Wheeze (whistling noise caused by a narrowed airway)
	Circulation:
	  Feeling dizzy or faint
	  Collapse
	  In babies and young children this may look like the sudden onset of paleness and floppiness
	  Loss of consciousness (unresponsive)
	May include symptoms of a mild to moderate allergic reaction including 1 or more of the following:
	Rash/hives (red raised, itchy bumps)
	Swelling of the lips, eyes, or face
	Itchy or tingling mouth
	Stomach pain, nausea, vomiting
	In the case of sting or bites, localized swelling at sting site
		Immediately when anaphylaxis is recognized; if in doubt, give it

(continued on next page)

	Symptoms and Signs of	
	Anaphylaxis after an	When to Administer
Organization	Exposure to an Allergen	Epinephrine

Table 2
(continued)

Organization	Symptoms and Signs of Anaphylaxis after an Exposure to an Allergen	When to Administer Epinephrine
European Academy of Allergy and Clinical Immunology – Patients[31]	At least 2 body systems should simultaneously be involved: Skin: itching, urticaria, generalized redness or angioedema Respiratory system: acute rhinitis, asthma, or upper airway angioedema Digestive track: nausea, vomiting, stomach cramps, or diarrhea Cardiovascular system: palpitations, increased heart rate, or drop in blood pressure Other: dizziness, loss of consciousness, cardiac or respiratory arrest	If they have developed symptoms suggestive of anaphylaxis (always according to their personalized management action plan)
Asthma Allergy Foundation of America[32]	Symptoms usually involve more than 1 organ system (part of the body), such as the skin or mouth, the lungs, the heart, and the gut; some symptoms include: Skin rashes, itching, or hives Swelling of the lips, tongue, or throat Shortness of breath, trouble breathing, or wheezing (whistling sound during breathing) Dizziness and/or fainting Stomach pain, bloating, vomiting, or diarrhea Uterine cramps Feeling like something awful is about to happen	At the first sign of an anaphylactic reaction Otherwise it should be determined through discussions with a doctor for an allergy emergency care plan or anaphylaxis emergency action plan
The Mast Cell Disease Society[33]	Mouth: itching, swelling of lips and/or tongue Throat: itching, tightness, closure, hoarseness Skin: itching, hives, redness, swelling, flushing Gut: nausea, vomiting, diarrhea, cramps Lung: shortness of breath, cough, wheeze Heart: weak pulse, dizziness, passing out	Determined through an emergency plan with the primary mast cell physician

(continued on next page)

Table 2
(continued)

Organization	Symptoms and Signs of Anaphylaxis after an Exposure to an Allergen	When to Administer Epinephrine
Australian Society of Clinical Immunology and Allergy[34]	Abdominal pain, vomiting (these are signs of anaphylaxis for insect allergy) Difficult/noisy breathing Swelling of tongue Swelling/tightness in throat Wheeze or persistent cough Difficulty talking and/or hoarse voice Persistent dizziness or collapse Pale and floppy (young children)	For any of the symptoms listed or if someone with known asthma and allergy to food, insects, or medication has sudden breathing difficulty (including wheeze, persistent cough, or hoarse voice)
Food Allergy Canada[35,36]	Generally includes 2 or more of the following body systems: Skin: hives, swelling (face, lips, tongue), itching, warmth, redness Respiratory (breathing): coughing, wheezing, shortness of breath, chest pain/tightness, throat tightness, hoarse voice, nasal congestion or hay fever–like symptoms (runny itchy nose and watery eyes, sneezing), trouble swallowing Gastrointestinal (stomach): nausea, pain/cramps, vomiting, diarrhea Cardiovascular (heart): paler than normal skin color/blue color, weak pulse, passing out, dizziness or lightheadedness, shock Other: anxiety, sense of doom (the feeling that something bad is about to happen), headache, uterine cramps, metallic taste However, a drop in blood pressure without other symptoms may also indicate anaphylaxis	At the first sign of a known or suspected anaphylactic reaction

(continued on next page)

Table 2 *(continued)*		
Organization	**Symptoms and Signs of Anaphylaxis after an Exposure to an Allergen**	**When to Administer Epinephrine**
Global Allergy & Airways Patient Platform[37]	Skin reactions, including hives along with itching Flushed or pale skin A feeling of warmth The sensation of a lump in your throat Wheezing, shortness of breath, throat tightness, cough, hoarse voice, chest pain/tightness, trouble swallowing, itchy mouth/throat, nasal stuffiness/congestion A weak and rapid pulse Nausea, vomiting or diarrhea Dizziness Headache Anxiety Low blood pressure Loss of consciousness	During an anaphylactic attack
Anaphylaxis Campaign[38]	Any 1 or more of the following ABC symptoms: Airway: Persistent cough Vocal changes (hoarse voice) Difficulty in swallowing Swollen tongue Breathing: Difficult or noisy breathing Wheezing (like an asthma attack) Circulation/consciousness: Feeling lightheaded or faint Clammy skin Confusion Unresponsive/unconscious (caused by a drop in blood pressure) In addition to the ABC symptoms listed above, the following, less severe symptoms may occur: Widespread flushing of the skin	The injection should be given as soon as any ABC symptoms of anaphylaxis are present; if in doubt, give it

(continued on next page)

Table 2
(*continued*)

Organization	Symptoms and Signs of Anaphylaxis after an Exposure to an Allergen	When to Administer Epinephrine
	Nettle rash (otherwise known as hives or urticaria) Swelling of the skin (known as angioedema) anywhere on the body (eg, lips, face) Abdominal pain, nausea, and vomiting	
Allergy Foundation of South Africa[39]	Can range from mild skin changes and swelling of the face to life-threatening lung and heart involvement Skin signs: flushing, redness, itching, hives, and local swelling especially of the face Abdominal symptoms: cramps, nausea, vomiting, and diarrhea Respiratory involvement: can cause swelling of the upper airways, such as the tongue, the back of the throat and the area of the voice box or larynx. This may start with a hoarse voice and a persistent dry cough and then progress to throat tightness causing difficulty breathing. The airways of the lung may be involved causing chest tightness and a wheezing noise. Heart and circulation: a sudden drop in blood pressure, irregular heartbeat, and general collapse	As soon as anaphylaxis occurs

(*continued on next page*)

Table 2
(continued)

Organization	Symptoms and Signs of Anaphylaxis after an Exposure to an Allergen	When to Administer Epinephrine
Allergy and Immunology Awareness Program-Qatar[40,41]	Includes 2 or more of the following body systems: skin, respiratory, gastrointestinal and/or cardiovascular; however, low blood pressure alone (ie, cardiovascular system), in the absence of other symptoms, can also represent anaphylaxis Skin: hives, swelling (face, lips, tongue), itching, warmth, redness Respiratory (breathing): coughing, wheezing, shortness of breath, chest pain or tightness, throat tightness, hoarse voice, nasal congestion or hay fever–like symptoms (runny, itchy nose and watery eyes, sneezing), trouble swallowing Gastrointestinal (stomach): nausea, pain or cramps, vomiting, diarrhea Cardiovascular (heart): paler than normal skin color/blue color, weak pulse, passing out, dizziness or lightheadedness, shock Other: anxiety, sense of doom (the feeling that something bad is about to happen), headache, uterine cramps, metallic taste	It is recommended that epinephrine be given at the start of a known or suspected anaphylactic reaction

(continued on next page)

Table 2 *(continued)*		
Organization	Symptoms and Signs of Anaphylaxis after an Exposure to an Allergen	When to Administer Epinephrine
American Academy of Pediatrics[42]	Shortness of breath, wheezing, or coughing Skin color is pale or has a bluish color Weak pulse Fainting or dizziness Tight or hoarse throat Trouble breathing or swallowing Swelling of lips or tongue that bother breathing Vomiting or diarrhea (if severe or combined with other symptoms) Many hives or redness over body Feeling of "doom," confusion, altered consciousness, or agitation	After any of these severe symptoms Action plan after discussion with physician may include epinephrine being given for MILD symptoms after a sting or eating these foods if child has a history of a severe reaction

Derived and adapted from each respective organization's public Web site, most of which are directed toward patients, as individually cited.

& Asthma Network recommends using epinephrine at the first symptoms and signs of SAR and anaphylaxis.[28] However, the Food Allergy Research & Education recommends administering it for severe symptoms or mild symptoms from more than one organ system.[29] Allergy UK recommends it as soon as anaphylaxis is recognized, but describes anaphylaxis as severe symptoms involving airway, breathing, and circulation.[30] A fourth example is the European Academy of Allergy and Clinical Immunology–Patient site, which recommends administering it at symptoms suggestive of anaphylaxis, but further goes to clarify that it should always be according to their personalized management action plan.[31] The recommendations of the other organizations fall within a spectrum of these four examples.

In summary, using the modified WAO definition of SAR and anaphylaxis, the authors recommend that verbal and written instructions be given to the affected subject, parent, or caregiver and that they administer IM epinephrine at the appropriate doses at the first symptoms and signs of SAR and anaphylaxis as illustrated in **Table 1**.

SUMMARY

IM epinephrine is the treatment of choice for SAR and anaphylaxis.[2,3,16] It is safe when given in the appropriate doses and route.[16] Severe adverse reactions are extremely unusual and occur most commonly with inappropriate intravenous administration.[16] Its early administration can prevent progression of SAR to anaphylaxis and thereby avoid the serious problems of hypotension, respiratory difficulties, and ultimately a fatal reaction.[4] Despite its safety and efficacy, its underuse continues to be a major problem among affected subjects, parents, and caregivers and physicians and other health care professionals.[3,14] The modified WAO definition of SAR and anaphylaxis is an excellent way to guide its early and appropriate administration. The recommendation of the authors is to instruct subjects to administer IM epinephrine at the first symptoms and signs of any grades 1 to 5 SAR and anaphylaxis. It is also appropriate to educate the affected individual or parent or caregiver on its use and instructions as to when and how it should be administered at least on a yearly basis.

CLINICS CARE POINTS

- IM epinephrine is extremely safe at the recommended doses.
- Early administration of IM epinephrine in the treatment of any symptoms and signs of SAR or anaphylaxis is critical to prevent progression to a more serious reaction and death.
- Subjects, parents, and caregivers should be provided with clear verbal and written instructions as to how and when to administer IM epinephrine at the first symptoms and signs of SAR and anaphylaxis.
- Subjects, parents, and caregivers should have the educational process of when and how to administer epinephrine repeated at least yearly.

DISCLOSURE

Dr J.C. Collie has nothing to disclose. Dr R.F. Lockey is a consultant for ARS Pharmaceuticals, Inc.

REFERENCES

1. Cox LS, Sanchez-Borges M, Lockey RF. World Allergy Organization systemic allergic reaction grading system: is a modification needed? J Allergy Clin Immunol Pract 2017;5(1):58–62 e55.
2. Sampson HA, Munoz-Furlong A, Campbell RL, et al. Second symposium on the definition and management of anaphylaxis: summary report–Second National Institute of Allergy and Infectious Disease/Food Allergy and Anaphylaxis Network symposium. J Allergy Clin Immunol 2006;117(2):391–7.
3. Cardona V, Ansotegui IJ, Ebisawa M, et al. World Allergy Organization anaphylaxis guidance 2020. World Allergy Organ J 2020;13(10):100472.
4. Shaker MS, Wallace DV, Golden DBK, et al. Anaphylaxis: a 2020 practice parameter update, systematic review, and Grading of Recommendations, Assessment, Development and Evaluation (GRADE) analysis. J Allergy Clin Immunol 2020; 145(4):1082–123.
5. Ma L, Danoff TM, Borish L. Case fatality and population mortality associated with anaphylaxis in the United States. J Allergy Clin Immunol 2014;133(4):1075–83.
6. Pumphrey RS. Lessons for management of anaphylaxis from a study of fatal reactions. Clin Exp Allergy 2000;30(8):1144–50.
7. Turner PJ, Jerschow E, Umasunthar T, et al. Fatal anaphylaxis: mortality rate and risk factors. J Allergy Clin Immunol Pract 2017;5(5):1169–78.
8. Lieberman P. Biphasic anaphylactic reactions. Ann Allergy Asthma Immunol 2005;95(3):217–26 [quiz 226, 258].
9. Passalacqua G, Baena-Cagnani CE, Bousquet J, et al. Grading local side effects of sublingual immunotherapy for respiratory allergy: speaking the same language. J Allergy Clin Immunol 2013;132(1):93–8.
10. Simons FE, Ardusso LR, Bilo MB, et al. International consensus on (ICON) anaphylaxis. World Allergy Organ J 2014;7(1):9.

11. SCIT risk factors, Bernstein DI, Epstein TEG. Safety of allergen immunotherapy in North America from 2008-2017: lessons learned from the ACAAI/AAAAI National Surveillance Study of adverse reactions to allergen immunotherapy. Allergy Asthma Proc 2020;41(2):108–11.

12. Stewart GE 2nd, Lockey RF. Systemic reactions from allergen immunotherapy. J Allergy Clin Immunol 1992;90(4 Pt 1):567–78.

13. Phillips JF, Lockey RF, Fox RW, et al. Systemic reactions to subcutaneous allergen immunotherapy and the response to epinephrine. Allergy Asthma Proc 2011; 32(4):288–94.

14. Prince BT, Mikhail I, Stukus DR. Underuse of epinephrine for the treatment of anaphylaxis: missed opportunities. J Asthma Allergy 2018;11:143–51.

15. Cardona V, Ferre-Ybarz L, Guilarte M, et al. Safety of adrenaline use in anaphylaxis: a multicentre register. Int Arch Allergy Immunol 2017;173(3):171–7.

16. Kemp SF, Lockey RF, Simons FE, World Allergy Organization ad hoc Committee on Epinephrine in A. Epinephrine: the drug of choice for anaphylaxis. A statement of the World Allergy Organization. World Allergy Organ J 2008;1(7 Suppl): S18–26.

17. Brown JC, Tuuri RE, Akhter S, et al. Lacerations and embedded needles caused by epinephrine autoinjector use in children. Ann Emerg Med 2016;67(3):307–15.e8.

18. Peyko V, Shams D, Lauver AR. Epinephrine auto-injection after allergic reaction leading to gas gangrene of the leg. Am J Case Rep 2021;22:e930889.

19. Fryar CD, Carroll MD, Afful J. Products - health E Stats - prevalence of overweight, obesity, and Extreme obesity among adults aged 20 and over: United States, 1960–1962 through 2017–2018. Centers for Disease Control and Prevention; 2021. Available at: https://www.cdc.gov/nchs/data/hestat/obesity-adult-17-18/obesity-adult.htm#Citation. Accessed June 29, 2021.

20. Tanno LK, Simons FER, Sanchez-Borges M, et al. Applying prevention concepts to anaphylaxis: a call for worldwide availability of adrenaline auto-injectors. Clin Exp Allergy 2017;47(9):1108–14.

21. Pepper AN, Westermann-Clark E, Lockey RF. The high cost of epinephrine auto-injectors and possible alternatives. J Allergy Clin Immunol Pract 2017;5(3): 665–668 e661.

22. Kassel L, Jones C, Mengesha A. Epinephrine drug degradation in autoinjector products. J Allergy Clin Immunol Pract 2019;7(7):2491–3.

23. Boswell B, Rudders SA, Brown JC. Emerging therapies in anaphylaxis: alternatives to intramuscular administration of epinephrine. Curr Allergy Asthma Rep 2021;21(3):18.

24. Srisawat C, Nakponetong K, Benjasupattananun P, et al. A preliminary study of intranasal epinephrine administration as a potential route for anaphylaxis treatment. Asian Pac J Allergy Immunol 2016;34(1):38–43.

25. Rawas-Qalaji MM, Simons FE, Simons KJ. Sublingual epinephrine tablets versus intramuscular injection of epinephrine: dose equivalence for potential treatment of anaphylaxis. J Allergy Clin Immunol 2006;117(2):398–403.

26. Simons FE, Clark S, Camargo CA Jr. Anaphylaxis in the community: learning from the survivors. J Allergy Clin Immunol 2009;124(2):301–6.

27. Turner PJ, DunnGalvin A, Hourihane JO. The Emperor Has No Symptoms: The Risks of a Blanket Approach to Using Epinephrine Autoinjectors for All Allergic Reactions. J Allergy Clin Immunol Pract 2016;4(6):1143–6.

28. Anaphylaxis. Allergy & Asthma Network. Available at: https://allergyasthmanetwork.org/anaphylaxis/. Accessed June 29, 2021.

29. Food Allergy & Anaphylaxis Emergency Care Plan. Food Allergy Research & Education; 2020. Available at: https://www.foodallergy.org/living-food-allergies/food-allergy-essentials/food-allergy-anaphylaxis-emergency-care-plan. Accessed June 29, 2021.

30. Brown T, Fox A, Waddell L, et al. Anaphylaxis and severe allergic reaction. Anaphylaxis | Would you know what to do? | Allergy UK. 2018. Available at: https://www.allergyuk.org/information-and-advice/conditions-and-symptoms/33-anaphylaxis-and-severe-allergic-reaction#download_access. Accessed June 29, 2021.

31. Anaphylaxis. EAACI Patients. 2018. Available at: https://patients.eaaci.org/anaphylaxis/. Accessed June 29, 2021.

32. ANAPHYLAXIS: A severe allergic reaction. Asthma and Allergy Foundation of America; 2017. Available at: https://www.aafa.org/anaphylaxis-severe-allergic-reaction/. Accessed June 29, 2021.

33. Emergency care for patients with mast cell diseases. The Mast Cell Disease Society. Available at: https://tmsforacure.org/wp-content/uploads/TMS_EmergencyCare_Brochure_2019_v1.pdf. Accessed June 29, 2021.

34. ASCIA Guidelines - Acute management of anaphylaxis. Australasian Society of Clinical Immunology and Allergy (ASCIA). Available at: https://www.allergy.org.au/hp/papers/acute-management-of-anaphylaxis-guidelines. Accessed June 29, 2021.

35. Reaction signs and symptoms. Food Allergy Canada; 2021. Available at: https://foodallergycanada.ca/food-allergy-basics/preventing-and-treating-allergic-reactions/reaction-signs-and-symptoms/. Accessed June 29, 2021.

36. Treating reactions. Food Allergy Canada; 2021. Available at: https://foodallergycanada.ca/food-allergy-basics/preventing-and-treating-allergic-reactions/treating-reactions/. Accessed June 29, 2021.

37. Anaphylaxis. Global Allergy &; Airways Patient Platform. Available at: https://gaapp.org/anaphylaxis/. Accessed July 1, 2021.

38. Anaphylaxis: The Facts. Anaphylaxis Campaign. 2019. Available at: https://www.anaphylaxis.org.uk/wp-content/uploads/2019/07/Anaphylaxis-The-Facts-Feb-2019.pdf. Accessed June 29, 2021.

39. Anaphylaxis and how to treat it. AFSA. 2019. Available at: https://www.allergyfoundation.co.za/patient-information/en/allergic-diseases/anaphylaxis/. Accessed June 29, 2021.

40. Signs and Symptoms. Hamad Medical Corporation. Available at: https://www.hamad.qa/EN/your%20health/allergy-and-immunology/allergy/anaphylaxis/signs-and-symptoms/Pages/default.aspx. Accessed June 29, 2021.

41. Emergency Protocol. Hamad Medical Corporation. Available at: https://www.hamad.qa/EN/your%20health/allergy-and-immunology/allergy/anaphylaxis/emergency-protocol/Pages/default.aspx. Accessed June 29, 2021.

42. Allergy and Anaphylaxis Emergency Plan. American Academy of Pediatrics. 2019. Available at: https://www.aap.org/en-us/Documents/AAP_Allergy_and_Anaphylaxis_Emergency_Plan.pdf. Accessed June 29, 2021.

Moving?

Make sure your subscription moves with you!

To notify us of your new address, find your **Clinics Account Number** (located on your mailing label above your name), and contact customer service at:

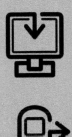

Email: journalscustomerservice-usa@elsevier.com

800-654-2452 (subscribers in the U.S. & Canada)
314-447-8871 (subscribers outside of the U.S. & Canada)

Fax number: 314-447-8029

Elsevier Health Sciences Division
Subscription Customer Service
3251 Riverport Lane
Maryland Heights, MO 63043

*To ensure uninterrupted delivery of your subscription, please notify us at least 4 weeks in advance of move.